Roshan Lall Gupta's
Recent Advances in
SURGERY

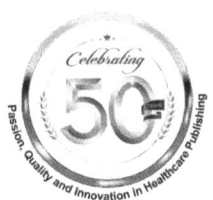

Roshan Lall Gupta's
Recent Advances in
SURGERY

Volume 17

Editor

Puneet MS DNB (Surg) MNAMS FACS
Professor and Head
Department of Surgery
Institute of Medical Sciences
Banaras Hindu University
Varanasi, Uttar Pradesh, India

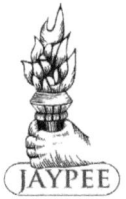

JAYPEE BROTHERS MEDICAL PUBLISHERS
The Health Sciences Publisher
New Delhi | London

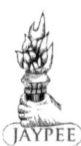 **Jaypee Brothers Medical Publishers (P) Ltd**

Headquarters

Jaypee Brothers Medical Publishers (P) Ltd
EMCA House, 23/23-B
Ansari Road, Daryaganj
New Delhi 110 002, India
Landline: +91-11-23272143, +91-11-23272703
+91-11-23282021, +91-11-23245672
E-mail: jaypee@jaypeebrothers.com

Corporate Office

Jaypee Brothers Medical Publishers (P) Ltd
4838/24, Ansari Road, Daryaganj
New Delhi 110 002, India
Phone: +91-11-43574357
Fax: +91-11-43574314
E-mail: jaypee@jaypeebrothers.com

Overseas Office

JP Medical Ltd
83 Victoria Street, London
SW1H 0HW (UK)
Phone: +44 20 3170 8910
Fax: +44 (0)20 3008 6180
E-mail: info@jpmedpub.com

Website: www.jaypeebrothers.com
Website: www.jaypeedigital.com

© 2021, Jaypee Brothers Medical Publishers

The views and opinions expressed in this book are solely those of the original contributor(s)/author(s) and do not necessarily represent those of editor(s) of the book.

All rights reserved. No part of this publication may be reproduced, stored or transmitted in any form or by any means, electronic, mechanical, photocopying, recording or otherwise, without the prior permission in writing of the publishers.

All brand names and product names used in this book are trade names, service marks, trademarks or registered trademarks of their respective owners. The publisher is not associated with any product or vendor mentioned in this book.

Medical knowledge and practice change constantly. This book is designed to provide accurate, authoritative information about the subject matter in question. However, readers are advised to check the most current information available on procedures included and check information from the manufacturer of each product to be administered, to verify the recommended dose, formula, method and duration of administration, adverse effects and contraindications. It is the responsibility of the practitioner to take all appropriate safety precautions. Neither the publisher nor the author(s)/editor(s) assume any liability for any injury and/or damage to persons or property arising from or related to use of material in this book.

This book is sold on the understanding that the publisher is not engaged in providing professional medical services. If such advice or services are required, the services of a competent medical professional should be sought.

Every effort has been made where necessary to contact holders of copyright to obtain permission to reproduce copyright material. If any have been inadvertently overlooked, the publisher will be pleased to make the necessary arrangements at the first opportunity. The **CD/DVD-ROM** (if any) provided in the sealed envelope with this book is complimentary and free of cost. **Not meant for sale.**

Inquiries for bulk sales may be solicited at: jaypee@jaypeebrothers.com

Roshan Lall Gupta's Recent Advances in Surgery (Volume 17)

First Edition: **2021**

ISBN: 978-93-90595-58-7

Dedicated to
My wife, Ritu Ragini
Son, Akshat and daughter, Aanya

Contributors

Ajay N Gangopadhyay
Professor
Department of Pediatric Surgery
Institute of Medical Sciences
Banaras Hindu University
Varanasi, Uttar Pradesh, India

Akash Singh
Junior Research Fellow
Department of Hepatology
Postgraduate Institute of
Medical Education and Research
Chandigarh, India

Amit Agarwal
Professor
Department of
Endocrine Surgery
Sanjay Gandhi Postgraduate
Institute of Medical Sciences
Lucknow, Uttar Pradesh, India

Anu Behari
Professor
Department of Surgical
Gastroenterology
Sanjay Gandhi Postgraduate
Institute of Medical Sciences
Lucknow, Uttar Pradesh, India

Arindam Mondal
Consultant
Department of Surgical Oncology
Mahavir Cancer Sansthan
Patna, Bihar, India

Arun Kumar Singh
Professor and Head
Department of
Plastic Surgery
King George's Medical University
Lucknow, Uttar Pradesh, India

Arunima Verma
Senior Consultant and Head
Department of Surgery
Tata Motors Hospital
Jamshedpur, Jharkhand, India

Ashok Kumar
Professor
Department of Surgical
Gastroenterology
Sanjay Gandhi Postgraduate
Institute of Medical Sciences
Lucknow, Uttar Pradesh, India

Chintamani
Professor and Head
Department of Surgery
Vardhman Mahavir Medical College
Safdarjang Hospital
New Delhi, India

Garvit Chitkara
Assistant Professor
Department of Surgical Oncology
Consultant Breast Surgeon
Tata Memorial Hospital
Mumbai, Maharashtra, India

Harsha Vardhan
Senior Resident
Department of Plastic Surgery
King George's Medical University
Lucknow, Uttar Pradesh, India

Jayanta Samanta
Assistant Professor
Department of Gastroenterology
Postgraduate Institute of
Medical Education and Research
Chandigarh, India

JV Divatia
Professor and Head
Department of Anesthesia
Critical Care and Pain
Tata Memorial Hospital
Mumbai, Maharashtra, India

Kailash Chand Kurdia
Assistant Professor
Department of Surgery
Postgraduate Institute of
Medical Education and Research
Chandigarh, India

Manish Suresh Bhandare
Consultant Surgeon
Gastrointestinal and
HPB Surgical Oncology
Associate Professor
Department of Surgical Oncology
Tata Memorial Centre
Homi Bhabha National Institute
Mumbai, Maharashtra, India

Manoj Gowda
Senior Resident
Department of Surgical Oncology
Dr BRA Institute Rotary Cancer Hospital
All India Institute of
Medical Sciences
New Delhi, India

Mansi Sharma
Consultant
Department of Medical Oncology
Rajiv Gandhi Cancer Institute and
Research Centre
New Delhi, India

Megha Tandon
Associate Professor
Department of Surgery
Vardhman Mahavir Medical College
Safdarjang Hospital
New Delhi, India

N Ananthakrishnan
Professor
Department of Surgery
Mahatma Gandhi Medical College and
Research Institute
Sri Balaji Vidyapeeth
Puducherry, India

Nishanth Baliga
Assistant Professor
Division of Critical Care
Department of Anesthesia
Critical Care and Pain
Tata Memorial Hospital
Mumbai, Maharashtra, India

R Kalayarasan
Associate Professor, Department of
Surgical Gastroenterology
Jawaharlal Institute of
Postgraduate Medical Education and
Research
Puducherry, India

R N Meena
Professor, Department of Surgery
Institute of Medical Sciences
Banaras Hindu University
Varanasi, Uttar Pradesh, India

Rahul
Assistant Professor
Department of Surgical
Gastroenterology
Sanjay Gandhi Postgraduate Institute of
Medical Sciences
Lucknow, Uttar Pradesh, India

Richa Sinha
Assistant Professor
Department of Microbiology
Indira Gandhi Institute of
Medical Sciences
Patna, Bihar, India

Roma Pradhan
Assistant Professor
Department of Endocrine Surgery
Dr Ram Manohar Lohia Institute of
Medical Sciences
Lucknow, Uttar Pradesh, India

S K Gupta
Professor, Department of Surgery
Institute of Medical Sciences
Banaras Hindu University
Varanasi, Uttar Pradesh, India

S Suresh Kumar
Additional Professor
Department of Surgery
Jawaharlal Institute of
Postgraduate Medical Education and
Research
Puducherry, India

Sabby Dias
Senior Resident
Department of Urology
Institute of Medical Sciences
Banaras Hindu University
Varanasi, Uttar, Pradesh, India

Sameer Trivedi
Professor and Head
Department of Urology
Institute of Medical Sciences
Banaras Hindu University
Varanasi, Uttar Pradesh, India

Sankha Shubhra Chakrabarti
Associate Professor
Department of Geriatric Medicine
Institute of Medical Sciences
Banaras Hindu University
Varanasi, Uttar Pradesh, India

Shailesh V Shrikhande
Professor and Head
Gastrointestinal and Hepato-Pancreato-Biliary Service
Department Surgical Oncology
Deputy Director
Tata Memorial Hospital
Mumbai, Maharashtra, India

Sharad Kumar
Consultant Anesthesiologist
Tata Main Hospital
Jamshedpur, Jharkhand, India

Sunil Kumar
Hon. Professor and Former Head
Department of Surgery
Tata Main Hospital
Jamshedpur, Jharkhand, India

Supriya Sharma
Associate Professor
Department of Surgical Gastroenterology
Sanjay Gandhi Postgraduate Institute of Medical Sciences
Lucknow, Uttar Pradesh, India

SVS Deo
Professor and Head
Department of Surgical Oncology
All India Institute of Medical Sciences
New Delhi, India

Vaibhav Pandey
Associate Professor
Department of Pediatric Surgery
Institute of Medical Sciences
Banaras Hindu University
Varanasi, Uttar Pradesh, India

Vani Parmar
Professor
Department of Surgical Oncology
Breast Services
Advanced Centre for Treatment Research and Education in Cancer (ACTREC)
(Tata Memorial Centre and Homi Bhabha National Institute) Kharghar
Navi Mumbai, Maharashtra, India

Vikram Anil Chaudhari
Consultant Surgeon
Gastrointestinal and
HPB Surgical Oncology
Associate Professor
Department of Surgical Oncology
Tata Memorial Centre
Homi Bhabha National Institute
Mumbai, Maharashtra, India

Vikram Kate
Professor
Department of General and Gastrointestinal Surgery
Jawaharlal Institute of Postgraduate Medical Education and Research
Puducherry, India

Vinita Singh
Chief Consultant and Head
Department of Obstetrics and Gynecology
Tata Main Hospital
Jamshedpur, Jharkhand, India

Virendra Singh
Professor and Head
Department of Hepatology
Postgraduate Institute of Medical Education and Research
Chandigarh, India

Preface

The edition of *Roshan Lall Gupta's Recent Advances in Surgery (Vol. 17)* has covered advances in various surgical specialties. The selected topics cover recent aspects of investigative and management modalities. The chapters also include the current guidelines and surgical practices, as well as complications and follow up of the patients. The current edition will help postgraduates and practicing surgeons to update themselves and utilize knowledge in patient care.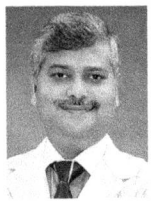

The contents of the book have been presented in an extremely simplified manner so as to help students preparing for MS/DNB (Surgery) exit exam. The year 2020 has been challenging due to COVID-19 pandemic and has changed the surgical practice. The chapter on COVID elaborates the presentation, challenges and precautions required with realistic facts and figures. The compilation of chapters are evidence based, done by eminent surgeons in their field. It is important for surgeons to keep themselves abreast with the current knowledge and surgical practices. Hope this edition will be step changing to many surgeons.

Puneet

Acknowledgments

I thank all the authors for their contribution to this edition. The text is in simple language and student-friendly for easy understanding, and appropriate for young surgeons to adapt in clinical practice. I am quite hopeful that this edition will be informative. I am thankful to M/s Jaypee Brothers Medical Publishers (P) Ltd, New Delhi, India, for publishing this book.

Contents

1. Biomarkers of Sepsis 1
   Nishanth Baliga, JV Divatia

2. Surgery for Gastric Cancer 13
   Arindam Mondal, Manish Suresh Bhandare,
   Vikram Anil Chaudhari, Shailesh V Shrikhande

3. Prenatal Surgery 34
   Vaibhav Pandey, Ajay N Gangopadhyay

4. Etiopathogenesis and Management of
   Fecal Incontinence 48
   Ashok Kumar, Kailash Chand Kurdia

5. Targeted Therapy in Gastrointestinal Malignancy 69
   Rahul, Mansi Sharma, Richa Sinha

6. Recent Advances in Endoscopy 92
   Jayanta Samanta, Akash Singh, Virendra Singh

7. Evaluation of Incidental Dilated Bile Duct 118
   Supriya Sharma, Anu Behari

8. Antibiotics in Abdominal Surgery:
   Current Guidelines and Practices 137
   S Suresh Kumar, R Kalayarasan, Vikram Kate, N Ananthakrishnan

9. Malignant Melanoma 159
   SVS Deo, Manoj Gowda

10. Surgical Safety Checklist 182
    Arunima Verma, Sharad Kumar, Vinita Singh, Sunil Kumar

11. Management of Penile Carcinoma 192
    Sameer Trivedi, Sabby Dias

12. Microvascular Surgery 217
    Arun Kumar Singh, Harsha Vardhan

13. Inflammatory Breast Cancer 232
    Vani Parmar, Garvit Chitkara

14. Phyllodes Tumors of the Breast 244
    Chintamani, Megha Tandon

15. Management of Thyroid Nodule 256
    Roma Pradhan, Amit Agarwal

16. Surgical Practice in COVID Era 273
    Sankha Shubhra Chakrabarti, RN Meena, SK Gupta

Index *295*

CHAPTER 1

Biomarkers of Sepsis

Nishanth Baliga, JV Divatia

INTRODUCTION

Sepsis remains the major cause of acute illness and death in all age groups worldwide. Early diagnosis and treatment influence the morbidity and mortality. The definition of sepsis has evolved over the years. In 1914, Schottmuller defined sepsis as a state which is caused by microbial invasion from a local infectious source into the bloodstream which leads to signs of systemic illness in remote organs. Subsequently, sepsis was defined as an uncontrolled host response to injury in the presence of infection. This systemic inflammatory response syndrome (SIRS) was diagnosed clinically by the presence of at least two features: tachycardia, tachypnea, leukocytosis or leukopenia, and fever or hypothermia **(Box 1)**. This definition was neither sensitive nor specific for sepsis. Several of these features are present in patients in the hospital, especially in postoperative patients. Many noninfective conditions such as burns, pancreatitis, trauma, and ischemia-reperfusion may also have features of SIRS. However, the presence or absence of infection is difficult to prove in these patients. The major dilemma was the diagnosis of infection. In addition, several patients with SIRS and suspected infection (postoperative patient with fever, or a patient with influenza) fitted the definition of sepsis, but had an excellent outcome. Thus, the SIRS plus infection criteria did not identify patients at a higher risk of death.

In 2016, sepsis was redefined as life-threatening organ dysfunction caused by dysregulated host response to infection. The focus shifted from inflammation to organ dysfunction in the presence of infection. Organ dysfunction was defined in terms of sequential organ failure assessment (SOFA) score increase in 2 points from baseline **(Table 1)**. One of the main components of this definition is the presence of infection. Present day methods

---

BOX 1: Systemic inflammatory response syndrome (SIRS). More than or equal to 2 of these features constitutes SIRS.

Systemic inflammatory response syndrome
- Temperature <36°C or >38°C
- Tachycardia >90 beats/minute
- Tachypnea >20 breaths/minute
- Leukocytosis >12 × 10^9/L, leukopoenia <4 × 10^9/L or bandemia >10%

TABLE 1: Sequential organ failure assessment (SOFA) score.

Points variables	0	1	2	3	4
Respiratory PaO_2/FiO_2	>400	≤400	≤300	≤200 with respiratory support	≤100 with respiratory support
Coagulation platelets ($\times 10^3$ cells/mm³)	>150	≤150	≤100	≤50	≤20
Liver Bilirubin (mg/L)	<1.2	1.2–1.9	2.0–5.9	6.0–11.9	>12.0
Cardiovascular Hypotension or Vasopressor doses (µg/kg/min>1 h)	MAP ≥70 mm Hg	MAP <70 mm Hg	Dopamine <5 or Dobutamine (any dose)	Dopamine 5.1–15 Or Adrenaline ≤0.1 or Noradrenaline ≤0.1	Dopamine >15 or Adrenaline >0.1 or Noradrenaline >0.1
Central nervous system GCS	15	13–14	10–12	6–9	<6
Renal Creatinine (mg/dL) or Urine output (mL/24 h)	<1.2	1.2–1.9	2.0–3.4	3.5–4.9 <500	>5.0 <200

(MAP: mean arterial pressure; GCS: Glasgow Coma Scale)

for identification of pathogens such as blood culture take time and are not helpful for rapid recognition. Early and rapid recognition could lead to early institution of therapy, reduce morbidity and mortality and improve outcome. Hence, there is a role for biomarkers for early recognition of sepsis.[1]

BIOMARKERS

The human body's response to sepsis is complex, comprising of inflammatory and anti-inflammatory processes, cellular and humoral responses. Biomarkers are naturally occurring molecules, genes, or other characteristics by which particular physiologic or pathologic processes can be identified. The characteristics of an ideal biomarker are: it should be an objective parameter, easy to measure, reproducible, inexpensive, have fast kinetics, high sensitivity and specificity, have a short turnaround time, show appropriate response to therapy (decline with response to therapy). However, no such ideal biomarker exists. Clinical biomarkers can be divided into two types: (1) diagnostic and (2) prognostic markers. Diagnostic biomarkers for sepsis are those which differentiate infectious from noninfectious causes as well as possible causative organisms or classes of organisms. Hence, diagnostic biomarkers can be used for prevention of unnecessary use of antibiotics. Prognostic biomarkers help in stratifying patients into risk groups and predict outcome. Biomarkers have also been used for differentiating local infection, disseminated infection and sepsis. They have been evaluated for the differentiation of viral and fungal from bacterial infection. Other potential uses of biomarkers include their role in prognostication, guidance of antibiotics, determine response to therapy, and prediction of organ dysfunction and complications.[2]

Initial biomarkers investigated in sepsis were white blood cell (WBC) counts, lactate, erythrocyte sedimentation rate (ESR) and C-reactive protein (CRP). The presence of leukocytosis or leukopenia was considered as response of infection and is a part of the SIRS criteria. However, noninfectious causes also lead to leukocytosis and hence it is not specific. Lactate, a byproduct of glycolysis has been investigated as a marker of sepsis. Several factors affect hyperlactatemia and lactate kinetics. Hypoperfusion leading to anaerobic glycolysis is an important mechanism. Currently, septic shock is defined as subset of sepsis in which underlying circulatory and cellular/metabolic abnormalities are profound enough to substantially increase mortality. It is clinically identified as sepsis with persisting hypotension requiring vasopressors to maintain mean arterial pressure >65 mm Hg and having a serum lactate level >2 mmol/L despite adequate volume resuscitation. Lactate levels are elevated in hypovolemia and hemorrhage during trauma and surgery. Lactate clearance is used as marker of adequate resuscitation. Thus, lactate levels are not useful biomarkers of sepsis, but are important indicators of the severity of shock and hypoperfusion, and the adequacy of resuscitation.

Erythrocyte sedimentation rate is an indicator of inflammation and utility as a marker of sepsis is limited. It can be influenced by the presence of anemia, immunoglobulins, and changes in erythrocyte size, shape and number. It can be elevated in malignant neoplasms, tissue injury, and in trauma. Hence it has limited utility in sepsis.[3]

C-reactive Protein

C-reactive protein (CRP) is an acute phase reactant protein which is synthesized in the liver in response to inflammation or tissue injury. Interleukin-6 (IL-6) upregulates the synthesis of CRP by hepatocytes. Normal CRP levels vary according to age, sex and race. CRP reference range varies from one laboratory to another. In general, levels less than 0.3-0.6 mg/L are considered normal. Its level can rise up to 1,000 times in response to an acute phase stimulus. CRP starts to rise after around 6 hours of the inciting stimulus, peaks at about 48 hours and has a plasma half-life of 19-20 hours. The role of CRP in acute inflammation is not clear. It has been found to bind to phospholipid components of microorganisms facilitating removal of necrotic and apoptotic cells by macrophages. CRP can also activate the complement system leading to binding to phagocytic cells and hence elimination. CRP levels can be elevated in both infectious and noninfectious inflammatory disorders. Modest elevations in CRP may be seen in noninflammatory or low-grade inflammatory conditions such as atherosclerosis, obesity, hypertension, diabetes and obstructive sleep apnea. Marked elevations in CRP are usually associated with infection, especially bacterial, however, modest elevations may be seen in viral infections. The primary drawback is its poor specificity although sensitivity is quite high. It appears to a better marker of inflammation rather than infection.[4]

PROCALCITONIN

Procalcitonin (PCT) is a 116 long amino acid peptide with a molecular weight of approximately 13 kDa. It is a precursor of calcitonin, produced by the C-cells of thyroid under the control of the calcitonin gene-related peptide 1 *(CALC-1)* gene. Under normal conditions C cells of thyroid secrete calcitonin after intracellular protoeolysis of the prohormone PCT. During microbial infections there is increase in *CALC-1* gene expression in various extra-thyroid tissues and cells which is mediated by pro-inflammatory cytokines such as tumor necrosis factor-alpha (TNF-α) and IL-6. Parenchymal tissues such as lung, liver and kidney are the principal sources of circulating PCT in sepsis. Either microbial toxins directly or the host response by humoral or cell-mediated indirectly can lead to inflammatory release of PCT. Procalcitonin starts rising by 2 hours after a stimulus, peaks at around 6 hours, and maintains a plateau through 8 and 24 hours and decreases to baseline values after 2 days. The half-life of PCT is around 20–24 hours. Usually in normal healthy individuals, PCT is detectable in very low concentrations. Low or negligible rise in PCT levels may be seen in localized infections. However, it can increase 1000-fold during active infection and sepsis. Interferon-gamma released during viral infections suppresses PCT; hence high levels are not observed in viral sepsis. Gram-negative bacteremia causes higher elevation of PCT than that caused by gram-positive pathogens. The release of PCT is determined only in systemic infection. Therefore, local bacterial colonizations, encapsulated abscesses and localized and limited infections do not cause PCT release. In addition to bacterial infections, plasma PCT concentration has been shown to increase in acute forms of malaria and fungal infections.[5]

Procalcitonin may also be elevated in absence of bacterial infections in neonates <48 hours age, first days after major surgery, trauma, burns, pancreatitis, treatment with OKT3 antibodies, interleukins, TNF-α, invasive fungal infections, acute falciparum malaria, severe cardiogenic shock, malignancies, e.g., medullary C-cell carcinoma of thyroid, small cell Ca lung,

TABLE 2: Interpretation of procalcitonin levels.

Procalcitonin values (ng/mL)	Interpretation
<0.05	Normal
0.05–0.5	Localized infection possible. Retest after 6–24 hours
0.5–2	Systemic bacterial infection possible. Retest after 6–24 hours
2–10	Systemic bacterial infection highly likely. High risk for severe sepsis
>10	Severe bacterial sepsis

bronchial carcinoid. Procalcitonin levels may be falsely low in presence of bacterial infection in early course of infection, localized infections and subacute bacterial endocarditis. **Table 2** summarizes the significance of PCT values in various conditions.

Utility of Procalcitonin

Diagnosis of Bacterial Infection and Sepsis

Procalcitonin has been evaluated as a biomarker for infection and sepsis. Assicot et al. in 1993 first described that PCT values may be considerably increased in patients with sepsis and infections.[6] Muller et al. studied whether biomarkers increased diagnostic and prognostic accuracy in community acquired pneumonia and found that procalcitonin indeed increased the accuracy and was useful in severity assessment.[7] A prospective controlled trial concluded that procalcitonin is a reliable diagnostic and prognostic marker in patients with septic shock compared to nonseptic shock.[8] In another study, PCT, CRP, IL-6 and lactate were evaluated for diagnosis of sepsis and PCT was found to be the most reliable marker for the diagnosis of sepsis, with 89% sensitivity and 94% specificity.[9] However few studies found that PCT could not accurately differentiate infection from inflammation.[10,11] A systematic review and meta-analysis on PCT as a diagnostic marker of sepsis found sensitivity of 0.77 (95% CI 0.72–0.81) and specificity of 0.79 (95% CI 0.74–0.84) with area under receiver operating curve to be 0.85 (95% CI 0.81–0.88). The authors concluded that PCT is helpful for early diagnosis of sepsis in critically ill patients. However, they also warned that the results of the test must be interpreted carefully in the context of medical history, physical examination, and microbiological assessment.[12]

Differentiation of Bacterial and Viral Infections

Procalcitonin is produced in response to endotoxin or few inflammatory mediators released by human body through humoral or cell-mediated immune response such as ILs, TNF. This sort of a response is classically seen in bacterial infections. On the other hand, in viral infections there is release of interferon (IF), a cytokine which attenuates PCT production. Hence, PCT levels rarely increase in response to viral infections, indicating that PCT may be useful for discrimination between bacterial and viral infections.[13,14]

De-escalation of Antibiotics

Due to rampant usage of antibiotics in past few decades, there is emergence of antibiotic resistance and development of multidrug resistance in pathogens. The concept of antibiotic stewardship for optimal usage of antibiotics and early de-escalation of antibiotics is accepted and encouraged. This helps prevent unnecessary usage of antibiotics and development of drug resistance. Due to favorable kinetics of PCT (in the presence of systemic bacterial infections, levels start rising by 2 hours after stimulus, peak at around 6 hours, and maintain a plateau through 8 and 24 hours and decrease to their baseline values after 2 days), PCT has been evaluated for discontinuation of antibiotics. Several studies have studied PCT as an aid for de-escalation of antibiotics after clinical stabilization. Initial single center studies found significant reduction of usage of antibiotics by using PCT based algorithms where antibiotics were stopped when PCT decreased 90% from the initial value.[15] Few studies considered cut-off value of PCT <1 μg/L or reduction by 25–35% of initial values over 3 days.[16,17] A large multicenter RCT—the PROcalcitonin to Reduce Antibiotic Treatments in Acutely ill patients (PRORATA) trial randomized 621 adult patients with suspected bacterial infection and utilized an algorithm in which initial procalcitonin was used to assess whether to start antibiotics. Subsequent daily procalcitonin levels were used to help decide when to stop antibiotics. Antibiotics were discontinued when PCT levels were <0.5 μg/L or decreased from peak value by ≥80%. They found that the PCT group had significantly fewer days on antibiotics and mortality was noninferior to control group with no significant complications.[18] ProGUARD, an RCT done in 11 Australian ICUs used an algorithm in which antibiotics were stopped if PCT levels were <0.1 μg/L or levels decreased by >90% from baseline. They enrolled 400 patients with suspected sepsis and did not find significant reduction in antibiotic use in PCT group. Probably the cut-off was too low and the study was under-powered which led to negative results.[19] Subsequently, a multicenter randomized trial—Stop Antibiotics on Procalcitonin guidance Study (SAPS) was done in Netherlands. The algorithm used was similar to PRORATA where antibiotics was stopped when PCT decreased to ≥80% of peak value, or ≤0.5 μg/L and they found significant reduction in antibiotic requirement with no increased rates of complications or mortality. However, there was mild increase in reinfection rates in PCT arm. The study provides a strong evidence for use of PCT based algorithms in sepsis.[20] Hence, the current evidence on PCT suggests utilization of PCT values as trends and de-escalation of antibiotics when there is significant reduction of PCT from baseline. Guidelines from the Infectious Diseases Society of America (IDSA) and the Surviving Sepsis Campaign (SSC) suggest utilization of PCT for cessation of antibiotics.

Procalcitonin in the Postoperative Period

The body's response to surgery consists of a complex inflammatory response to promote healing. Following cell disruption, hemorrhage or ischemia-reperfusion injury there occurs activation of the innate proinflammatory response as well as adaptive anti-inflammatory response. The proinflammatory response helps in destruction of harmful molecules whereas the anti-inflammatory response promotes healing by restricting inflammatory process. Apart from usual mediators which are released following tissue injury such as oxygen reactive species, cytokines and nitric oxide, molecules such as high-mobility group B1 (HMGB1), mitochondrial DNA, glycosaminoglycans, heat shock protein (HSP), adenosine triphosphate (ATP), protein S100 and uric acid collectively called damage associated molecular patterns (DAMPs) are also released. The activation of innate immunity leads to release of cytokines such as IL-6, IL-1b, IL-8, TNF, etc. IL-6 stimulates production of PCT. Depending on the degree of tissue injury during surgery, levels of PCT rise in the postoperative period based on inflammatory response. Normally levels rise up to 9 ng/mL in the postoperative period.[21] Usually in postoperative period PCT levels start rising few hours after surgery, peak around 24 hours and start declining to normal levels. However, persistently high levels should raise suspicion of postoperative infection.[22] Any PCT more than 10 ng/mL in the postoperative non-transplant patient is considered to be abnormal. Site of surgery influences levels of PCT. Typically, PCT elevations are greatest with abdominal and retroperitoneal surgery. Other sites such as thoracotomies lead to minor elevations in PCT.[23] PCT has been used for detection of postoperative complications and has been found to be more useful than CRP, white cell count, and IL6 in detecting infections.[24] Some studies have utilized PCT kinetics for detection of postoperative infection and sepsis. Trásy et al. used delta-PCT (PCT level from preceding day subtracted from PCT level on day of suspected infection) and found that patients with an infection exhibited a significantly higher delta PCT than those without an infection.[25] Tsangaris et al. in their study concluded that a twofold increase in PCT within a 24-hour period together with fever was useful to detect infections in an intensive care unit (ICU) population.[26] Few studies have looked at PCT kinetics for appropriateness of initial antibiotic therapy as well as adequacy of source control after abdominal surgery; however more studies and RCTs are required to reach conclusions.[27]

Guide Antibiotic Therapy in Respiratory Infections

Several studies have been done looking at PCT as a guide for initiation and discontinuation of antibiotics in respiratory infections. An initial study PROCAP trial done in a single hospital in Switzerland first demonstrated that in patients who presented to the emergency department with suspected lower respiratory tract infections, use of procalcitonin to determine whether not to initiate antibiotics, a cut-off threshold of 0.25 µg/L had a 47% reduced rate of antibiotic exposure in the procalcitonin group with no difference in laboratory or clinical outcomes.[28] Subsequent RCTs on respiratory tract infections have explored PCT levels for initiation and discontinuation of antibiotics. Prominent among them is the PROHOSP study which was a multicenter RCT which explored whether PCT based algorithm could reduce antibiotic exposure in patients with lower respiratory tract infections. Patients were randomized into either PCT based algorithm group—antibiotics were strongly discouraged if procalcitonin was <0.1, discouraged if 0.1–0.25, encouraged if 0.25–0.5, strongly encouraged if >0.5. They found that antibiotic exposure and antibiotic associated adverse events were significantly decreased in the PCT group while adverse outcomes were similar in both groups.[29] Hence in patients with suspected respiratory tract infections, procalcitonin can help differentiating between infectious and noninfectious causes as well as differentiating bacterial from viral causes. However, if patients present with features of lower respiratory tract infections, clinical picture and radiology is suggestive of bacterial infections, antibiotics are initiated without procalcitonin levels, as delay in initiation has been found to increase mortality. In these cases, procalcitonin is used primarily after initiation and trends of procalcitonin are used for discontinuation of antibiotics.

Prognostication

Several studies have looked at levels of PCT as well as PCT clearance as prognostic markers and found varying results. A systematic review and meta-analysis which evaluated prognostic value of procalcitonin in adult patients with sepsis found that an elevated PCT was associated with higher risk of death, initial PCT value had limited prognostic value and PCT nonclearance was significant prognostic factor for mortality. However, the optimal cut-offs and definition of procalcitonin clearance is not yet defined.[30]

Procalcitonin in Renal Failure

In patients with renal dysfunction and on renal replacement therapy, basal PCT may be raised as half-life increases, however kinetics is not altered and hence PCT decline rates may be unaltered.[31,32]

NEWER BIOMARKERS

Several other biomarkers are investigated for sepsis. Some of them are triggering receptor expressed on myeloid cells-1 (TREM-1), interleukin 27 (IL-27), presepsin, cell free DNA, miRNA. Biomarkers related to the symptoms of sepsis rather than the mechanisms of inflammation have also been tested, such as CT-pro-AVP (C-terminal segment of pro-arginine vasopressin), which aids in regulation of blood pressure; however, these biomarkers have not proven effective in diagnostic testing.[33] TREM 1, an immunoglobulin induces inflammatory process by activation of production of chemokines, cytokines and reactive oxygen species. Levels of its soluble form sTREM-1 can be detected by enzyme linked immunosorbent assay (ELISA). A recent review and meta-analysis by Jiyong et al. showed that elevated sTREM-1, sampled and measured from the location of infection, is highly predictive of bacterial infection. However further studies are required for validation and to be used clinically.[34]

Interleukin 27 is a cytokine produced upon exposure to microbial products and inflammatory stimuli which has found to have both pro- and anti-inflammatory effects. Initial studies done in pediatric population was found to have good specificity and positive predictive value however similar results through subsequent studies in adults could not be reproduced. Combination of IL-27 along with PCT is being explored but yet not validated.[35] CD64 is an immunoglobulin which when activated by proinflammatory cytokines leads to phagocytosis of bacteria. Studies have found that CD64 is specific to bacterial infection hence used as a biomarker in sepsis. A systematic review and meta-analysis by Cid et al., found sensitivity and specificity of CD64 to be 79% and 91% respectively, however authors concluded that methodological quality of studies to be poor.[36] Hence, further studies are required to confirm its validity.

Presepsin is a soluble form of CD14 which is expressed on monocytes and macrophages leading to activation of toll-like receptors and TNF alpha. A multicenter study was done to evaluate utilization of presepsin in SIRS without infection, sepsis, severe sepsis and septic shock. It was noted that presepsin was consistently elevated with higher degrees of sepsis and was significantly lower in noninfected patients and concluded to be a good diagnostic biomarker.[37] A recent systematic review and meta-analysis which compared diagnostic accuracy of presepsin and procalcitonin for sepsis in critically ill adults concluded that both were useful for early detection of sepsis and lead to reduction of mortality in critically ill patients.[38] Cell-free plasma DNA (cfDNA) are fragments of DNA that are released because of cell necrosis or apoptosis. This is being explored as a prognostic biomarker of sepsis and is usually associated with cell death. Observational studies found that nonsurvivors of sepsis and septic shock had higher levels of cfDNA compared to survivors. Hence, it is being explored as a prognostic biomarker[35] miRNAs are a newly identified class of biomarkers that may serve as diagnostic or prognostic role in various human pathologic conditions, including sepsis. miRNAs are short sequences of endogenous RNAs that are involved in translational gene regulation.

The combination of three sentinel biomarkers, IL-6, PCT, and sTREM-1, is uncommon, but pairs within the three have been attempted before to predict and/or prognosticate sepsis: sTREM-1 and PCT or sTREM-1 and IL-6.[39]

Finally, it is being increasingly recognized that while sepsis is often thought of as an exaggerated proinflammatory state, there may be a significant anti-inflammatory and immunosuppressive component, especially in late sepsis or sepsis occurring in elderly patients. New biomarkers to estimate the degree of immunosuppression include circulating blood monocyte expression of HLA-DR, monocyte expression of programmed cell-death ligand-1 (PD-L1), and low absolute lymphocyte counts. These could help identify patients who might require immunostimulating or immunomodulating therapy rather than anti-inflammatory therapies in the immunosuppressed stages.[40] However, this is still experimental.

CONCLUSION

Biomarkers are naturally occurring molecules, genes, or other characteristics by particular physiologic or pathologic processes can be identified. Several biomarkers such as WBC count, ESR, lactate, CRP and procalcitonin have been investigated. CRP has been found to have high sensitivity but poor specificity for infection. It has been found to be a better indicator of inflammation than infection. Procalcitonin (PCT), a precursor of calcitonin which is usually undetectable has been found to be increased several fold in sepsis. PCT is used in diagnosis of sepsis, de-escalation of antibiotics, and differentiation of bacterial and viral infections. In postsurgical patients, PCT levels raise on first postoperative day depending on degree of injury. PCT levels start rising few hours after surgery, peak around 24 hours and start declining to normal levels by 48 hours. Persistent elevations of PCT especially >10 ng/L in nontransplant postsurgery patients should raise suspicion of postoperative infection. PCT is recommended for de-escalation of antibiotics when PCT reduces significantly from baseline. Newer biomarkers such as triggering receptor expressed on myeloid cells-1 (sTREM-1), interleukin 27 (IL-27), presepsin, cell free DNA, miRNA are being evaluated for sepsis but are not yet validated.

REFERENCES

1. Gül F, Arslantaş MK, Cinel İ, Kumar A. Changing definitions of sepsis. Turkish J Anesthesiol. 2017;45:129-38.
2. van Engelen TSR, Wiersinga WJ, Scicluna BP, Poll TVD. Biomarkers in sepsis. Crit Care Clin. 2018;34:139-52.
3. Barati M, Alinejad F, Bahar MA, Tabrisi MS, Shamshiri AR, Bodouhi NO, et al. Comparison of WBC, ESR, CRP and PCT serum levels in septic and non-septic burn cases. Burns. 2008;34:770-4.
4. Faix JD. Biomarkers of sepsis. Crit Rev Clin Lab Sci. 2013;50:23-36.
5. Iskandar A, Susianti H, Anshory M, Di Somma S. Biomarkers utility for sepsis patients management. London: Intechopen; 2018.
6. Assicot M, Gendrel D, Carsin H, Raymond J, Guilbaud J, Bohuon C. High serum procalcitonin concentrations in patients with sepsis and infection. Lancet. 1993;341:515-8.

7. Müller B, Harbarth S, Stolz D, Bingisser R, Mueller C, Leuppi J, et al. Diagnostic and prognostic accuracy of clinical and laboratory parameters in community-acquired pneumonia. BMC Infect Dis. 2007;7:10.
8. Clec'h C, Ferriere F, Karoubi P, Fosse JP, Cupa M, Hoang P, et al. Diagnostic and prognostic value of procalcitonin in patients with septic shock. Crit Care Med. 2004;32:1166-9.
9. Müller B, Becker KL, Schächinger H, Rickenbacher PR, Huber PR, Zimmerli W, et al. Calcitonin precursors are reliable markers of sepsis in a medical intensive care unit. Crit Care Med. 2000;28:977-83.
10. Ugarte H, Silva E, Mercan D, De Mendonça A, Vincent JL. Procalcitonin used as a marker of infection in the intensive care unit. Crit Care Med. 1999;27:498-504.
11. Ruokonen E, Ilkka L, Niskanen M, Takala J. Procalcitonin and neopterin as indicators of infection in critically ill patients. Acta Anaesthesiol Scand. 2002;46:398-404.
12. Wacker C, Prkno A, Brunkhorst FM, Schlattmann P. Procalcitonin as a diagnostic marker for sepsis: a systematic review and meta-analysis. Lancet Infect Dis. 2013;13:426-35.
13. Delèvaux I, André M, Colombier M, Albuisson E, Meylheuc F, Bègue RJ, et al. Can procalcitonin measurement help in differentiating between bacterial infection and other kinds of inflammatory processes? Ann Rheum Dis. 2003;62:337-40.
14. Lee H. Procalcitonin as a biomarker of infectious diseases. Korean J Intern Med. 2013;28:285-91.
15. Nobre V, Harbarth S, Graf JD, Rohner P, Pugin J. Use of procalcitonin to shorten antibiotic treatment duration in septic patients: a randomized trial. Am J Respir Crit Care Med. 2008;177:498-505.
16. Hochreiter M, Köhler T, Schweiger AM, Keck FS, Bein B, von Spiegel T, et al. Procalcitonin to guide duration of antibiotic therapy in intensive care patients: a randomized prospective controlled trial. Crit Care. 2009;13:R83.
17. Schroeder S, Hochreiter M, Koehler T, Schweiger AM, Bein B, Keck FS, et al. Procalcitonin (PCT)-guided algorithm reduces length of antibiotic treatment in surgical intensive care patients with severe sepsis: results of a prospective randomized study. Arch Surg. 2009;394:221-6.
18. Bouadma L, Luyt CE, Tubach F, Cracco C, Alvarez A, Schwebel C, et al. Use of procalcitonin to reduce patients' exposure to antibiotics in intensive care units (PRORATA trial): a multicentre randomised controlled trial. Lancet. 2010;375:463-74.
19. Shehabi Y, Sterba M, Garrett PM, Rachakonda KS, Stephens D, Harrigan P, et al. Procalcitonin algorithm in critically ill adults with undifferentiated infection or suspected sepsis. A randomized controlled trial. Am J Respir Crit Care Med. 2014;190:1102-10.
20. Jong EA, Lange DW, Van Oers JA, Nijsten MW, Twisk JW, Beishuizen A. Stop Antibiotics on guidance of procalcitonin Study (SAPS): A randomised prospective multicenter investigator-initiated trial to analyse whether daily measurements of procalcitonin versus a standard-of-care approach can safely shorten antibiotic duration in intensive care unit patients. BMC Infect Dis. 2013;13:178.
21. Paruk F, Chausse JM. Monitoring the postsurgery inflammatory host response. J Emerg Crit Care Med. 2019;3:47.
22. Lindberg M, Hole A, Johnsen H, Asberg A, Rydning A, Myrvold HE, et al. Reference intervals for procalcitonin and C-reactive protein after major abdominal surgery. Scand J Clin Lab Invest. 2002;62:189-94.
23. Meisner M, Tschaikowsky K, Hutzler A, Schick C, Schüttler J. Postoperative plasma concentrations of procalcitonin after different types of surgery. Intensive Care Med. 1998;24:680-4.
24. Domínguez-Comesaña E, Estevez-Fernández SM, López-Gómez V, Ballinas-Miranda J, Domínguez-Fernández R. Procalcitonin and C-reactive protein as

early markers of postoperative intra-abdominal infection in patients operated on colorectal cancer. Int J Colorectal Dis. 2017;32:1771-4.
25. Trásy D, Tánczos K, Németh M, Hankovszky P, Lovas A, Mikor A, et al. Delta procalcitonin is a better indicator of infection than absolute procalcitonin values in critically ill patients: a prospective observational study. J Immunol Res. 2016;2016:3530752.
26. Tsangaris I, Plachouras D, Kavatha D, Gourgoulis GM, Tsantes A, Kopterides P, et al. Diagnostic and prognostic value of procalcitonin among febrile critically ill patients with prolonged ICU stay. BMC Infect Dis. 2009;9:213.
27. Novotny AR, Emmanuel K, Hueser N, Knebel C, Kriner M, Ulm K, et al. Procalcitonin ratio indicates successful surgical treatment of abdominal sepsis. Surgery. 2009; 145:20-6.
28. Christ-Crain M, Jaccard-Stolz D, Bingisser R, Gencay MM, Huber PR, Tamm M, et al. Effect of procalcitonin-guided treatment on antibiotic use and outcome in lower respiratory tract infections: cluster-randomised, single-blinded intervention trial. Lancet. 2004;363:600-7.
29. Schuetz P, Christ-Crain M, Thomann R, Falconnier C, Wolbers M, Widmer I, et al. Effect of procalcitonin-based guidelines vs standard guidelines on antibiotic use in lower respiratory tract infections: the ProHOSP randomized controlled trial. JAMA. 2009;302:1059-66.
30. Liu D, Su L, Han G, Yan P, Xie L. Prognostic value of procalcitonin in adult patients with sepsis: a systematic review and meta-analysis. PLoS One. 2015;10(6):e0129450.
31. Meisner M, Lohs T, Huettemann E, Schmidt J, Hueller M, Reinhart K. The plasma elimination rate and urinary secretion of procalcitonin in patients with normal and impaired renal function. Eur J Anaesthesiol. 2001;18:79-87.
32. Grace E, Turner RM. Use of procalcitonin in patients with various degrees of chronic kidney disease including renal replacement therapy. Clin Infect Dis. 2014;59: 1761-7.
33. Laribi S, Lienart D, Castanares-Zapatero D, Collienne C, Wittebole X, Laterre P. CT-proAVP is not a good predictor of vasopressor need in septic shock. Shock. 2015;44(4):330-5.
34. Jiyong J, Tiancha H, Wei C, Huahao S. Diagnostic value of the soluble triggering receptor expressed on myeloid cells-1 in bacterial infection: a meta-analysis. Intensive Care Med. 2009; 35:587-95.
35. Sandquist M, Wong HR. Biomarkers of sepsis and their potential value in diagnosis, prognosis and treatment. Expert Rev Clin Immunol. 2014;10:1349-56.
36. Cid J, Aguinaco R, Sanchez R, García-Pardo G, Llorente A. Neutrophil CD64 expression as marker of bacterial infection: a systematic review and meta-analysis. J Infect. 2010;60:313-9.
37. Ulla M, Pizzolato E, Lucchiari M, Loiacono M, Soardo F, Forno D, et al. Diagnostic and prognostic value of presepsin in the management of sepsis in the emergency department: a multicenter prospective study. Crit Care. 2013;17(4):R168.
38. Kondo Y, Umemura Y, Hayashida K, Hara Y, Aihara M, Yamakawa K. Diagnostic value of procalcitonin and presepsin for sepsis in critically ill adult patients: a systematic review and meta-analysis. J Intensive Care. 2019;7:22.
39. Gibot S, Béné MC, Noel R, Massin F, Guy J, Cravoisy A, et al. Combination biomarkers to diagnose sepsis in the critically ill patient. Am J Resp and Crit Care Med. 2012;186(1):65-71.
40. Hotchkiss RS, Monneret G, Payen D. Immunosuppression in sepsis: a novel understanding of the disorder and a new therapeutic approach. Lancet Infect Dis. 2013;13:260-8.

Surgery for Gastric Cancer

Arindam Mondal, Manish Suresh Bhandare,
Vikram Anil Chaudhari, Shailesh V Shrikhande

INTRODUCTION

Gastric cancer (GC) is the third leading cause of cancer-related deaths worldwide,[1] after lung and colorectal cancers. The highest incidence of GC is reported in Japan, China, Korea, Costa Rica, and Russia. Its incidence and mortality has shown a decline in the western hemisphere. However, the same is not true in the Indian context which has seen an increase in its incidence, with the highest recorded incidence in the North-Eastern state of Mizoram according to National Cancer Registry Programme (NCRP) 2013. Surgery has remained as the primary weapon in the armamentarium for the treatment of GC. However, advances in chemotherapy and radiotherapy have also contributed to improvement in survival of patients with GC.[2] Studies to assess the applicability of these western treatment protocols to Indian patients are still awaited. A study from Tata Memorial Centre, Mumbai, India has confirmed the safety of GC surgery in experienced high-volume centers, with an overall major morbidity of 8.9% and mortality of 1.5%.[3] With surgery and neoadjuvant or adjuvant chemotherapy, the 5 years' survival of GC is around 51%.

The histological classification of GC was first described by Lauren in 1965, and divided adenocarcinoma into two types: intestinal and diffuse types. Intestinal type is common in older individual and common in male gender. It is also seen in endemic area, associated with atrophic gastritis and environmental factors. It usually spreads hematogenously and the most common site is the liver. Correa et al.[4] suggested multistep progression in *Helicobacter pylori*-induced gastritis to intestinal type GC. This model explains progression of intestinal type GC, not applied for diffuse type, suggesting that the histological type has different molecular and pathological behavior. The diffuse variety is common in younger individual and has no gender predilection. It is characterized by the submucosal infiltrative growth resulting in thick rigid leather bottle appearance (Linitis plastica). The other differences in the two histological type are enumerated in **Table 1**.

CLINICAL PRESENTATION

The most common symptoms of early stages of GC are nonspecific dyspepsia, bloating, and early satiety. These are often overlooked by patients resulting

TABLE 1: Various characteristic features of Lauren classification.

Characteristics	Intestinal type	Diffuse type
Age	Older individual	Younger individual
Gender	Common in male	Equal
Associated with	Environmental factor	Hereditary
Preexisting condition	Atrophic gastritis	Blood type A
Site of stomach	Distal part	Proximal part
Common mode of spread	Hematogenous	Lymphatic and transmural
The most common site of metastases	Liver	Peritoneal
Histology	Well-differentiated glands, intestinal metaplasia	Poor glandular differentiation
Gross appearance	Exophytic lesions	Ulcerated

in diagnosis at an advanced stage in most cases. The symptoms which bring the patient to medical notice are mostly abdominal pain, vomiting, bleeding (hematemesis and/or melena), lump in the abdomen, loss of appetite, or unexplained weight loss. Proximal tumors, especially at the gastroesophageal (GE) junction, present with early symptom of dysphagia. For advanced tumors, clinically evident signs can be present, such as, a palpable mass in the epigastrium, left supraclavicular or axillary lymphadenopathy (Virchow node/Irish node), umbilical nodule (Sister Mary Joseph node), ovarian masses (Krukenberg tumor), deposits in the Blumer's shelf on rectal examination, nodular hepatomegaly, or ascites. When present, these signs can help direct precise investigations and avoid extensive workup, especially in patients with poor general condition.

Diagnosis and Staging

A suspected GC patient should be evaluated to confirm the diagnosis, accurately stage the disease, and evaluate fitness for treatment (surgery/chemotherapy). The investigations include:

- *Routine blood investigations:* Complete hemogram, renal function tests, liver function tests and coagulation profile
- *Upper gastrointestinal endoscopy (UGIE) and biopsy:* For mapping the disease, and obtaining tissue for biopsy confirmation. Multiple (n = 6–8) biopsies are recommended. In patients with impending gastric outlet obstruction (GOO), a nasojejunal feeding tube can be placed during an UGIE.
- *Endoscopic ultrasonography (EUS):* When available, EUS should be considered in the following situations, after contrast-enhanced computed tomography (CT) scan shows suspected early disease:

- To confirm T1/T2 N0 status to offer upfront surgery versus local treatment
- Doubtful T3 disease, to differentiate from T2 disease to decide between neoadjuvant chemotherapy (NACT) and upfront surgery
- For patients with advanced/metastatic disease, biopsy from the suspected metastatic disease sites is an acceptable alternative to endoscopic biopsy. HER2 neu status evaluation on biopsy specimens is recommended in such situations.
- Contrast-enhanced CT scan of thorax, abdomen, and pelvis is the most valuable staging investigation. Abdominal CT is used to determine the site, bulk, and extent of the gastric wall thickening **(Fig. 1)**, involvement of surrounding structures such as pancreas, transverse colon, and extent of nodal involvement **(Fig. 2)**, evidence of metastatic disease such as ascites, liver metastases or omental nodules, any variation in vasculature, and evidence of GOO or perforation. A CT scan of the chest is also required as a part of staging evaluation, to rule out metastatic disease.
- *Staging laparoscopy:* Staging laparoscopy is recommended for all patients with radiologically suspected stage II/III disease. Staging laparoscopy has been shown to upstage approximately 30% of GC.[5-7] Its advantages include detection of peritoneal disease which can be easily missed in conventional imaging (e.g., small peritoneal nodules), and it allows collection of peritoneal fluid/washings for cytology.
- *CEA and CA 19.9:* These tumor markers are not essential or diagnostic for GC. However, if their baseline levels are elevated, they can be used during follow-up for early detection of recurrences.[8,9]
- Magnetic resonance imaging (MRI) of the liver can be used as a problem-solving tool in cases with doubtful liver metastases on CT scan.[10]

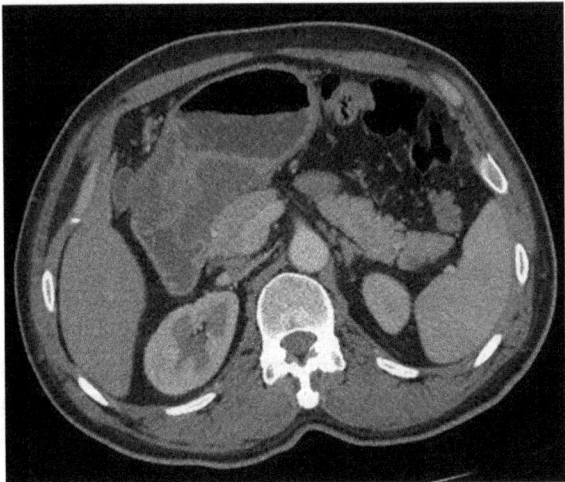

Fig. 1: Bulky pyloric growth abutting head of pancreas and causing gastric outlet obstruction (GOO).

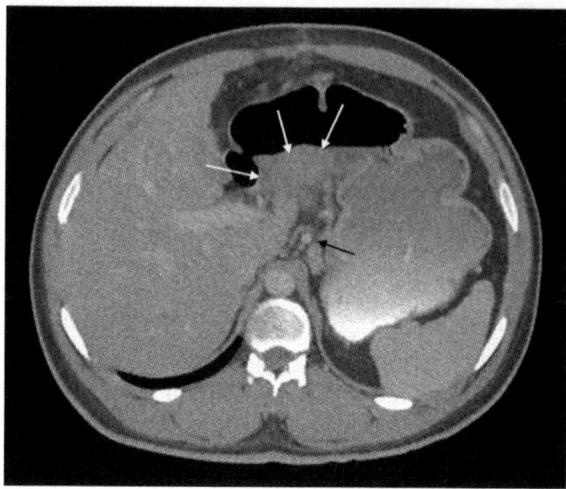

Fig. 2: Thickening of posterior wall of antrum (white arrows) with enlarged coeliac axis node (black arrow).

- Positron emission tomography (PET) scan is not routinely recommended since around 50% of the GCs have reduced numbers of glucose transporter 1 (GLUT1) transporters rendering them fluorodeoxyglucose (FDG)-negative. However, it is more sensitive than CT scan for detecting distant metastases,[11] but less sensitive than staging laparoscopy for peritoneal disease. It has also been recently studied for directing treatment changes based on response to treatment.[12]

With these baseline investigations, the patient should be staged as per the American Joint Committee on Cancer Staging manual (8th edition) and a TNM stage assigned. Nutritional assessment is an important part of the workup for patients of GC before planning any treatment, since most patients are nutritionally challenged owing to cancer cachexia per se, or mechanical GOO. Collecting a dietary history, assessing clinical signs of malnutrition, performing a physical examination and obtaining anthropometric data, laboratory data such as blood albumin levels, A:G ratio, and evaluating the functional status can all contribute to provide an estimate of the nutritional status of the patient.

Management

Broadly, GC is managed with a curative intent if the disease is confined to stages I to III, whereas for stage IV disease, the intent is palliative. The treatment of the curative stages also differs based on early or locally advanced disease. The following are three scenarios to elucidate the different management principles:
1. *Early gastric cancers (EGCs) (T1a/T1b N0/N1 M0):* The management options include:
    a. Endoscopic resection (based on certain criteria):[13]
        i. Endoscopic mucosal resection (EMR)
        ii. Endoscopic submucosal dissection (ESD)

b. Surgery (gastrectomy/local resection)[14-16]
   c. Eradication of *H. pylori*[17]

   Node-positive patients are treated with radical surgery and chemotherapy.

2. *Locally advanced GC (resectable, T2-T4 N+ M0):* The management options include:
   a. Perioperative chemotherapy (as per FLOT/MAGIC protocol)[18,19]
   b. Upfront surgery followed by adjuvant chemoradiotherapy [20-22]
   c. Upfront surgery followed by adjuvant chemotherapy [23-25]

3. *Advanced GCs [unresectable T3/T4 N+ or M1]:* Management is palliative in nature and depends on the patient's performance status. The options are:
   a. *Surgery:* Palliative gastrojejunostomy, palliative gastrectomy (in select patients with obstruction or bleeding not responding to nonsurgical treatment)
   b. *Palliative chemotherapy:* Can improve quality of life and increase survival
   c. *Palliative radiotherapy:* For control of bleeding or pain from bone metastasis
   d. *Targeted therapy:* Like trastuzumab in HER2 positive tumors or the vascular endothelial growth factor receptor (VEGFR) inhibitor, ramucirumab[26,27]
   e. Pain management
   f. Palliation of ascites

ENDOSCOPIC RESECTION

The endoscopic resection is recommended for the EGC, it includes EMR and ESD.[28-30] In EMR, suction through an endoscope creates a pseudopolyp of the mucosa and then the removal is done through snare. It often results in piecemeal resection and higher local recurrence rates (2.3–36.5%) because of incorrect pathological assessment.[31] The major limitation of this procedure is incomplete resection for lesions larger than 2 cm in diameter due to the size limitations of accessories. According to the Japanese Gastric Cancer Association (JGCA), EMR is recommended for: well-differentiated adenocarcinoma, limited to the mucosa, tumor ≤ 2 cm in elevated type or depressed lesions ≤ 1 cm without ulceration. 5-year overall survival (OS) rates and recurrence rates are almost similar in EMR and surgery groups (93.6 vs. 94.2% and 1.2 vs. 1.1%).[32] However, the metachronous lesions are reported higher in the EMR than in surgery group (5.8 vs. 1.1%).[31]

Endoscopic submucosal dissection involves dissection and excision with cutting instrument following submucosal injection of viscous fluid. It allows en bloc resection of the specimen, improved pathological assessment, and is associated with lower recurrence rate. The major advantage of ESD has complete resection of lesion irrespective of size. 5-year OS rates and recurrence-free rates are 93.6-100% and 98.7-100%, respectively.[31] The complication includes perforation (3.6-4.5%) and bleeding (7-15.6%).[31] This procedure is mostly practiced in Japan and Asia; however, data from West are limited. ESD is superior to EMR as it enables precise pathologic staging for large EGC. With the development of ESD technique, expanded indications of endoscopic resection for EGC are differentiated type cancers without evidence of lymphovascular invasion, including: (1) mucosal cancer without ulceration, irrespective of tumor size; (2) mucosal cancer with ulceration, <3 cm in diameter; and (3) minimal (500 μm from the muscularis mucosae) submucosal invasive cancer <3 cm in size.[29,30]

Another issue with the endoscopic procedure is the nodal staging. Early gastric carcinomas are defined as lesions confined to mucosa or submucosa irrespective to nodal metastases; however, they carry 10-20% risk of lymph node metastases.[33] Soetikno et al.[34] addressed the risk of lymph nodal metastases and has justified the expanded criteria. The various key pathological assessments should be performed in the specimen. The precise negative lateral and vertical margin status should be confirmed for completion of resection. In presence of undifferentiated type tumor mixed within the differentiated type, it is important to evaluate the proportion of undifferentiated type to predict the vascular and lymph node metastases. In presence of submucosal invasive, the extent of invasion and histologic type determines additional surgery. The muscularis mucosae is identified by using the immunohistochemistry of desmin, as risk of lymph nodal metastases is higher when the tumor depth is 500 μm or more from the lower edge of muscularis mucosae (≥sm2) than sm1. The microscopic examination of vascular and lymphatic invasion should be performed.[34,35]

PRINCIPLES OF RADICAL GASTRECTOMY

Surgery is the only curative treatment for GC. The primary aim of GC surgery is to achieve complete removal of the primary tumor and regional nodal tissues with histological confirmation of tumor-free (R0) surgical margins. A grossly normal margin of 5 cm on either side of the gastric tumor should be aimed for during surgical resections. Stomach has extensive lymphatic network, causing tumor spread, more aggressive in diffuse than intestinal GC. Thus, larger resection margin required for diffuse than intestinal type (5 vs. 3 cm). However, this rule does not hold true for tumors on either extremes- distal tumors or lesions in the cardia, where a shorter distal and proximal margins respectively are acceptable. In such cases, a minimum negative margin of 1 cm is considered acceptable when confirmed by intraoperative frozen section analysis. Given the adverse nutritional and quality of life implications of a total gastrectomy, preservation of a remnant stomach should be aimed for if deemed safe oncologically.

Depending on the location of the tumor in stomach, three surgeries have been defined, namely subtotal (distal), proximal, and total gastrectomy.
- *Total gastrectomy:* Complete removal of stomach, including the GE junction and the pylorus
- *Subtotal gastrectomy:* Removal of the pylorus, antrum, entire lesser curve till GE junction and variable portions of the gastric body. The remnant stomach is supplied by the short gastric vessels and hence these should be preserved.
- *Proximal gastrectomy:* Removal of GE junction, cardia, fundus, the lesser curve till the incisura angularis and variable portions of the body depending on distal tumor extent. Significant nodal disease along the greater curvature (i.e., stations 4 and 6) is a contraindication to proximal gastrectomy and these patients are best treated with total gastrectomy for adequate nodal clearance. The remnant stomach is supplied by the right gastroepiploic and right gastric vessels and should be adequate for a tension-free esophagogastric anastomosis. Some form of pyloric drainage, either pyloric dilatation or pyloroplasty, is necessary in view of inevitable complete vagal denervation of the gastric remnant.

SURGERY BY SITE OF TUMOR

Proximal Tumors

Gastric cancer in proximal part stomach has poor prognosis than distal part. Proximal gastrectomy is an alternative to total gastrectomy in very early stage tumors.[36] But it can be an option even in locally advanced proximal GCs after treatment with NACT, provided the tumor size and location permit preservation of an adequate remnant without compromising oncological margins.[37] However, total gastrectomy is preferred for proximal tumors by most surgeons for the following reasons:
- The Roux-en-Y reconstruction performed following a total gastrectomy has an extremely low incidence of reflux esophagitis, as compared to approximately one-third of patients of proximal subtotal gastrectomy who develop reflux esophagitis.[38] The role of jejunal J pouch reconstruction may be used by few authors in patients undergoing R0 resection with long-term expected survival.
- Proximal subtotal gastrectomy may leave behind lymph nodes along the lesser curvature of the stomach, which is the most common site of nodal metastases.

A meta-analysis comparing proximal and total gastrectomy,[39] comprising of two randomized controlled trials (RCTs) and nine retrospective studies, showed no difference in 5-year survival (61 vs. 64%) but more cancer recurrences (39 vs. 24%) in the proximal gastrectomy group. Also, the incidence of complications, including anastomotic stenosis (27 vs. 7%) and reflux esophagitis (20 vs. 2%), was more with a proximal subtotal gastrectomy. Therefore, total gastrectomy remains the preferred surgery for proximal tumors.

Distal Tumors

For distal tumors, the preferred surgery is a subtotal gastrectomy preserving the cardia and fundus. For tumors limited to the pylorus, antrum, and distal body, at least two trials show no added survival benefit for total compared to subtotal gastrectomy.[40,41] Also, subtotal gastrectomy has been reported to be associated with a better nutritional status and quality of life, and hence is widely accepted as the procedure of choice for distal tumors. Also, as discussed earlier, laparoscopic radical distal gastrectomy remains a safe alternative to open surgery for early distal tumors in experienced high volume centers.

CONTROVERSIES IN GASTRIC CANCER SURGERY

Role of Bursectomy

Bursectomy refers to the removal of the entire lesser sac peritoneal covering during surgery for GC. Popularized by the Japanese since the 1960s, it is recommended for tumors with invasion of the serosa, and advised to be avoided in T1/T2 tumors in order to prevent injury to the pancreas or adjacent blood vessels.[36] However, its role is debated. A meta-analysis by Shen et al., including two RCTs and three retrospective studies, showed that bursectomy had no survival benefit in GC patients.[42] Though a subgroup analysis suggested that bursectomy may improve survival in serosa-positive patients, this was statistically insignificant. Also, a large RCT, including over 1,200 patients from Japan, is evaluating the role of bursectomy in cT3/cT4a GC. The preliminary results showed no difference in 3 years' survival rates in the bursectomy and nonbursectomy groups [hazard ratio (HR) for bursectomy—1.075]. Hence, the authors concluded that, although technically feasible, bursectomy is not recommended routinely for cT3 or cT4 GC.[43]

Total Omentectomy for Early Tumors

Omentectomy is considered as an important part of radical gastrectomy for GC. But the incidence of omental involvement is only 2–8% as per various retrospective studies.[44,45] However, patients with omental disease have very poor outcomes with early recurrent metastatic disease. Though one study proposed avoiding omentectomy in early T1/T2 GC,[44] the absence of predictive factors for omental involvement and the prognostic value of omentectomy makes it an integral component of radical surgery for GC. Another study compared partial and total omentectomy for early-stage GC and concluded that partial omentectomy was a more useful procedure in this setting.[46] However, this needs further investigations for before any recommendations can be made.

Extent of Lymph Nodal Dissection

The lymph nodes involvement is the most important independent prognostic factor of GC. The lymph node stations of stomach have been classified by the JGCA, and four different extent of dissections have been described, D1, D2, D3, and D4.[47,48] D1 includes removal of stations 1–6 (perigastric lymph nodes), D2 includes removal of D1 with stations 7–11 (nodes along left gastric artery, common hepatic artery, celiac trunk, and splenic artery) **(Fig. 3)**, D3 includes removal of D2 with stations 12–14 (hepatoduodenal ligament and root of mesentery) **(Figs. 4A to C)**, and D4 includes removal of D3 with stations 15–16 (para-aortic and paracolic lymph nodes). D1 dissection is also classified as conservative lymph node dissection whereas D2 to D4 as extended lymph node dissection.

The differences between the surgical practice and outcomes between the west and the east are probably best exemplified in the nodal management of GC. In Japan, D2 lymphadenectomy has been a standard practice since the 1960s. But most Western surgeons perform gastrectomy with only limited lymph node dissection (D1), because of lack of survival benefit and the associated morbidity with D2 lymphadenectomy.[49,50] Indian data from Tata Memorial Hospital suggest that morbidity and mortality following D2 lymphadenectomy are low, i.e., <10 and <1.5%, respectively.[3,51] Cochrane collaboration meta-analysis including both randomized and nonrandomized trials showed no difference in the survival between D1 and D2 dissection in GC. However, data supported D2 dissection in T3/T4 tumors. The increased postoperative mortality noted following extended lymph node dissection attributed to the performance of pancreatectomy, splenectomy, and surgeons' inexperience.

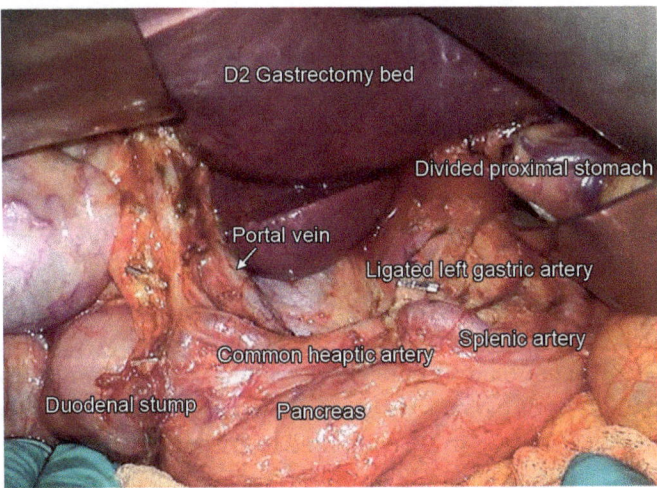

Fig. 3: Intraoperative image, post-D2 lymph node dissection.

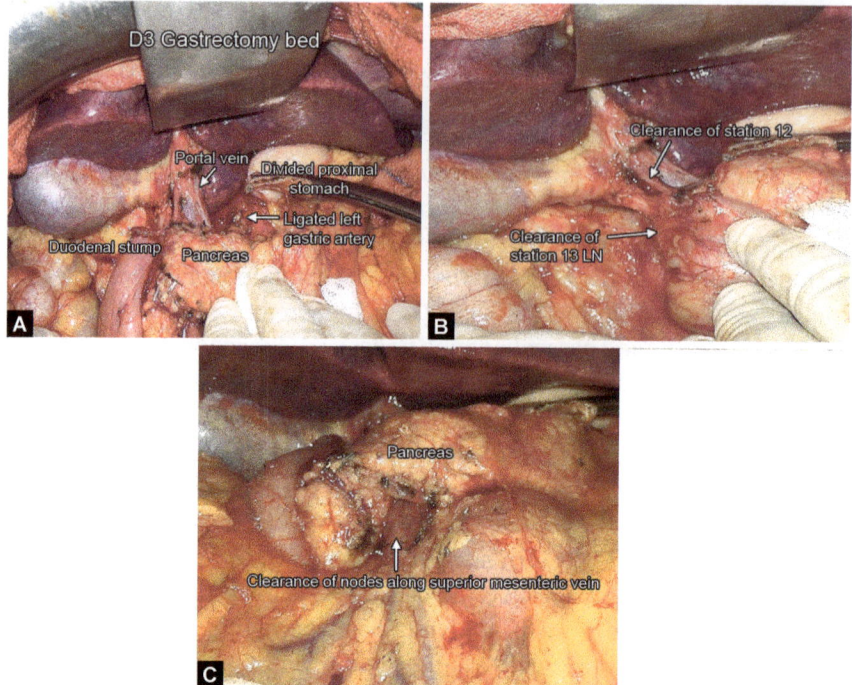

Figs. 4A to C: Intraoperative image, post-D3 lymph node dissection.

A randomized trial from Taiwan showed a significant benefit in OS and recurrence free survival (RFS) for a D2 or D3 procedure as compared with D1 lymphadenectomy, with no increase in operative mortality.[52] 15-year follow-up of the Dutch Trial, which had initially showed no benefit of D2 over a D1 lymphadenectomy, was published in 2010, and showed gastric-cancer-related deaths were significantly higher in the D1 group compared with the D2 group.[53] This difference was even higher after the exclusion of the perioperative mortalities. Subgroup analysis showed that distal pancreaticosplenectomy, a routine component of D2 lymphadenectomy as per the protocol, was associated with high perioperative mortality, and significantly lowered the OS in the D2 arm. However, the long-term local recurrences were lesser in the D2 arm compared to the D1 arm. These findings led the authors to recommend spleen and pancreas preserving D2 dissection in the patients with resectable GC.

Similar results were seen in a meta-analysis by Jiang L, which included 12 RCTs on different lymphadenectomies for resectable GC. It found no significant survival benefit between D1 and D2 lymphadenectomy, but subgroup analysis of patients without splenectomy and/or pancreatectomy had a trend for better OS in D2 compared to D1 patients.[54] Also, there was a significant RFS improvement in favor of D2 lymphadenectomy. There were no significant differences in OS and RFS between D2 group and D3 group.

At Tata Memorial Hospital, Mumbai, a "Phase III Randomized Trial Comparing D2 vs D3 Lymphadenectomy with Gastric Cancer Following Neoadjuvant Chemotherapy" (ELANCe trial) is ongoing (clinicaltrials.gov, trial ID - NCT02139605) to further evaluate the role of D3 lymphadenectomy in the era of perioperative chemotherapy.[55]

In summary, D2 lymphadenectomy offers survival advantage and is the current standard of care for nonmetastatic, resectable T3/T4 GC. Routine pancreaticosplenectomy is not recommended as a part of D2 dissection. Limited data suggest that D3 lymphadenectomy does not further improve survival outcome. Removal and histological examination of a minimum of 16 nodes is recommended for adequate lymph nodal staging.

Splenectomy

The splenic hilar nodes have shown metastatic disease in 15–27% patients of GC. For patients with proximal gastric tumor, splenectomy and distal pancreatectomy are sometimes performed to have nodal clearance. However, as mentioned above, concomitant splenectomy or pancreaticosplenectomy has higher postoperative morbidity as higher septic complication, pancreatic fistulae, and anastomotic leak. Thus, splenectomy should only be performed in patients with macroscopic disease involving perisplenic nodes or spleen.

Adequacy of Surgical Margins

Based on the studies in 1980s that illustrated a margin <3–6 cm from the gross tumor was related to increased risk of microscopically positive (R1) resection margins, the recommendation was to resect 5 cm of grossly normal stomach on either side of the tumor.[56] National Comprehensive Cancer Network (NCCN) practice guidelines recommend resection margins >4 cm from the gross tumor, whereas Japanese Gastric Cancer Treatment guidelines advise a >2 cm margin for T1 tumors and a 3–5 cm margin for T2–T4 tumors.[36,57] In this regard, the limiting factor is often the location of the tumor in stomach (proximal margin in tumors with close proximity to GE junction, and distal margins in tumors in close proximity to duodenum). Most studies on the margin in gastric adenocarcinoma, including the data on margin length, focus on the proximal margin, and there is limited data on the distal margin.

The Proximal Margin for Proximal Tumors

A study from Japan, which included only patients with R0 resection showed that a margin of >2.8 cm on gross measurement was independently associated with increased survival in Siewert type II/III tumors.[58] However, this study was before the advent of modern chemotherapy and neoadjuvant therapy strategies, and due to paradigm shifts in these regards, its conclusions cannot be compared to the present time period. In contrast to the Japanese study, the

US Gastric Cancer Collaborative Study and a study by Lee et al. showed no difference in local recurrence or OS based on the length of proximal margin.[59,60] Generally, for proximal tumors, a negative proximal margin of 1 cm confirmed on intraoperative frozen section is deemed acceptable.

The Distal Margin

As opposed to data on proximal margins, there is very limited data on the distal margin in GC. Kakeji et al. in their study on prognostic significance of duodenal invasion in patients with distal gastric carcinoma stated that duodenal invasion is associated with increased size, lymphovascular invasion, lymph node metastases, and decreased survival.[61] Few studies have reported that a positive distal margin is not related to OS, recurrence, or local recurrence.[62] In most instances, conversion to a negative margin is only possible by performing a pancreaticoduodenectomy (PD) and its role is discussed later. Generally, a negative distal margin of at least 1 cm confirmed on intraoperative frozen section is deemed acceptable.

Value of Intraoperative Frozen Section for Assessment of Margins

Intraoperative frozen section has a diagnostic accuracy of 93-98%, and does impact changes in operative management.[63,64] This practice is based on the premise that a microscopically positive margin is associated with increased recurrence, and by re-excising such a margin to a negative margin, patients would have better outcomes. A number of studies have shown that outcomes improved when margins were revised and the resection was converted from R1 to R0, only in patients where nodal burden was less, but had no effect on the outcomes in patients with extensive nodal disease.[65,66] If the recommended gross margin distance cannot be obtained, Japanese treatment guidelines endorse frozen section examination to optimize the chance of a negative margin resection.

Management of Positive Resection Margins

Margin positivity can be either microscopically positive or gross positive (R2 or R1), with different treatment implications. Between R2 and R1 margins, the intent of treatment changes from potentially curative to only palliative, with vastly different patient outcomes. R1 resection margins have been associated with proximal location, diffuse tumors, increased tumor size, poor differentiation, increased T stage, and increased N stage.[62,67,68] The options after R1 resection include chemotherapy, radiation therapy, and repeat surgical intervention with re-resection. The decision to choose one of these options must be taken after consideration of the clinical situation as a whole, weighing the risks and benefits of additional treatment. The performance status of the patient and the amount of disease burden are key factors in determining further intervention. In patients with earlier stage disease where a positive margin can influence the outcome, consideration of more aggressive management such as re-surgery is reasonable. However, in later stages of the disease where other pathologic factors such as T-stage or nodal metastases are likely to drive recurrence rather than the positive margin, one must exercise caution in choosing aggressive therapies to treat the margin.

ROLE OF EXTENDED RESECTIONS

Pancreaticoduodenectomy: For Duodenal Involvement or Pancreatic Infiltration

Traditionally, the operative risk of the PD has outweighed the potential benefit, but with advances in surgery and improvements in perioperative care, it has become a more viable option to attain long-term survival. The evidence for this comes from a systematic review of pancreaticoduodenectomies for locally advanced GC,[69] which comprised of eight retrospective case series, with 132 patients. The results showed that, in the absence of incurable factors (para-aortic lymph node metastasis, positive lavage cytology, and peritoneal dissemination), PD with gastrectomy had a median survival of 26 months, and 5-year survival of 47.4%, in comparison to a median survival of 6 months in patients with incurable factors. The authors concluded that PD for GC was associated with a higher morbidity; and defining exact selection criteria is difficult in view of the heterogeneity of the available data. Nonetheless, it can certainly improve survival in a very selected group of patients, in the hands of experienced surgeons at high volume centers for pancreatic and gastric surgery.

Multivisceral Resections

A systematic review on the role of extended resections in GC concluded that radical gastrectomy with multivisceral resection (colectomy, distal pancreaticosplenectomy, and PD) can be performed in advanced GCs, in highly selected patients, after NACT, in order to achieve R0 resection, and can attain long-term survival.[70] However, such extended surgeries may not benefit patients with extensive nodal disease.

Cytoreductive Surgery and Hyperthermic Intraperitoneal Chemotherapy

Peritoneal carcinomatosis (PC) associated with GC has a poor prognosis. Systemic chemotherapy is not very effective in patients with peritoneal involvement, therefore, regional therapies such as cytoreductive surgery (CRS) and hyperthermic intraperitoneal chemotherapy (HIPEC) have been investigated to improve survival of these patients. HIPEC can be used in three scenarios in the management of GC:

1. Prophylactic measure, to prevent peritoneal recurrence after a curative gastrectomy in high risk patients
2. Therapeutic measure, after CRS in patients with established PC
3. Palliation in patients with intractable ascites due to extensive PC not suitable for CRS

Patients with advanced T stage (especially serosal involvement), advanced nodal stage, large tumors, young age, female gender, signet ring cell, and diffuse-mixed histology are considered at high risk for peritoneal relapse. There is strong evidence from Asian countries regarding the survival benefit of prophylactic HIPEC in patients with GC at high risk for peritoneal recurrence.[71-73] The therapeutic role of CRS with HIPEC in GC with macroscopic PC is still evolving and is not recommended at present. Till now, the evidence is in the form of multiple nonrandomized studies,[74,75] which have shown benefit, although modest, of adding HIPEC when a complete CRS can be achieved in patients with GC and PC. Palliative HIPEC in patients with intractable malignant ascites may provide lasting symptomatic relief. Laparoscopic HIPEC has been successfully used to palliate patients with intractable ascites requiring repeated paracenteses.[76,77]

Laparoscopic Surgery

Minimally invasive surgery (MIS) is increasingly been performed for the GC due to new surgical tool and techniques. It has shown both short-term and long-term benefits. MIS has been reported oncologically equivalent to open gastrectomy with added advantage of less morbid, faster postoperative recovery.[78] Kitano et al.[79] performed the first laparoscopic-assisted gastrectomy in 1994. MIS procedure started in Korea and Japan as most of the gastric carcinomas are diagnosed early because of screening program. The first RCT published by Kitano et al. in 2002 comparing laparoscopic distal gastrectomy (LADG) and open distal gastrectomy (ODG) for EGC (n = 28) and has showed less intraoperative blood loss, less postoperative pain, early recovery, and equivalent oncologic procedure. In 2016, Korean Laparoscopic Study Group (KLASS) published multicenter, RCT in 1,426 patients underwent laparoscopic versus open distal gastrectomy. The overall complication rate was lower in LADG group. The number of lymph nodes retrieved in LADG group was significantly lower than ODG ($P > 0.001$).[80] However, nodal yields were adequate for pathological staging. The few nonrandomized reviews were published from West in selected patients, elaborating the safety and effectiveness of laparoscopic procedure.[80,81]

Cai et al.[82] published the first RCT of advanced GC patients comparing laparoscopic and open distal gastrectomy with no significant difference in overall postoperative morbidity rate (12.2 vs. 19.2%). No statistically significant difference was noted on OS among the two groups. Recently, RCTs on patients undergoing laparoscopic or open gastrectomy with D2 lymph adenectomy for locally advanced GC showed no significant differences in postoperative morbidity or mortality and justified the adoption of laparoscopic gastrectomy with extended lymphadenectomy for advanced GC.[83,84] The various multicenter trials evaluating the role of laparoscopic gastrectomy for GC are ongoing like KLASS-03, JLSSG0901, CLASS-01, and STOMACH trial.

Robotic Gastrectomy

The robotic radical gastrectomy for GC was first carried out at Severance Hospital, Yonsei University Health System in 2005. Initially, relatively early clinical stage GC patients were indicated; however, now it may be used for more advanced lesions and found to be a safe and feasible alternative to conventional laparoscopy. In Korea and Japan, neither robotic nor laparoscopic gastrectomy is indicated for the treatment of serosa-involved advanced GC. There are some reports on serosa-involved GC treated with robotics or laparoscopy, thus it is no more contraindication to a minimally invasive approach. However, limitations to a minimally invasive approach includes: bulky tumors, massive lymphadenopathy, or tumors that require multiorgan resection. The da Vinci Xi Surgical System (Intuitive Surgical Inc., Sunnyvale, CA, USA) is a new robotic system that has overcome the limitations of the previous platform. The use of a single-port system, semi-rigid instruments minimizes the external collision of instrument and camera arms. It has overcome the ergonomic disadvantages of conventional single-port laparoscopic surgery. Robotic system also allows the integration of functional imaging such as near infrared after injection of indocyanine green. This imaging acts as navigation tool for tumor localization and lymph node dissection and increased number of harvested lymph node. The use of new instruments in the robotic system such as multifiring clips, angulating ultrasonic sheers, and autonomous knot-tying would reduce operation time and also improve operative outcomes.[78,85]

ROLE OF SURGERY IN MANAGEMENT OF COMPLICATIONS OF GASTRIC CANCER

Bleeding

Bleeding from tumor can be the presenting symptom and it can be either acute or chronic. Endoscopic treatment[86] (injection therapy, mechanical therapy, ablative therapy, e.g., argon plasma coagulation) or angiographic embolization[87] is generally preferred as first-line therapy. However, patients with localized resectable disease can be offered upfront emergency gastrectomy[88] with lymph node dissection, after hemodynamic stabilization and adequate blood transfusions. For patients with advanced metastatic disease, surgery is not preferred and are instead offered angioembolization or palliative hemostatic radiotherapy (EBRT).[89] Patients with chronic blood loss can be managed with proton-pump inhibitors (PPIs), and/or EBRT till the time of definitive treatment.

Gastric Outlet Obstruction

Patients with localized resectable disease with GOO can be offered upfront gastrectomy with lymph node dissection, if the nutritional status is acceptable for postoperative recovery; else endoscopic placement of nasojejunal tube for nutritional rehabilitation and perioperative chemotherapy is an option. In advanced metastatic disease with GOO, palliative gastrojejunostomy or endoscopic placement of metal stents is offered.[90] In patients with good performance status, gastrojejunostomy is preferable over stenting.

Perforation

Small perforations with absence of signs of peritonitis can be managed conservatively with nasogastric tube placement and adequate antibiotic cover. Patients with peritonitis should undergo emergency exploration with lavage and gastrectomy (if feasible) or patch closure of the perforation.[88]

Postgastrectomy Care

After gastrectomy patients need to be taught certain lifestyle changes which are necessary to prevent or reduce the postgastrectomy complications. These include:

- *Posture*: After total gastrectomy or proximal gastrectomy, the absence of the lower esophageal sphincter mechanism makes these patients prone for biliary reflux esophagitis. Hence, they should be advised to maintain an upright posture after taking meals for at least an hour. Taking short frequent meals, no water with meals, elevating the head end of the bed from the waist up, avoiding alcohol, quitting smoking, regular exercises, and reducing excessive weight are other changes advised to these patients.
- *Nutritional supplements*: Post gastrectomy, patients are at a high risk of developing nutritional deficiencies, such as anemia (megaloblastic anemia due to intrinsic factor deficiency or iron deficiency anemia due to duodenal bypass) or steatorrhea, secondarily leading to calcium deficiency and weight loss. These nutrients need to be regularly supplemented and the blood investigations repeated at every follow-up to detect any abnormality and treat the same. A regular visit to a nutritionist is also advised for dietary modifications and supplements.
- *Follow-up*: Patients are generally followed up every 3 months for the first 2 years, and 6 monthly for the next 3 years. Thereafter yearly follow-up is adequate. At every follow-up, tumor markers (CEA, CA 19.9) are checked along with physical examination. Cross-sectional imaging is advised 6 monthly for the first 2 years and yearly for the next 3 years, unless suspicion of a recurrence arises. Patients need to be explained to visit their oncologist in case of any new symptom apart from the regular follow-up schedule.

REFERENCES

1. WHO 2018 update.
2. Noh SH, Park SR, Yang HK, Chung HC, Chung IJ, Kim SW, et al. Adjuvant capecitabine plus oxaliplatin for gastric cancer after D2 gastrectomy (CLASSIC): 5-year follow-up of an open-label, randomised phase 3 trial. Lancet Oncol. 2014;15(12):1389-96.
3. Bhandare MS, Kumar NA, Batra S, Chaudhari V, Shrikhande SV. Radical gastrectomy for gastric cancer at Tata Memorial Hospital. Indian J Cancer. 2017;54(4):605-8.
4. Correa P, Piazuelo MB, Camargo MC. Etiopathogenesis of gastric cancer. Scand J Surg. 2006;95(4):218-24.
5. Irino T, Sano T, Hiki N, Ohashi M, Nunobe S, Kumagai K, et al. Diagnostic staging laparoscopy in gastric cancer: a prospective cohort at a cancer institute in Japan. Surg Endosc. 2018;32(1):268-75.
6. Huang J, Luo H, Zhou C, Zhan J, Rao X, Zhao G, et al. Yield of staging laparoscopy for incurable factors in Chinese patients with advanced gastric cancer. J Laparoendosc Adv Surg Tech A. 2018;28(1):19-24.
7. Machairas N, Charalampoudis P, Molmenti EP, Kykalos S, Tsaparas P, Stamopoulos P, et al. The value of staging laparoscopy in gastric cancer. Ann Gastroenterol. 2017;30(3):287-94.
8. Takahashi Y, Takeuchi T, Sakamoto J, Touge T, Mai M, Ohkura H, et al. The usefulness of CEA and/or CA19-9 in monitoring for recurrence in gastric cancer patients: a prospective clinical study. Gastric Cancer Off J Int Gastric Cancer Assoc Jpn Gastric Cancer Assoc. 2003;6(3):142-5.
9. Bagaria, B, Sood S, Sharma R, Lalwani S. Comparative study of CEA and CA19-9 in esophageal, gastric and colon cancers individually and in combination (ROC curve analysis). Cancer Biol Med. 2013;10(3):148-57.
10. Namasivayam S, Martin DR, Saini S. Imaging of liver metastases: MRI. Cancer Imaging. 2007;7(1):2-9.
11. Smyth E, Schöder H, Strong VE, Capanu M, Kelsen DP, Coit DG, et al. A prospective evaluation of the utility of 2-deoxy-2-[(18) F] fluoro-D-glucose positron emission tomography and computed tomography in staging locally advanced gastric cancer. Cancer. 2012;118(22):5481-8.
12. Lordick F, Ott K, Krause BJ, Weber WA, Becker K, Stein HJ, et al. PET to assess early metabolic response and to guide treatment of adenocarcinoma of the oesophagogastric junction: the MUNICON phase II trial. Lancet Oncol. 2007;8(9):797-805.
13. Uedo N, Iishi H, Tatsuta M, Ishihara R, Higashino K, Takeuchi Y, et al. Long term outcomes after endoscopic mucosal resection for early gastric cancer. Gastric Cancer Off J Int Gastric Cancer Assoc Jpn Gastric Cancer Assoc. 2006;9(2):88-92.
14. Morita S, Katai H, Saka M, Fukagawa T, Sano T, Sasako M. Outcome of pylorus-preserving gastrectomy for early gastric cancer. Br J Surg. 2008;95(9):1131-5.
15. Mochiki E, Kamiyama Y, Aihara R, Nakabayashi T, Asao T, Kuwano H. Laparoscopic assisted distal gastrectomy for early gastric cancer: Five years' experience. Surgery. 2005;137(3):317-22.
16. Hiki N, Nunobe S, Kubota T, Jiang X. Function-preserving gastrectomy for early gastric cancer. Ann Surg Oncol. 2013;20(8):2683-92.
17. Kwon YH, Heo J, Lee HS, Cho CM, Jeon SW. Failure of Helicobacter pylori eradication and age are independent risk factors for recurrent neoplasia after endoscopic resection of early gastric cancer in 283 patients. Aliment Pharmacol Ther. 2014;39(6):609-18.
18. Cunningham D, Allum WH, Stenning SP, Thompson JN, Van de Velde CJ, Nicolson M, et al. Perioperative chemotherapy versus surgery alone for resectable gastroesophageal cancer. N Engl J Med. 2006;355(1):11-20.
19. Al-Batran SE, Homann N, Pauligk C, Goetze TO, Meiler J, Kasper S, et al. Perioperative chemotherapy with fluorouracil plus leucovorin, oxaliplatin, and docetaxel versus fluorouracil or capecitabine plus cisplatin and epirubicin for locally advanced,

resectable gastric or gastro-oesophageal junction adenocarcinoma (FLOT4): a randomised, phase 2/3 trial. T. Lancet. 2019;393(10184):1948-57.
20. Macdonald JS, Smalley SR, Benedetti J, Hundahl SA, Estes NC, Stemmermann GN, et al. Chemoradiotherapy after surgery compared with surgery alone for adenocarcinoma of the stomach or gastroesophageal junction. N Engl J Med. 2001;345(10):725-30.
21. Lee J, Lim DH, Kim S, Park SH, Park JO, Park YS, et al. Phase III trial comparing capecitabine plus cisplatin versus capecitabine plus cisplatin with concurrent capecitabine radiotherapy in completely resected gastric cancer with D2 lymph node dissection: the ARTIST trial. J Clin Oncol. 2012;30(3):268-73.
22. Mari E, Floriani I, Tinazzi A, Buda A, Belfiglio M, Valentini M, et al. Efficacy of adjuvant chemotherapy after curative resection for gastric cancer: A meta-analysis of published randomised trialsA study of the GISCAD (Gruppo Italiano per lo Studio dei Carcinomi dell'Apparato Digerente). Ann Oncol. 2000;11(7):83743.
23. Bang Y-J, Kim Y-W, Yang H-K, Chung HC, Park Y-K, Lee KH, et al. Adjuvant capecitabine and oxaliplatin for gastric cancer after D2 gastrectomy (CLASSIC): a phase 3 open-label, randomised controlled trial. Lancet. 2012;379(9813):315-21.
24. Sakuramoto S, Sasako M, Yamaguchi T, Kinoshita T, Fujii M, Nashimoto A, et al. Adjuvant chemotherapy for gastric cancer with S-1, an oral fluoropyrimidine. N Engl J Med. 2007;357(18):1810-20.
25. GASTRIC (Global Advanced/Adjuvant Stomach Tumor Research International Collaboration) Group; Paoletti X, Oba K, Burzykowski T, Michiels S, Ohashi Y, et al. Benefit of adjuvant chemotherapy for resectable gastric cancer: a meta-analysis. JAMA. 2010;303(17):1729-37.
26. Fu X, Zhang Y, Yang J, Qi Y, Ming Y, Sun M, et al. Efficacy and safety of trastuzumab as maintenance or palliative therapy in advanced HER2-positive gastric cancer. Onco Targets Ther. 2018;11:6091-100.
27. Fuchs CS, Shitara K, Di Bartolomeo M, Lonardi S, Al-Batran S-E, Cutsem EV, et al. Ramucirumab with cisplatin and fluoropyrimidine as first-line therapy in patients with metastatic gastric or junctional adenocarcinoma (RAINFALL): a double-blind, randomised, placebo-controlled, phase 3 trial. 2019;20(3):420-35.
28. Sano T, Kobori O, Muto T. Lymph node metastasis from early gastric cancer: endoscopic resection of tumour. British J Surg. 1992;79(3):241-4.
29. Patel SH, Kooby DA. Gastric adenocarcinoma surgery and adjuvant therapy. Surg Clin North Am. 2011;91(5):1039-77.
30. Ko WJ, Song GW, Kim WH, Hong SP, Cho JY. Endoscopic resection of early gastric cancer: current status and new approaches. Transl Gastroenterol Hepatol. 2016;1:24.
31. Nakamoto S, Sakai Y, Kasanuki J, Kondo F, Ooka Y, Kato K, et al. Indications for the use of endoscopic mucosal resection for early gastric cancer in Japan: a comparative study with endoscopic submucosal dissection. Endoscopy. 2009;41(9):746-50.
32. Choi KS, Jung HY, Choi KD, Lee GH, Song HJ, Kim DH, et al. EMR versus gastrectomy for intramucosal gastric cancer: comparison of long-term outcomes. Gastrointest Endosc. 2011;73(5):942-8.
33. Kwee RM, Kwee TC. Predicting lymph node status in early gastric cancer. Gastric Cancer. 2008;11(3):134-48.
34. Soetikno R, Kaltenbach T, Yeh R, Gotoda T. Endoscopic mucosal resection for early cancers of the upper gastrointestinal tract. J Clin Oncol. 2005;23(20):4490-8.
35. Kaneko S, Yoshimura T. Time trend analysis of gastric cancer incidence in Japan by histological types, 1975-1989. Br J Cancer. 2001;84(3):400-5.
36. Japanese Gastric Cancer Association. Japanese gastric cancer treatment guidelines 2010 (ver. 3). Gastric Cancer. 2011;14(2):113-23.
37. Sugoor P, Shah S, Dusane R, Desouza A, Goel M, Shrikhande SV. Proximal gastrectomy versus total gastrectomy for proximal third gastric cancer: total gastrectomy is not always necessary. Langenbecks Arch Surg. 2016;401(5):687-97.

38. Buhl K, Schlag P, Herfarth C. Quality of life and functional results following different types of resection for gastric carcinoma. Eur J Surg Oncol. 1990;16(4):404-9.
39. Pu YW, Gong W, Wu YY, Chen Q, He TF, Xing CG. Proximal gastrectomy versus total gastrectomy for proximal gastric carcinoma. A meta-analysis on postoperative complications, 5-year survival, and recurrence rate. Saudi Med J. 2013;34(12):1223-8.
40. Bozzetti F, Marubini E, Bonfanti G, Miceli R, Piano C, Gennari L. Subtotal versus total gastrectomy for gastric cancer: five-year survival rates in a multicenter randomized Italian trial. Italian Gastrointestinal Tumor Study Group. Ann Surg. 1999;230(2):170-8.
41. Gouzi JL, Huguier M, Fagniez PL, Launois B, Flamant Y, Lacaine F, et al. Total versus subtotal gastrectomy for adenocarcinoma of the gastric antrum. A French prospective controlled study. Ann Surg. 1989;209(2):162-6.
42. Shen W-S, Xi H-Q, Wei B, Chen L. Effect of gastrectomy with bursectomy on prognosis of gastric cancer: A meta-analysis. World J Gastroenterol. 2014;20(40):14986-91.
43. Terashima M, Doki, Y, Kurokawa Y, Mizusawa J, Katai H, Yoshikawa T. et al. Primary results of a phase III trial to evaluate bursectomy for patients with subserosal/serosal gastric cancer (JCOG1001). J Clin Oncol. 2017;35:4_suppl, 5-5.
44. BARCH LC, Ramos MF, Dias AR, Yagi OK, Ribeiro-Júnior U, Zilberstein B, et al. Total omentectomy in gastric cancer surgery: is it always necessary? Arq Bras Cir Dig. 2019;32(1):e1425.
45. Haverkamp L, Brenkman HJ, Ruurda JP, Ten Kate FJW, van Hillegersberg R. The oncological value of omentectomy in gastrectomy for cancer. J Gastrointest Surg. 2016;20(5):885-890.
46. Kim M-C, Kim K-H, Jung GJ, Rattner DW. Comparative study of complete and partial omentectomy in radical subtotal gastrectomy for early gastric cancer. Yonsei Med J. 2011;52(6):961-6.
47. Japanese Gastric Cancer Association. Japanese classification of gastric carcinoma: 3rd English edition. Gastric Cancer Off J Int Gastric Cancer Assoc Jpn Gastric Cancer Assoc. 2011;14(2):101-12.
48. Association JGC. Japanese gastric cancer treatment guidelines 2014 (ver. 4). Gastric Cancer. 2017;20(1):1-19.
49. Bonenkamp JJ, Hermans J, Sasako M, van de Velde CJ, Welvaart K, Songun I, et al. Extended lymph-node dissection for gastric cancer. N Engl J Med. 1999;340(12):908-14.
50. Cuschieri A, Fayers P, Fielding J, Craven J, Bancewicz J, Joypaul V, et al. Postoperative morbidity and mortality after D1 and D2 resections for gastric cancer: preliminary results of the MRC randomised controlled surgical trial. The Surgical Cooperative Group. Lancet Lond Engl. 1996;347(9007):995-9.
51. Shrikhande SV, Shukla PJ, Qureshi S, Siddachari R, Upasani V, Ramadwar M, et al. D2 lymphadenectomy for gastric cancer in Tata Memorial Hospital: Indian data can now be incorporated in future international trials. Dig Surg. 2006;23(3):192-7.
52. Wu C-W, Hsiung CA, Lo S-S, Hsieh M-C, Chen J-H, Li AF-Y, et al. Nodal dissection for patients with gastric cancer: a randomised controlled trial. Lancet Oncol. 2006;7(4):309-15.
53. Songun I, Putter H, Kranenbarg EM-K, Sasako M, van de Velde CJH. Surgical treatment of gastric cancer: 15-year follow-up results of the randomised nationwide Dutch D1D2 trial. Lancet Oncol. 2010;11(5):439-49.
54. Jiang L, Yang K-H, Guan Q-L, Zhao P, Chen Y, Tian J-H. Survival and recurrence free benefits with different lymphadenectomy for resectable gastric cancer: a meta-analysis. J Surg Oncol. 2013;107(8):807-14.
55. ClinicalTrials.gov. (2018). Phase III Randomized Trial Comparing D2 vs D3 Lymphadenectomy With Gastric Cancer Following Neoadjuvant Chemotherapy - Full Text View. Available from: https://clinicaltrials.gov/ct2/show/NCT02139605
56. Bozzetti F, Bonfanti G, Bufalino R, Menotti V, Persano S, Andreola S, et al. Adequacy of margins of resection in gastrectomy for cancer. Ann Surg. 1982; 196(6):685-90.

57. National Comprehensive Cancer Network. Gastric Cancer (Version 1.2017). Available from: http://www.nccn.org/professionals/physician_gls/pdf/gastric.pdf.
58. Mine S, Sano T, Hiki N, Yamada K, Kosuga T, Nunobe S, et al. Proximal margin length with transhiatal gastrectomy for Siewert type II and III adenocarcinomas of the oesophagogastric junction. Br J Surg.2013;100:1050-4.
59. Postlewait LM, Squires MH, Kooby DA, Poultsides GA, Weber SM, Bloomston M et al. The importance of the proximal resection margin distance for proximal gastric adenocarcinoma: A multi-institutional study of the US Gastric Cancer Collaborative. J Surg Oncol. 2015;112(2):203-7.
60. Lee CM, Jee YS, Lee JH, Son SY, Ahn SH, Park DJ, et al. Length of negative resection margin does not affect local recurrence and survival in the patients with gastric cancer. World J Gastroenterol. 2014;20(30):10518-24.
61. Kakeji Y, Tsujitani S, Baba H, Moriguchi S, Mori M, Maehara Y, et al. Clinicopathologic features and prognostic significance of duodenal invasion in patients with distal gastric carcinoma. Cancer. 1991;68(2):380-4.
62. Bickenbach KA, Gonen M, Strong V, Brennan MF, Coit DG Association of positive transection margins with gastric cancer survival and local recurrence. Ann Surg Oncol. 2013;20(8):2663-8.
63. Shen JG, Cheong JH, Hyung WJ, Kim J, Choi SH, Noh SH. Intraoperative frozen section margin evaluation in gastric cancer of the cardia surgery. Hepatogastroenterology. 2006;53(72):976-8.
64. Spicer J, Benay C, Lee L, Rousseau M, Andalib A, Kushner Y, et al. Diagnostic accuracy and utility of intraoperative microscopic margin analysis of gastric and esophageal adenocarcinoma. Ann Surg Oncol. 2014;21(8):2580-6.
65. Kim SH, Karpeh MS, Klimstra DS, Leung D, Brennan MF. Effect of microscopic resection line disease on gastric cancer survival. J Gastrointest Surg. 1999;3(1):24-33.
66. Chen JD, Yang XP, Shen JG, Hu WX, Yuan XM, Wang LB. Prognostic improvement of reexcision for positive resection margins in patients with advanced gastric cancer. Eur J Surg Oncol. 2013;39(3):229-34.
67. Cho BC, Jeung HC, Cho HJ, Rha SY, Hyung WJ, Cheong JH, et al. Prognostic impact of resection margin involvement after extended (D2/D3) gastrectomy for advanced gastric cancer: A 15-year experience at a single institute. J Surg Oncol. 2007;95(6):461-8.
68. Nagata T, Ichikawa D, Komatsu S, Inoue K, Shiozaki A, Fujiwara H, et al. Prognostic impact of microscopic positive margin in gastric cancer patients. J Surg Oncol. 2011;104(6):592-7.
69. Roberts P, Seevaratnam R, Cardoso R, Law C, Helyer L, Coburn N. Systematic review of pancreaticoduodenectomy for locally advanced gastric cancer. Gastric Cancer. 2012;15(1):108-15.
70. Brar SS, Seevaratnam R, Cardoso R, Yohanathan L, Law C, Helyer L, et al. Multivisceral resection for gastric cancer: a systematic review. Gastric Cancer. 2012;15(1):100-7.
71. Sun J, Song Y, Wang Z, Gao P, Chen X, Xu Y, et al. Benefits of hyperthermic intraperitoneal chemotherapy for patients with serosal invasion in gastric cancer: a meta-analysis of the randomized controlled trials. BMC Cancer. 2012;12(1):526.
72. Glehen O, Passot G, Villeneuve L, Vaudoyer D, Bin-Dorel S, Boschetti G, et al. GASTRICHIP: D2 resection and hyperthermic intraperitoneal chemotherapy in locally advanced gastric carcinoma: a randomized and multicenter phase III study. BMC Cancer. 2014; 14(1):183.
73. Garofalo A, Valle M, Garcia J, Sugarbaker PH. Laparoscopic intraperitoneal hyperthermic chemotherapy for palliation of debilitating malignant ascites. Eur J Surg Oncol. 2006;32(6):682-5.
74. Bonnot PE, Piessen G, Kepenekian V, Decullier E, Pocard M, Meunier B, et al. Cytoreductive surgery with or without hyperthermic intraperitoneal chemotherapy for gastric cancer with peritoneal metastases (CYTO- CHIP study): A propensity score analysis. J Clin Oncol. 2019;37(23):2028-40.

75. Hotopp T. HIPEC and CRS in peritoneal metastatic gastric cancer - who really benefits? Surg Oncol. 2019;28:159-66.
76. Roviello F, Caruso S, Neri A, Marrelli D. Treatment and prevention of peritoneal carcinomatosis from gastric cancer by cytoreductive surgery and hyperthermic intraperitoneal chemotherapy: overview and rationale. Eur J Surg Oncol J Eur Soc Surg Oncol Br Assoc Surg Oncol. 2013;39(12):1309-16.
77. Facchiano E, Scaringi S, Kianmanesh R, Sabate JM, Castel B, Flamant Y, et al. Laparoscopic hyperthermic intraperitoneal chemotherapy (HIPEC) for the treatment of malignant ascites secondary to unresectable peritoneal carcinomatosis from advanced gastric cancer. Eur J Surg Oncol. 2008;34(2):154-8.
78. Costantino CL, Mullen JT. Minimally invasive gastric cancer surgery. Surg Oncol Clin N Am. 2019;28(2):201-13.
79. Kitano S, Iso Y, Moriyama M, Sugimachi K. Laparoscopy-assisted Billroth I gastrectomy. Surg Laparosc Endosc. 1994;4(2):146-8. Erratum in: Surg Laparosc Endosc. 2013;23(5):480.
80. Kitano S, Shiraishi N, Fujii K, Yasuda K, Inomata M, Adachi Y. A randomized controlled trial comparing open vs laparoscopy-assisted distal gastrectomy for the treatment of early gastric cancer: an interim report. Surgery. 2002;131(1 Suppl):S306-11.
81. Kim W, Kim HH, Han SU, Kim MC, Hyung WJ, Ryu SW, et al. Decreased morbidity of laparoscopic distal gastrectomy compared with open distal gastrectomy for stage I gastric cancer: Short-term outcomes from a multicenter randomized controlled trial (KLASS-01). Ann Surg. 2016;263(1):28-35.
82. Cai J, Wei D, Gao CF, Zhang CS, Zhang H, Zhao T. A prospective randomized study comparing open versus laparoscopy-assisted D2 radical gastrectomy in advanced gastric cancer. Dig Surg. 2011;28(5-6):331-7.
83. Hu Y, Huang C, Sun Y, Su X, Cao H, Hu J, et al. Morbidity and mortality of laparoscopic versus open D2 distal gastrectomy for advanced gastric cancer: A randomized controlled trial. J Clin Oncol. 2016;34 (12):1350-7.
84. Shi Y, Xu X, Zhao Y, Qian F, Tang B, Hao Y, et al. Short-term surgical outcomes of a randomized controlled trial comparing laparoscopic versus open gastrectomy with D2 lymph node dissection for advanced gastric cancer. Surg Endosc. 2018;32(5):2427-33.
85. Alhossaini RM, Altamran AA, Seo WJ, Hyung WJ. Robotic gastrectomy for gastric cancer: Current evidence. Ann Gastroenterol Surg. 2017;1(1):82-9.
86. Kim YI, Choi IJ. Endoscopic management of tumor bleeding from inoperable gastric cancer. Clin Endosc. 2015;48(2):121-7.
87. Lee HJ, Shin JH, Yoon HK, Ko GY, Gwon DI, Song HY, et al. Transcatheter arterial embolization in gastric cancer patients with acute bleeding. Eur Radiol. 2009;19(4): 960-5.
88. Kasakura Y, Ajani JA, Fujii M, Mochizuki F, Takayama T. Management of perforated gastric carcinoma: a report of 16 cases and review of world literature. Am Surg. 2002;68(5):434-40.
89. Lee JA, Lim DH, Park W, Ahn YC, Huh SJ. Radiation therapy for gastric cancer bleeding. 2009;95(6):726-30.
90. No JH, Kim SW, Lim CH, Kim JS, Cho YK, Park JM, et al. Long-term outcome of palliative therapy for gastric outlet obstruction caused by unresectable gastric cancer in patients with good performance status: endoscopic stenting versus surgery. Gastrointest Endosc. 2013;78(1):55-62.

CHAPTER 3

Prenatal Surgery

Vaibhav Pandey, Ajay N Gangopadhyay

INTRODUCTION

Prenatal surgery or fetal surgery is simply the surgery of unborn or yet to born. The concept of prenatal surgery came with the understanding that some problems in fetus can hamper its growth and development. This can progress to an extent that it effects the viability or development. Further, even if the fetus crosses all the hurdles and delivers, the underlying problems have advanced to the extent that no treatment is beneficial. This frustrating situation led to the evolution of fetal therapy. It was also realized that fetal healing could better or even scar less. Though the concept is old, its development and realization were limited by uterus which acted as a barrier for observation and intervention on the developing fetus. This barrier was crossed with the advent of prenatal ultrasound and other advances in imaging and instrumentation. The whole concept of fetal surgery revolves around the safety of mother as fetal interventions are maternal-fetal interventions.

HISTORY

The first intrauterine intervention is credited to AW Liley, who in 1963, transfused blood in the peritoneum of fetus suffering from hemolytic disease.[1] Freda and Adamson performed open fetal transfusion a year later.[2] The fetal interventions were limited to fetal transfusion till Dr Michael R Harison and colleagues performed the intrauterine intervention in fetuses with hydronephrosis and congenital diaphragmatic hernia (CDH) in the year 1981. For his enormous efforts and innovations, Dr Harrison is regarded as the *Father of Fetal Medicine*.[2,3] A year later, the International Fetal Surgical Society was founded, and in 1983, it was transformed into the International Fetal Medicine and Surgery Society (IFMSS) with a primary motive of elaborating preliminary directives concerning intrauterine surgery.[4,5] A timeline of important events in the history of fetal surgery is listed in **Table 1**.

COMPONENTS OF FETAL SURGERY

Prenatal surgery has following components:
- *Diagnosis*: Pin-point diagnosis of cases which will be benefited by the surgery is a prerequisite.

TABLE 1: History of fetal surgery.	
Year	Event
1980	First in utero surgical technique employed in animal model
1981	First successful ultrasound-guided vesicoamniotic shunt performed in a fetus for vesical outflow obstruction
1984	First successful congenital cyst resection in congenital cystic adenoid malformation of lung
1991	Radioemitters implemented for the first time in fetal physiological parameters monitoring during in utero procedures
1994	First large clinical studies on open in utero operation for congenital diaphragmatic hernia
1995	Ex utero intrapartum therapy (EXIT) procedure developed and performed for the first time in fetal upper airway obstruction
1996	First successful sacrococcygeal teratoma (SCT) resection
1997	First open in utero operation in meningomyelocele (MMC)
2003	Management of Myelomeningocele study (MOMS) trial in utero and neonatal MMC treatment outcomes comparative study launched

- *Multidisciplinary approach*: After an accurate diagnosis, different team members are involved for their different roles. Success is only possible with a well-coordinated multidisciplinary team approach.
- *Surgical intervention*: Different types of surgical interventions can be performed depending upon the indication.

Diagnosis

The prerequisite for a fetal intervention is a pinpoint diagnosis. An accurate diagnosis will enable the interventionist to make sure that the procedure involving both the mother and fetus is worth or not. The progress of fetal surgery has been mostly dependent on the advances in the imaging. Any diagnostic modality utilized for the evaluation of fetus should not be damaging and so any kind of ionizing radiation is discouraged. The main diagnostic modalities are ultrasound and magnetic resonance imaging (MRI).

Ultrasound

The development of ultrasound has been the backbone of prenatal diagnosis and management. Obstetric ultrasound employs transducer frequencies of 2–10 MHz. Higher frequency transducers have a higher spatial resolution. This means they can better differentiate two closely located side-by-side spots in the region of interest. The penetration of high-frequency wave is however limited. Therefore, high-frequency probes are used to look at near structures and lower frequency probes are used to study tissues at depth. Abdominal transducers use a frequency of 2–6.5 MHz and transvaginal transducers use frequencies of 5–15 MHz. Most obstetric ultrasound use an abdominal approach. Transvaginal scanning is used in the first trimester for more accurate information on early pregnancy complications, delineation of fetal morphology, assessing the cervical length and other features of incompetence, delineation of cranial anatomy in the deeply engaged head and in some situations of suspected placental anomalies.[6,7]

Development in ultrasound:
- *A-mode or amplitude modulation:* A-mode studies were the most primitive forms of ultrasound imaging and consisted of a graph indicating reflectors at the level of their depth. These are no longer used in obstetrics.
- *B-mode or brightness modulation or 2D:* B-mode ultrasounds are currently most commonly used and are the conventional ultrasound. Unlike A-Mode, B-Mode is based on brightness with the absence of vertical spikes. Therefore, the brightness depends upon the amplitude or intensity of the echo. B-Mode will display an image of large and small dots, which represent strong and weak echoes, respectively. The other advantage of B-mode study is it being a real-time study.
- *M-mode, or motion mode (also called time motion or TM-mode):* It is the display of a one-dimensional image that is used for analyzing moving body parts commonly in fetal cardiac imaging. This can be accomplished by recording the amplitude and rate of motion in real-time by repeatedly measuring the distance of the object from the single transducer at a given moment. The single sound beam is transmitted and the reflected echoes are displayed as dots of varying intensities thus creating lines across the screen.
- *3D and 4D ultrasound:* Three-dimensional image in ultrasounds can be recoded. A special transducer and computer software arrangement is made to the conventional ultrasound, and is referred to as 3D ultrasound. Real-time 3D ultrasound is known as 4D ultrasound.

The utility of ultrasound advances: Three-dimensional ultrasound is now widely available and is commonly applied in the diagnosis of craniofacial, neural tube, and skeletal abnormalities. Assessment of volumetric measurements of fetal organs, such as lung volume to determine the degree of pulmonary hypoplasia in a fetus with a congenital lung malformation (CLM) is one of the major developments. Application of 3D/4D echocardiography allows heart monitoring and helps in supervising the changes in the capacity of ventricles in real-time. Spatiotemporal image correlation and reconstruction of the fetal cardiac cycle is utilized to isolate images of five classic planes of fetal echocardiography at any point in the cycle. Ultrasound can be used to identify markers of fetal distress and indicators of imminent fetal demise. This allows for stratification of fetal distress to determine if and when intrauterine intervention is necessary. Ultrasound is used intraoperatively to map the placental location and select the hysterotomy site during ex utero intrapartum treatment (EXIT) procedures as well as myelomeningocele (MMC) repair and other open fetal surgeries. Intraoperative ultrasound is also used to guide needle and instrument placement in fetoscopy and other procedures such as laser ablation for twin-twin transfusion. Four-dimensional ultrasound provides real-time images and multiplanar views as opposed to two dimensional ultrasounds. Although improvement in resolution is still needed to improve the technique, 4D ultrasound has been used to guide the cauterization of an umbilical cord in twin-twin transfusion syndrome.[7,8]

Limitations of ultrasound: More than 80% of the most common fetal anomalies develop before the twelfth week of gestation and unfortunately, this is when visualization of the developing fetus is most difficult. Beam attenuation by maternal adipose tissue, poor image quality in oligohydramnios, and obscuration of the fetal head by the maternal pelvic bones limits the scope of ultrasound. Relatively subjective observation of real-time ultrasound findings by sonologist sometimes creates confusion and thus delays intervention at a suitable time.

Magnetic Resonance Imaging

Magnetic resonance imaging is the other non-ionizing modality which has become very useful in prenatal surgery. Initially, the use of MRI was limited by the frequent and rapid movements of the developing fetus. With the advent of ultrafast MRI, this has been overcome as the sequences can be recorded in a span of 20 seconds.

Advantages of MRI: Compared with ultrasound, MRI affords higher soft-tissue imaging contrast and greater anatomic delineation of deep soft-tissue structures. Better soft-tissue contrast, precise volumetric measurements, a larger field of view, and better imaging of intracranial structures are few among several technical sophistications offered by MRI. Further, MRI is less operator-dependent. Advances in imaging technology and the approach of combining ultrasound with fetal MRI in prenatal evaluations have led to improved accuracy and precision in the early diagnosis of congenital malformations.[9,10]

Risks of MRI: Maternal risks are same as for non-pregnant. But prolonged supine positioning of gravid uterus of significant size can lead to hypotension due to compression of the inferior vena cava. The hypotension can be avoided by placing the patient in a lateral oblique or lateral decubitus position. There are theoretical risks of adverse effects with regard to neonatal hearing or fetal growth with 3 Tesla MRI. But now studies are showing that even 3T MRI have no adverse effect.

Multidisciplinary Approach in Fetal Surgery (Fig. 1)

Prenatal surgery needs a multidisciplinary approach. Each member of the team should work in coordination with others to identify the potential cases, those who will benefit from surgery, potential risks to mother, risks to the fetus and postnatal management of the fetus with prenatal surgery.[11]

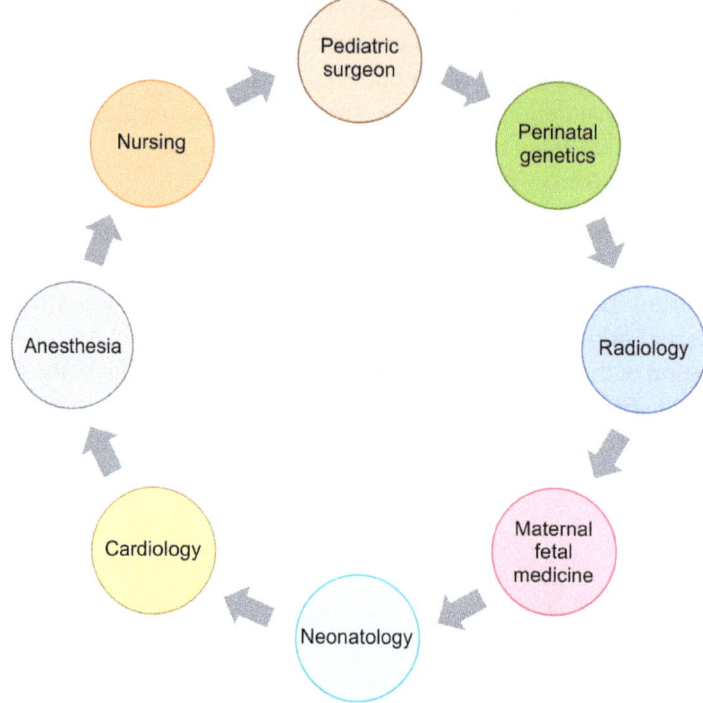

Fig. 1: Multidisciplinary approach for fetal surgery.

Indications

Fetal surgery is indicated in conditions which interfere with the normal development of the fetus and correction of the abnormality will allow the normal development of the fetus.

Contraindications

Prenatal surgery is contraindicated in conditions that are incompatible with life, conditions with severe affliction or pain. It is also contraindicated in conditions associated with other life-threatening abnormalities, and chromosomal and genetic abnormalities.

Techniques of Fetal Intervention

Principles of operation in utero in humans were elaborated based on long-term experiences with animals, mainly sheep and Rhesus monkeys. Patterns of anesthesia for mother and child, principles of prenatal diagnosis, operations in multidisciplinary teams, and methods of fighting the most common and severe complications of intrauterine operations, i.e., premature labor have been established from research models.

Intrauterine procedures might be performed by applying one of the methods: open surgery with hysterotomy or other less-invasive techniques.

At present, the tendency to favor less-invasive techniques is strong as it is associated with a lower number of complications, such as premature childbirth or fetal injury during shorter or less-traumatic procedures. Owing to fetal tissue's fragility and fetus size, the performance of operation before the 18th week of pregnancy is technically difficult. So, the majority of operations are performed between the 18th and 30th weeks of pregnancy.[11]

Types of Fetal Surgery

- Fetal image-guided surgery (FIGS)
- Fetal endoscopic surgery (FETENDO)
- Ex utero intrapartum treatment procedure (EXIT)
- Open surgery.

Fetal image-guided surgery: It is the least invasive method of fetal intervention. It does not involves any incision of endoscopic view inside the uterus. The intervention is performed under ultrasound guidance. There is real-time cross-sectional view under which working needle or needles are passed through the abdominal wall of the mother and then the uterus **(Table 2)**. While the

TABLE 2: Examples of fetal image guided surgery.

Diagnostics	Therapeutic
• Chorion villus sampling • Amniocentesis • Cordocentesis • Fetal skin biopsy	• Radiofrequency ablation (RFA) of sacrococcygeal teratoma **(Fig. 2)** or anomalous twins • Cord cauterization in twins • Vesical/pleural shunts • Balloon dilatation of aortic stenosis

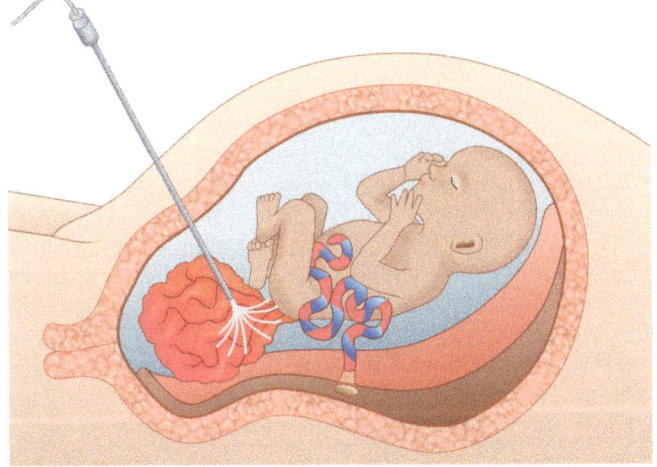

Fig. 2: Radiofrequency ablation of sacrococcygeal teratoma performed by image guided surgery. The tumor is localized under USG guidance and radiofrequency probe is inserted under its guidance.

procedure is being carried out, the fetus is continuously monitored through the ultrasound.[12,13]

Advantages: FIGS is the least invasive mode of prenatal surgery. It has got minimum risk of amniotic fluid leak and has minimum risk of preterm labor.

Disadvantage: The image-guided intervention can be utilized on a small number of procedures and requires a specialized setup.

Minimally invasive fetal endo-surgery: This technique involves access to fetus via an endoscope. This gives a real time visualization of the fetus. As this is a minimal access technique, it is associated with lower percentage of complications for the mother and the fetus.[13,14]

Technique: FETENDO intervention is done by accessing the uterus either percutaneously or via mini-laparotomy. One or multiple ports can be inserted **(Table 3)**. For creation of space, helium or isotonic sodium chloride solution is used (Carbon dioxide is not used) **(Fig. 3)**.

TABLE 3: Examples fetoendoscopic surgery.	
Congenital diaphragmatic hernia (CDH)	Balloon occlusion of trachea
Twin-to-twin transfusion syndrome (TTTS)	Laser coagulation of vessels
Acardiac Twins	Cord ligation in cases of acardiac
Amniotic bands	Amniotic bands division

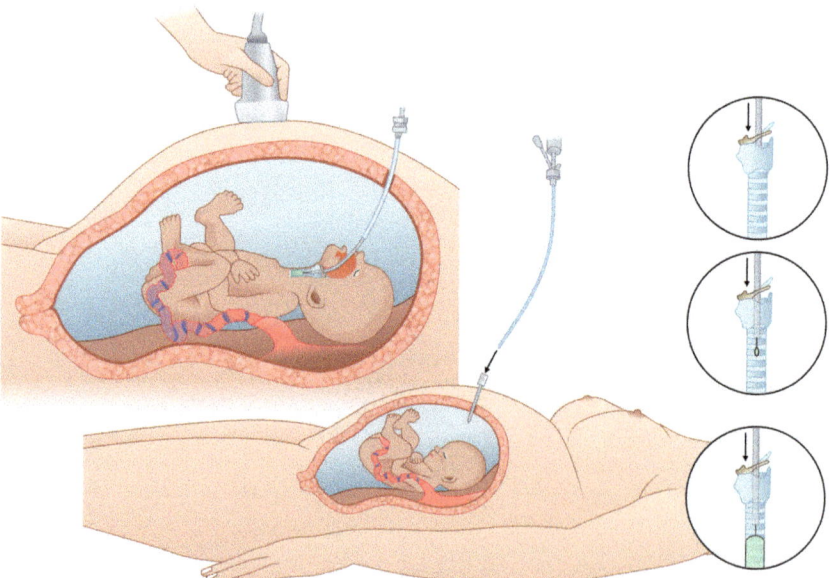

Fig. 3: Fetoscopic endoluminal tracheal occlusion for congenital diaphragmatic hernia. Monitoring is performed by ultrasound and single fetoscope with working channel is used.

Advantages: The biggest advantage of the FETENDO technique is the direct visualization of the fetus. During procedure multiple functions can be performed using one port only with multiple instruments. Further as it is a minimal access technique, there is minimal handling of the fetus.

Disadvantages: The most common complication with FETENDO is premature rupture of membrane (PROM). The rate of PROM increases with the use of multiple ports and longer duration of surgery. Due to the introduction of ports and handling of fetus hemorrhage is an important complication. Amniotic membrane detachment can also occur, rarely during the insertion of ports or during the handling.

EXIT technique (Ex utero intrapartum treatment or therapy): Ex utero intrapartum therapy is not a fetal surgery in true terms. It stands for the intervention in a fetus at term, at the time of cesarean section. The fetus is delivered outside the uterus but is it attached to placental circulation. The circulation provides the fetus with a mean of anesthesia and gaseous exchange. While the fetus is on placental circulation, procedures can be performed. The main indication for EXIT procedure is antenatally diagnosed potential airway abnormality which exposes the fetus to hypoxia immediately after the delivery.[15]

There are four types of EXIT procedures:
1. EXIT to airway
2. EXIT to resection
3. EXIT to ECMO (extracorporeal membrane oxygenation)
4. EXIT to separation.

The EXIT procedure involves different specialties and experts at the time of the procedure. The team includes about 15-30 specialists from the fetal anesthesiologist, scrub nurses, circulators, anesthesia technician, maternal-fetal medicine specialist, fetal cardiologist, pediatric surgeons, and the ECMO team at minimum. The procedure is usually performed at term, around 34-37 weeks **(Table 4)**.

Open fetal surgery: Open fetal surgery is the most invasive form of fetal surgery. It is in true terms a preterm surgery as it involves both a maternal laparotomy and a hysterotomy.[16]

TABLE 4: Example of ex utero intrapartum therapy (EXIT).	
EXIT to airway	Congenital high airway obstruction syndrome (CHAOS) **(Figs. 4A and B)**
	Severe micrognathia, lymphatic malformation, vascular malformation, cervical teratoma
EXIT to resection	Thoracic clip or Balloon
EXIT to ECHMO	Severe congenital heart disease or severe congenital diaphragmatic hernia
EXIT to separation	Conjoined twin

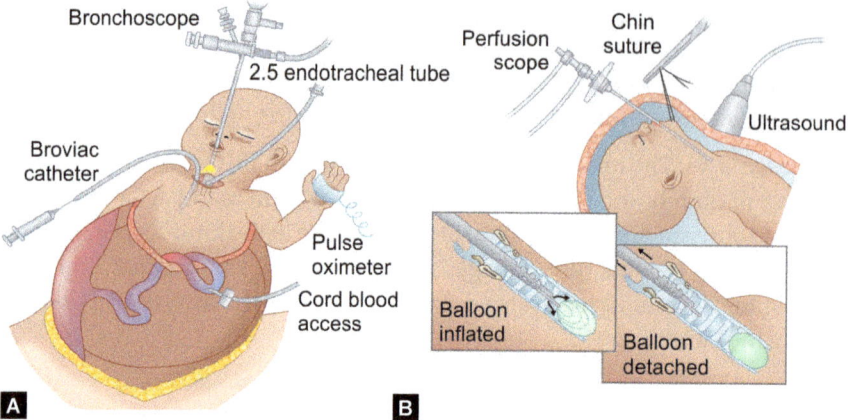

Figs. 4A and B: Ex utero intrapartum therapy (EXIT) treatment procedures for congenital high airway obstruction syndrome (CHAOS). The fetus is attached to the placental circulation. Balloon is inflated at the site of tracheal stenosis.

TABLE 5: Example of open fetal surgery.	
Malformation of lung: Congenital cystic adenomatoid (CCAM)	Lobectomy
Sacrococcygeal teratoma (SCT)	Resection
Meningomyelocele (MMC)	Repair

Indications: Life-threatening conditions: Life-threatening indications historically included fetuses with hydrops, meningomyelocele **(Table 5)**.

Procedure: Isoflurane with epidural anesthesia is most commonly used. Postoperative maternal pulmonary edema is a real risk. The uterus is exposed through a low, transverse abdominal incision. The hysterotomy is made as far away as possible from the placental edge (at least 4 cm), in order to minimize bleeding. The uterus is displaced to the left to avoid compression of the inferior vena cava. Intraoperative ultrasound locates the placenta and identifies the fetal position. The fetus is injected with a narcotic and a paralytic agent. Absorbable staples compress the myometrium and control the membranes, maintaining hemostasis. A rapid infusion replenishes lost amniotic fluid with warm Ringer's lactate solution along with an antibiotic. Only the part of the fetus undergoing surgery is brought out, the rest remains submerged in amniotic fluid. During the procedure and exposure to the outer environment, the fetus is washed with warm normal saline solution to counteract the drying out and cooling down. There is a range of fetus hemodynamic monitoring methods: constant electrocardiography, pulse oximetry, venous access, arterial blood pressure monitoring, and evaluating of hemoglobin level.

After surgery, the uterus is closed in two layers retaining the staples. During the closure, magnesium sulfate bolus followed by continuous infusion is given.

The tocolytic regimen with indomethacin is started 4 hours after surgery. Both these agents are continued for 48-72 hours after surgery. Uterine irritability and amniotic fluid volume are monitored and fetal well being assessed by its movements and echocardiography.

Complications: Open fetal surgery is most invasive form of prenatal surgery. It can be associated with significant complication to mother and fetus. Premature labor is one of the most important complications. After surgery and repair there are higher chance of premature detachment and rupture of fetal membranes. Due to laparotomy and hysterotomy there is a significant chance of maternal and fetal bleeding and infection to both.

CHALLENGES IN FETAL SURGERY

- *Ethical dilemma:* The most common ethical dilemma is that whether we should perform a procedure which is not guaranteed to produce results only because the mother is insisting. This is enhanced by the increased risk to both the mother and fetus. But the other side of the same questions is whether a procedure should not be done as it does not guarantee to produce results or as a mother is refusing the procedure.[17]
- *Complication:* Different prenatal surgical procedures have different complication. These can pose risk to both to mother and the fetus. The complication can affect the ongoing pregnancy and also possible future pregnancies. These also pose variable risk to fetus also.
- *Potential of fetal surgery:* Deliver stem cells or DNA to treat sickle cell anemia or other genetic disorders. Potential conditions which can be cured by fetal stem cell intervention include hemoglobinopathies, Immunodeficiency diseases, mucopolysaccharidoses, mucolipidoses, Diamond-Blackfan syndrome, and Fanconi anemia.

APPLICATIONS OF FETAL SURGERY

Congenital Diaphragmatic Hernia

Congenital diaphragmatic hernia is characterized by herniation of bowel in the thoracic cavity and underlying hypoplasia of the lungs, less mature airway branches and abnormal vasculature development. Initially an attempt of thoracotomy with reduction and repair of the defect was performed in the hope of improving the lung development. But this approach does not improve overall survival. Further, there was kinking of the umbilical vein while reduction of the liver in the abdomen which was incompatible with life. So, this approach was abandoned.

It was observed that fetus with laryngeal atresia had a markedly increased lung volume and alveolar number. This happened because when the trachea is blocked the fluid in lung stays in the lungs and as it builds up, the lung fluid expands the lungs stimulate their growth, and pushes the abdominal contents (liver, intestine) out of the chest and into the abdomen. This approach was utilized in the balloon occlusion of the trachea by fetoscopy endoluminal tracheal occlusion (FETO). The occlusion of the trachea was also tried with hemoclips. A reversal of the clipping was performed at 34 weeks as it stimulated the surfactant production. This is only approach approved in CDH for the antennal management. But it has also not shown the absolute reversal of persistent pulmonary hypertension.[18]

Congenital Pulmonary Airway Malformation

This term is used for a rare developmental disorder characterized by abnormal airway patterning and branching during lung morphogenesis resulting in the formation of multiple lung cysts. Previously it was known as congenital cystic adenomatoid malformation (CCAM). CPAM can be divided as macrocystic (>5 mm) in size and microcystic (<5 mm) in size. The macrocystic lesions are usually solitary and grow slowly, and have a good prognosis. The microcystic lesions are multiple and grow rapidly. This causes inferior vena caval compression, mediastinal shift, and fetal hydrops. The development of hydrops is typically limited to those fetuses with very large chest masses with mediastinal shift and vena cava obstruction.

The indication of fetal intervention depends on the degree of severity. Ultrasound is used to differentiate between the microcystic or macrocystic variants and the presence of hydrops. Further, CPAM volume ratio (CVR) is utilized to estimate the severity. It is CPAM volume divided by the head circumference. A CVR greater than 1.6 predicts an increased risk for hydrops fetalis and is the indication of prenatal intervention. Minimally invasive procedures or open fetal surgery can be performed apart from maternal steroids. The aim of surgery is to alleviate the mass effect and prevent the progression of complications. A thoracoamniotic shunt (TAS) can decompress the lesion. By fetal surgery segmentectomy or lobectomy can be performed.[19]

Lower Urinary Tract Obstructions

Lower urinary tract obstructions (LUTO) is also is known as obstructive uropathy and is common in male fetuses. The obstruction in urethra causes complete or partial blockage to the passage of urine. This leads to gradual dilation and other pressure change in the upper tract. Gradually, the renal parenchyma of both sides gets destroyed in severe cases. The pathological process can be reversed by relieving the obstruction.

The prognosis depends on the type of obstruction and its severity. Most important anomaly is posterior urethral valves (PUV). Poor prognostic factors are: detection before 24 weeks gestation, oligohydramnios, loss of corticomedullary differentiation, renal cortical cysts, increased cortical echogenicity and fetal urine values of calcium >8 mg/L, sodium >100 mEq/L, chloride >90 mEq/L, beta-2 microglobulin >4 mg/L, and urine osmolality >200 mOsm/L. Only fetuses with bilateral (both kidneys) urinary obstruction and evidence of good kidney function by ultrasound, electrolyte and protein levels are candidates for fetal intervention.

The goal of fetal intervention is to allow the urine to pass the obstruction and exit from the fetus into the amniotic fluid. This can be achieved by minimally invasive placement of vesicoamniotic shunts **(Fig. 5)**. The urine is able to exit the fetus through this opening and drain into the amniotic fluid. There is a high risk of preterm labor. Open fetal vesicostomy can also be performed as catheters tend to displace.[20]

Spina Bifida

Spina bifida is a congenital defect consisting of an opening in the spinal column with fetus having many disabilities, including paralysis, difficulty with bowel and bladder control, Chiari II malformation and hydrocephalus. The continuous exposure of neural elements to amniotic fluid damages the neural elements. Further, CSF leak leads to the formation of Chiari II malformation.

The Management of Myelomeningocele Study (MOMS) trial is a landmark trial which proved that prenatal repair of MMC leads to improvement in motor power, decrease hydrocephalus, decreased incidence of shunt surgery and decreased bladder and bowel involvement. Open fetal surgery is performed between 19 and 25 weeks' gestation. An incision is made in the mother's abdomen and uterus just large enough for the spinal defect to be operated upon. The neural tube and other layers of the back are surgically closed **(Fig. 6)**.[21]

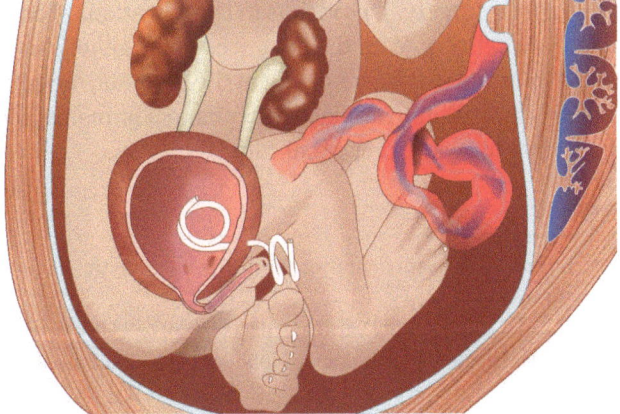

Fig. 5: Vesicoamniotic shunt for posterior urethral valve. The shunt drains fluid into the amniotic cavity and urinary bladder is decompressed.

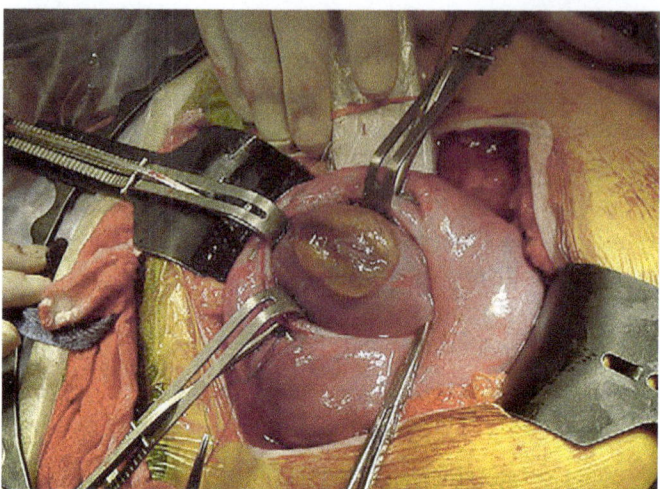

Fig. 6: Open fetal surgery for meningomyelocele. The back is exposed by hysterotomy and the defect of the spinal cord is repaired in layers.

CONCLUSION

Fetal surgery has completed a journey of nearly two and half a decade from its inception. There has been a long-standing debate regarding the patient selection, potential harm to mothers and optimal technical approach. The technological advances and advent of miniature scope have not been able to completely stop this debate. Fetal surgery has shown positive results in the conditions such as meningomyelocele, congenital diaphragmatic hernia, sacrococcygeal teratoma and others. On the one hand, the healing in the fetus is without much scarring has been the most important driving force making the physicians to believe in the potential scar less healing in these children but on the other hand, the nonhealing property of the amnion has been the main thorn in the progress of fetal surgery. This results in complications of amniotic fluid leak and premature delivery. With the advances in the genetic engineering it may be possible in future to trigger healing in the amniotic membrane which may overcome this limitation. The fetal surgery has got immense potential and is going to come in a big way in very near future.

REFERENCES

1. Liley AW. Intrauterine transfusion of foetus in haemolytic disease. Br Med J. 1963;2(5365):1107-9.
2. Harrison MR. Fetal surgery. Am J Obstet Gynecol. 1996;174(4):1255-64.
3. Jancelewicz T, Harrison MR. A history of fetal surgery. Clin Perinatol. 2009;36(2):227-36.
4. Harrison MR, Anderson J, Rosen MA, Ross NA, Hendrickx AG. Fetal surgery in the primate. Anesthetic, surgical, and tocolytic management to maximize fetal—neonatal survival. J Pediatr Surg. 1982;17(2):115-22.

5. Albanese CT, Harrison MR. Surgical treatment for fetal disease. The state of the art. Ann NY Acad Sci. 1998;847:74-85.
6. Hopkins LM, Feldstein VA. The use of ultrasound in fetal surgery. Clin Perinatol. 2009;36(2):255-72.
7. Yagel S, Cohen SM, Shapiro I, Valsky DV. 3D and 4D ultrasound in fetal cardiac scanning, a new look at the fetal heart. Ultrasound Obstet Gynecol. 2007;29; 81-95.
8. Coakley FV. Role of magnetic resonance imaging in fetal surgery. Top Magn Reson Imaging. 2001;12(1):39-51.
9. Pugash D, Brugger PC, Bettelheim D, Prayer D. Prenatal ultrasound and fetal MRI: the comparative value of each modality in prenatal diagnosis. Eur J Radiol. 2008;68(2):214-26.
10. Vander Wall KJ, Bruch SW, Meuli M, Kohl T, Szabo Z, Adzick NS, Harrison MR. Fetal endoscopic ('Fetendo') tracheal clip. J Pediatr Surg. 1996;31:1101-3.
11. Marwan A, Crombleholme T. The EXIT procedure: principles, pitfalls, and progress. Semin Pediatr Surg. 2006;15;107-15.
12. Cannon JW, Stoll JA, Salgo IS, Knowles HB, Howe RD, Dupont PE, et al. Real-Time Three-Dimensional Ultrasound for Guiding Surgical Tasks, Comput Aided Surg. 2003;8(2):82-90.
13. Maselli KM, Badillo A. Advances in fetal surgery. Ann Transl Med. 2016;4(20):394.
14. Deprest J, Jani J, Lewi L, Ochsenbein-Kölble N, Cannie M, Doné E, et al. Fetoscopic surgery: Encouraged by clinical experience and boosted by instrument innovation. Semin Fetal Neonatal Med. 2006;11;398-412.
15. Bouchard S, Johnson MP, Flake AW, Howell LJ, Myers LB, Adzick NS, et al. The EXIT procedure: experience and outcome in 31 cases. J Pediatr Surg. 2002;37(3):418-26.
16. Moron AF, Barbosa MM, Milani H, Sarmento SG, Santana E, Suriano IC, et al. Perinatal outcomes after open fetal surgery for myelomeningocele repair: a retrospective cohort study. BJOG. 2018;125(10):1280-6.
17. Albanese CT, Harrison MR. Surgical treatment for fetal disease. The state of the art. Ann NY Acad Sci.1998;847:74-85.
18. Grethel EJ, Nobuhara KK. Fetal surgery for congenital diaphragmatic hernia. J Paediatr Child Health. 2006;42(3):79-85.
19. Fan D, Wu S, Wang R, Huang Y, Fu Y, Ai W, et al. Successfully treated congenital cystic adenomatoid malformation by open fetal surgery: a care-compliant case report of a 5-year follow-up and review of the literature. Medicine (Baltimore). 2017;96(2):e5865.
20. Holmes N, Harrison MR, Baskin LS. Fetal surgery for posterior urethral valves: long-term postnatal outcomes. Pediatrics. 2001;108(1):e7.
21. Adzick NS, Thom EA, Spong CY, Brock JW 3rd, Burrows PK, Johnson MP, et al. A randomized trial of prenatal versus postnatal repair of myelomeningocele. N Engl J Med. 2011;17(364):993-1004.

CHAPTER 4

Etiopathogenesis and Management of Fecal Incontinence

Ashok Kumar, Kailash Chand Kurdia

INTRODUCTION

Fecal incontinence (FI) is defined as the involuntary loss of rectal contents (feces, gas) and inability to postpone an evacuation until socially convenient. It is a socially and psychologically devastating condition for the family and the patients. In India, its exact prevalence is not known. International population-based studies suggested a FI prevalence of 0.4–18%.[1,2] There are several mechanisms which plays role in continence, i.e., anatomical, neurological and mechanical. Injury to sphincter, pudendal nerve, and weakness of sphincter complex and age related changes may lead to FI. Several risk factors for sphincter injuries and weakness are obstetric trauma, road traffic accident or surgery, assault, pelvic radiotherapy for cancer, smoking, obesity, diabetes, and certain neurological conditions.

Fecal along with urinary incontinence is 12 times more common in geriatric patients than fecal incontinence alone. Proper management of fecal incontinence requires complete evaluation, including detailed history, physical examinations, and investigation. Majority of patients can be managed with conservative and nonsurgical treatment; however some patients may still require surgical intervention. The type of surgery and surgical outcome are variable.

ANATOMY OF THE ANAL SPHINCTER COMPLEX

Internal anal sphincter (IAS): It is the continuation of the smooth muscle of the rectum and is under control of the involuntary nervous system. IAS is tonically contracted and contributes 80% of the resting pressure.

External anal sphincter (EAS): It is striated muscle, which is under voluntary control. The muscle is innervated by pudendal nerve (S2, S3, S4), which remains partially contracted at rest. It generates approximately 20% of the resting pressure in the anal canal. Inhibition of EAS during defecation allows the passage of stool.

Puborectalis muscle (PRM): It is U-shaped sling around the anorectal junction with an angle of approximately 90 degrees, which obstructs the outlet and prevents the passage of solid stool. It also remains partially contracted at rest and derives nerves from S2, S3, and S4. During normal defecation, with relaxation of PRM and descent of pelvic floor, the anorectal angle widens approximately to 135 degrees, which facilitates the passage of stool **(Figs. 1 and 2)**.

Factors Responsible for Maintenance of Continence

- Internal and external anal sphincter
- Puborectalis muscle
- Anal canal sensation
- Neurogenic integrity
- Capacity and compliance of the rectum
- Stool consistency
- Colonic transit time
- Psychological motivation.

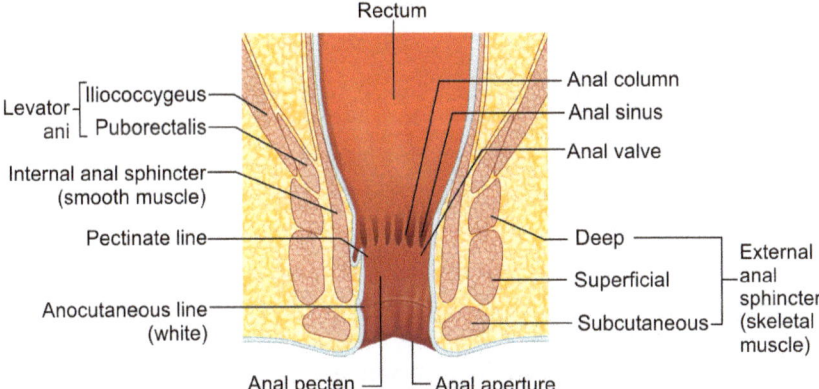

Fig. 1: Anatomy of the anal sphincter.

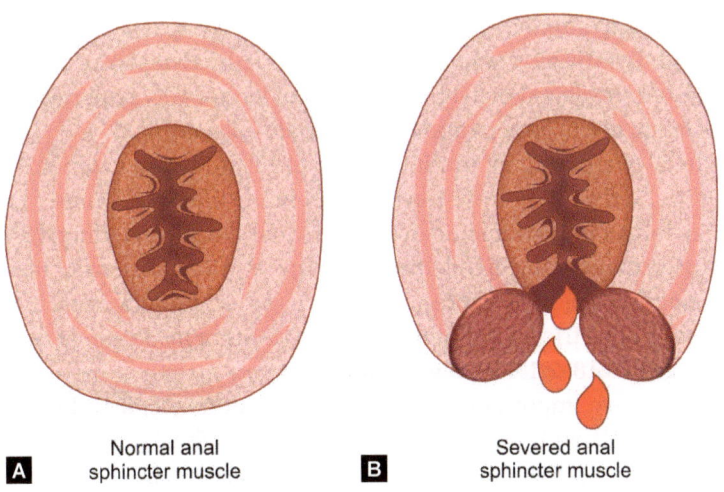

Figs. 2A and B: Normal and damaged sphincters.

COMMON CAUSES OF FECAL INCONTINENCE

- Trauma
  - Obstetrical injury
  - Accidental injury
  - Anorectal surgery
- Neurological conditions
  - Diabetes (autonomic dysfunction, bacterial overgrowth, ingestion of hexitols, pancreatic insufficiency)
  - Multiple sclerosis
  - Congenital anomalies
  - Tumor of brain and spinal cord
- Diarrheal states
  - Infectious diarrhea
  - Inflammatory bowel disease (IBD)
  - Short gut syndrome
- Congenital disease
  - Mega rectum
  - Hirschsprung's disease
- Pelvic floor denervation
  - Chronic straining at stool
  - Descending perineum syndrome
  - Rectal prolapse
  - Vaginal delivery
- Aging.

Obstetric Trauma and Fecal Incontinence

Fecal incontinence is more prevalent among females than males, which is attributed to obstetric injuries sustained during childbirth; however, other factors may play a role in late-onset FI, such as menopause, changes in the pelvic floor due to aging, and pudendal neuropathy. The risk of FI increases with number of vaginal deliveries, delivery of large baby, prolonged second stage of labor, use of forceps and inappropriate episiotomy.[3-6]

In developed country the incidence of FI following vaginal delivery appears to be declining from rates of 13% in primiparous women to 8%.[7,8] This may reflect improvements in obstetrical practices including decreased use of instrumented vaginal delivery (forceps and vacuum extraction), and more selective use of episiotomy. There is no exact data from India but incidence of obstetric anal sphincter injury (OASI) in institutional delivery is in the range of 0.18–2.1% for vaginal delivery.[9,10]

There are two important mechanism of incontinence, first disruption of sphincter muscle with neuropathy (cause for early fecal incontinence) and second is isolated pudendal neuropathy (late manifestation). Stretching of the pudendal nerve is one of the important reasons for the idiopathic incontinence in the middle-aged women. Electromyography (EMG) and histopathology study have shown 80% of denervation of puborectalis muscle and external anal sphincter.

Aging and Fecal Incontinence

- Sclerosis of IAS
- Increased fibers density in EAS and pelvic floor muscle
- Elderly and hospitalized patients
- Anatomical and functional outlet obstruction

CLASSIFICATION OF FECAL INCONTINENCE

- *Major incontinence:* Characterized by frequent and regular inability to control stool of any consistency, e.g., surgical or other trauma, pelvic floor neuropathy
- *Minor incontinence:* Inability to control passage of flatus or loose stool, e.g., surgical injury to IAS, overflow incontinence (fecal impaction)
- *Urge incontinence with increased frequency:* When compliance of the rectum is decreased, smaller volume of stool can cause increased pressure, e.g., IBD, radiation proctitis, coloanal anastomosis.

DIAGNOSIS AND EVALUATION

History and detailed physical examination is important and is sufficient in majority of patients for treatment decision making. A detailed history and examination often reveal the etiology and severity of the incontinence.

History

Following points to be emphasized while taking the history:
- Degree of incontinence (solid, liquid, flatus)
- Frequency of incontinence
- Urgency
- Diarrhea/constipation
- Perianal surgery (fistula, fissure, hemorrhoid, prolapse)
- Underlying medical disease [Irritable bowel syndrome (IBS), IBD, infectious colitis, diabetes)]
- Detailed obstetric history (number of deliveries, baby birth weight, episiotomy, use of forceps).

Physical Examination

Examination of the Perianal Area

Important findings on perineal examination are signs of moisture or fecal leakage, use of pad or diaper, scar from previous trauma or previous surgery. Special attention should be given to look for keyhole deformity. Female patients with previous obstetric injury may have thin perineal body, rectovaginal fistula or cloaca visible on examination. Patients with road traffic accident (RTA) usually have complex injury including anal sphincter complex, urethral injury and pelvic bone fracture.

Per rectal examination: Note for the following findings:
- Decrease resting sphincter tone, strength of squeeze
- Any mass or palpable defect
- Impacted stool
- Puborectalis muscle testing (appreciated posteriorly during squeeze)
- Perianal sensation
- Sacral reflex
- Any neurological defect in the spine.

Diagnostic Tools

Objective testing such as anal manometry, rectal distention testing, electromyography (EMG), pudendal nerve terminal motor latency (PNTML) endoanal ultrasound, magnetic resonance imaging (MRI) and defecography are useful investigations for documentation of the abnormalities of anorectal physiology, degree of anorectal dysfunction and delineation of sphincter loss.[11,12] These may further help in postoperative follow-up. For complete mapping of anal sphincter, investigations of choice are anorectal ultrasound or MRI.

Endorectal Ultrasonography

It is done to assess the integrity of the internal and external anal sphincter. When performed by experienced clinician, endoanal ultrasonography (USG) approaches 100% sensitivity and specificity in identifying the sphincter defects. A 15-mm diameter probe with 360-degree rotation, 10 MHz transducer is used to image the sphincter at the several levels in the anal canal. IAS is imaged as a hypoechoic ring, close to the transducer, surrounded by a hyperechoic ring representing the EAS. Sphincter defect is measured as a lateral break in the sphincter. Endo-USG sphincter abnormalities are seen in up to 90% of the women, whose sole risk factor for FI is obstetric trauma **(Figs. 3A and B)**.

Magnetic Resonance Imaging

Magnetic resonance imaging is a valuable alternative to endosonography. For detection of external sphincter defects the techniques have comparable results. However, visualization of the external sphincter at MRI is superior to endosonography, facilitating identification of external sphincter atrophy. External sphincter atrophy at MRI is related to poor outcome of anterior anal repair and therefore MRI should be considered in potential candidates

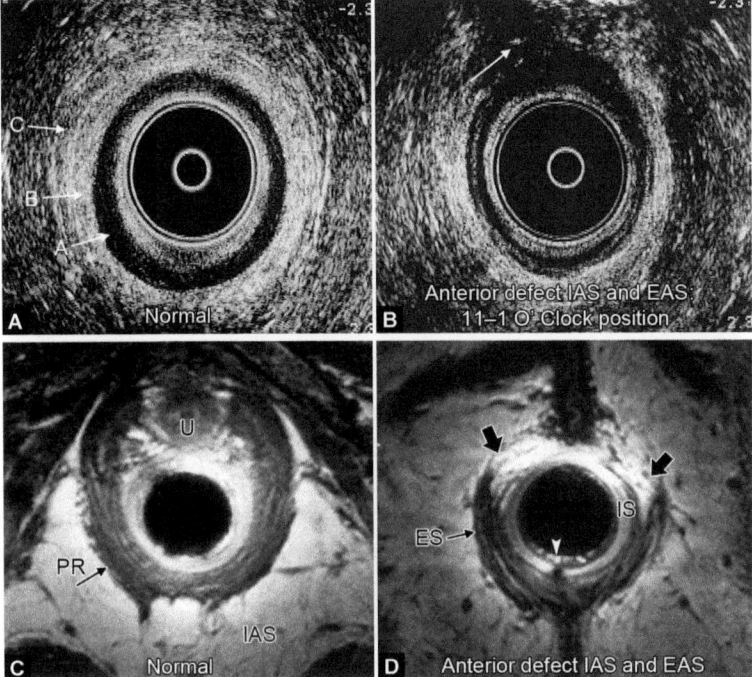

Figs. 3A to D: (A and B) Images of endoanal ultrasonography; (C and D) MRI of normal and damaged sphincter complex.

for anterior anal repair. External coil MRI is a widely available alternative to endoanal MRI and can be used as an alternative in experienced hands **(Figs. 3C and D)**.

Anorectal Manometry

It measures pressure in the anal canal and distal rectum, for functional assessment of the internal and external sphincters as well as anorectal reflexes. Following should be measured by the anorectal manometry:
- Resting pressure
- Squeeze pressure
- Sensation
- Compliance
- Sphincter response to distension

There are various techniques available, including using microtransducers, water perfused catheters, or solid state catheters. Microtransducers are the most reliable catheters because they minimize the distention of the anus. However, the cost and the fragility of these devices restrict their use. The most commonly used sensory devices are 4 to 8-mm in diameter, water perfused soft, plastic, multichannel catheters with radial array. Squeeze pressure can be measured by asking the patient to contract the sphincter as the catheter is positioned in the pressure zone. Normal values of both resting and squeeze pressures vary among patient population.

Rectal sensory testing includes volumetric measurement of first detectable sensation, sensation of fullness and the maximum tolerated volume by balloon distension. Hypersensitivity can be seen with inflammatory conditions and poor rectal compliance. Compliance is measured by inflating the rectal balloon with increasing volume of air or water. The result is expressed as the ratio of the pressure to the volume ($C = P/V$). The compliance decreases, with inflammation, fibrosis, drugs or surgery.

Pudendal Nerve Terminal Motor Latency

Pudendal nerve, containing fibers from sacral nerves S2-4, provides motor innervation to the external sphincter and receives sensory information from the perineum. PNTML measures the conduction time to external sphincter contraction, after the nerve stimulation at the level of the ischial spine. This is easily performed using a digitally mounted device with a stimulating electrode mounted at the fingertip and recording electrode mounted at the base of the finger. The mass production of a self-adhesive disposable electrode, which can easily be mounted on a gloved finger, has enabled this assessment to become routine in most centers. The normal latency is considered 2.1 ± 0.2 ms. Prolonged latency may be associated with obstetric injury, perineal descent, prolapse and medical neuropathies. The success rate after sphincter repair decreases from about 90% if the pudendal nerve is intact to 50% in the presence of pudendal neuropathy.

Electromyography

It can be used in different ways. It is done to record electrical activity in the muscle of continence during anorectal function. It is used to determine whether there is evidence of inappropriate puborectalis contraction during defecation or for sphincter mapping, especially in patients with ectopic anus, congenital anomalies, and after severe disruption. Needle EMG, either with concentric needle or with single fiber electrodes, had an important role in the clinical mapping of the EAS. Results of the needle EMG corroborate well with those of endoanal USG and with surgical or histological methods to identify the sphincter damage. Surface EMG, with an anal plug within the anal canal is without pain and less risk of infection and has a definite role in indicating and applying biofeedback training.

Defecography

Defecography or the dynamic proctogram is used to define the anatomy and changes of the pelvic floor muscle position with defecation. It can identify abnormalities such as prolapse, perineal descent and intussusceptum. This investigation utilizes the paste of barium and potato powder to simulate the fecal material. Video recording used during strain, squeeze and defecation into a radiolucent commode, allows real time assessment of anatomic changes during defecation. Sigmoidoscopy and stool examination may be also required.

INVESTIGATION AND ITS USEFULNESS

- *Transanal ultrasound:* Assess integrity of external and internal anal sphincter.
- *MRI:* Muscles of the pelvic floor, CNS or spinal cord lesions.
- *Defecography:* Descent, anorectal angle, prolapse, intussusceptum
- *Anal manometry:* Functional deficit
- *Electromyography:* Electrical activity (in muscle of continence)
- *PNTML:* Neural deficit.

TREATMENT

Management depends mainly on the symptomatology and also complexity of injury such as degree of perineal tear or associated injury (rectal, vaginal, bladder and bowel). Overall patient's subjective symptoms are important when the clinician is formulating a treatment plan; it is helpful to quantify the severity of incontinence in an objective manner. There are various scoring systems or severity indices but none of them is universally accepted. Commonly used scoring systems included fecal incontinence severity index (FISI),[13] and Wexner score.[14] Patients with mild to moderate symptoms, regardless of etiology, may improve enough to delay or preclude investigation. Many individuals can be managed adequately by noninvasive means.

Conservative Treatment

- *Dietary measures*: Fiber, bulking agents
- *Pharmacological agents*: Motility altering agents
- *Bowel management*: Disimpaction, use of enemas
- Biofeedback
- Strengthening exercise
- Procon device.

Dietary Measures

Counseling of patients regarding following:
- *Diarrhea-inducing foods*: Alcohol, caffeine, fruit juice, prunes, licorice beans, broccoli, cauliflower, cabbage
- *Source of food intolerance*: Lactose, gluten, sorbitol, fructose
- *Addition of bulking agent*: Daily fiber intake 20–25 g/day, methylcellulose, psyllium products

Pharmacological Agents

- *Antidiarrheals:* The most commonly used antidiarrheals are adsorbents and opium derivatives.
  - *Adsorbents*: Kaopectate useful for mild degree of incontinence.
  - *Opium derivatives*: Loperamide (Imodium)—commonly used.
  - Diphenoxylate, Diphenoxylate hydrochloride, atropine, codeine, tincture of opium
- *Tricyclic antidepressant:* Amitriptyline (20 mg, daily). It has anticholinergic and serotoninergic properties.
- *Bulking agents:* These are better, and used for patients of diarrheal variety of IBS.
- *Bile salt binders:* Cholestyramine and colestipol. These resins treat bile acid diarrhea by binding with bile salts in the small intestine.
- *Topical agents:* Acts on internal sphincter and increases the resting tone—10% phenylephrine.

Bowel Management

The aim is to allow the patients to produce a complete bowel movement at a schedule time by using an individualized combination of dietary measures, laxatives, suppositories, enemas or digitization. This method is useful for patients with neurological problems, diabetes, and congenital anorectal malformation. This is also useful for patients with overflow incontinence and pediatric patients with encopresis having symptoms of seepage of stool from full rectum. The aim is complete cleansing of colon by use of various combinations. Later, the use of the daily formulation of polyethylene glycol/laxative is better.

Biofeedback

Biofeedback has a broad acceptance as a useful treatment of fecal incontinence. The term "biofeedback" describes a therapeutic instrument that derives from psychological "theory of learning". This type of learning is also called instrumental learning or operant conditioning. A body function, which cannot or can only be perceived poorly by the subject under normal condition, is measured by a technical device and demonstrated (fed back) to the subject. There are two methods of biofeedback training:
1. Response to rectal distension using manometric techniques
2. Unrelated to rectal distension, muscle strengthening, using EMG or manometric technique.

A biofeedback therapist who evaluates patients during 6-8 weeks supervises the treatment. Both methods are effective, although, some patients may respond better to one system than the other. Biofeedback therapy is best applied to motivate patients with some ability to voluntarily contract the external anal sphincter (even if the muscle is partially disrupted) and an intact rectal sensation. Biofeedback is beneficial in patients with incontinence of variable etiology such as diabetes, after childbirth or after anorectal surgery. However, best results can be seen in patients who have primarily a sensory problem in the anal canal leading to insensible loss of feces. The results of biofeedback training in different patient groups suffering from incontinence vary from 64–89%, with an overall success rate of approximately 70%. Symptom improvement may sustain several years after treatment. The exact mechanism of success is unclear. Nevertheless, it is safe, effective, and does not preclude other treatments.

Sacral Nerve Stimulation

Recently, sacral nerve stimulation (SNS) has been developed as a minimally invasive and effective technique for idiopathic and acquired fecal incontinence. The technique uses chronic low-level electrical stimulation of the sacral nerve, or neuromodulation, to produce a clinically beneficial effect on the distal colon and rectum, the pelvic floor and the anal sphincter complex.

SNS is a two stage procedure:
1. A diagnostic stage—temporary percutaneous nerve evaluation (PNE)
2. Therapeutic stage—permanent SNS.

The procedure entails placing the electrode in a sacral foramen (S2, 3, or 4) to stimulate the nerve roots with the help of nerve stimulator. The desired effect is the maximum contraction of the pelvic muscles with minimal stimulation of the fiber to the lower extremity. Once the optimal site is elected, the lead is connected to the temporary external pulse generator for a test period of stimulation (4-6 weeks).

If the function improves adequately at the end of the test period, implantation of a permanent pulse generator is performed. Most published reports of the sacral nerve stimulation, for treatment of fecal incontinence were case studies and methods of assessing outcome were variable. Patient selection criteria are evolving and are to be defined. The initial assumption that a patient needs an intact sphincter and pudendal nerve is already being challenged. There is growing body of evidence that supports its use as a first line treatment for fecal incontinence in patients where conservative measures have failed. In a study from St. Marks Hospital London on 138 patients (FU in 95 patients) with a median follow-up was 139 months (range 60-242), the success rate of SNS was 48.4% **(Figs. 4A and B)**.

Anal Plug

The anal plug is a soft compliant hydrophilic plug, which expands after insertion and occluding the anorectal junction. Insertion is added by the use of lubricant jelly and extraction by means of attached ribbon. It provides tampons, those who able to retain tampons and tolerate its presence, it made substantial contributions to their quality of life. Although intolerance of the device and failure of retention are reported with adverse events.

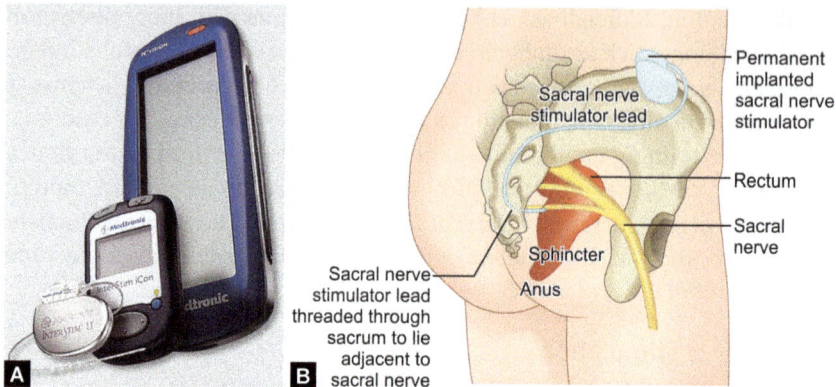

Figs. 4A and B: Sacral nerve stimulation (SNS) system. (A) Device; (B) Placement of device.

Injectable Biomaterials

Injected materials included autologous fat, crosslinked collagen, silicon, bioplastique and carbon coated beads. Silicone implant comprises medical-grade vulcanized silicone particles which are ductile and of irregular texture. These materials suspended in hydrogel low molecular weight; water soluble polyvinylpyrrolidone (povidone, PVP) carrier vehicle which is eliminated by the reticuloendothelial system and excreted through the kidney unchanged. Mechanism of action is still unclear. It is presumed to exert a "padding effect" in the submucosal plane to promote anal closure. Advantages of injectable therapy are simplicity and the ability to offer treatment in an outpatient setting, but it requires repeated injection and migration of the injectable material is reported.

Surgical Options

Surgical options are sphincteroplasty, artificial sphincter replacement, muscle transposition, Thiersch wiring and diversion stoma.[15,16]

- Sphincter repair
  - Direct apposition
  - Plication or reefing
  - Overlapping repair
- External sphincter alone or combined with internal sphincter
- Encirclement
  - *Muscle transfer procedures*: Skeletal muscle flaps [gluteus, gracilis (uni- or bilateral), Stimulated gracilis (uni- or bilateral), free muscle transplant]
  - *Synthetic material*: Thiersch procedure, Dacron-impregnated silastic sling, artificial bowel sphincter.

Surgical Treatment for Fecal Incontinence

Indications

- Incontinence refractory to medical therapy
- Failure of other modalities of treatment
  Results are usually better with incontinence for solid stool than liquid stool. Good for isolated sphincter defect.

Choice of Operation

The choice of operation is largely determined by the preoperative physiological and radiological findings.
- *Anterior repair*: Defect in the sphincter (iatrogenic or obstetric trauma)
- *Anterior repair + levatorplasty*: Anterior defect clinically or on investigation (obstetric trauma)
- *Postanal repair*: Patients with idiopathic or neurogenic incontinence
- *Total pelvic floor repair*: Complicated injury to EAS and PRM at one or more sites, neurogenic incontinence
- Augmentation procedures, complex anatomic defects, and artificial sphincter neurogenic incontinence

Bowel Preparation

The patient is kept on liquid diet for 2 days prior to surgery. A full mechanical bowel preparation a day before surgery or two phosphate enemas, one the evening before and one the morning of surgery, is adequate. A failed bowel preparation is worse than no bowel preparation at all with liquid stool trickling over the operation site. Antibiotic prophylaxis may be given as per protocol of the hospital.

Sphincter Repair

Sphincter repair is considered in patients with isolated sphincter defect because the remaining muscle usually maintains the ability to contract. There are three approaches to sphincter repair—apposition, plication, and overlapping. Surgical procedure is usually performed in lithotomy position or prone jackknife position. Postoperative complication rates are generally low. Rates for the most commonly reported complication of wound infection range from 6 to 35%. Success rates decline with time after the procedure.

Direct Apposition

This method involves mobilization of the external sphincter, excision of the scar tissue, and suture of the muscle ends in an end-to-end fashion, using non-absorbable or 2/0 polydioxanone (PDS) interrupted suture. Results of this repair are variable, ranging from 33.5 to 100%. The failed repairs with this technique have been attributed mostly to separation of the sutured ends of

TABLE 1: Result of direct sphincter repair.

Authors (year)	No. of patients	% with complete response
Manning, Pratt (1964),[18]	102	74%
Fang, et al. (1984),[19]	79	58

TABLE 2: Published series of long-term outcomes of overlapping sphincteroplasty.

Authors (year)	Study period	Total no. of patients (% F/U available)	F/U Duration (months, median)	Excellent/ Good results	Fair/Poor Results
Karoui et al. (2000),[17]	1990–1997	86 (86%)	40	34 (45%)	40 (55%)
Halverson et al. (2002),[20]	1989–1996	71 (69%)	69	18 (37%)	31 (63%)
Bravo et al. (2004),[21]	1985–1994	191 (54%)	120	24 (23%)	80 (77%)
Barisic et al. 2006),[22]	1990–2002	65 (86%)	80	15 (26%)	12 (21%)
Maslekar et al. (2007),[23]	1995–1999	72 (88%)	84	14 (22%)	41 (64%)
Chase et al. (2010)[24]	2004-2008	34 (94%)	NR	23 (67%)	9 (26%)

the muscle as a result of excision of scar. The results of direct sphincter repair are mentioned in **Table 1**.

Overlapping Repair

Overlapping sphincteroplasty is the most common delayed procedure performed to treat traumatic disruption of the sphincter. However, there is no randomized trial comparing sphincteroplasty with nonsurgical therapy such as biofeedback. A curvilinear incision is made in the perineal body over the anterior injury. Anterior vaginal and posterior anodermal flaps are created, and the sphincter muscle is dissected laterally on each side of the defect. Sphincter mobilization is not carried out posterior to the mid lateral line to avoid pudendal nerve injury. The anterior scar is divided in the midline but not excised, to aid in suture fixation. The flap muscles are then overlapped to form a snug anal opening. The repair is done either with 2/0 PDS or prolene mattress suture **(Table 2)**.

Plication procedures: Simple reefing procedure for the anal sphincter has been described for many years in the literature. The role of simple reefing of the external sphincter is limited. It is applied in cases where external sphincter is merely thinned out but not divided (such as obstetric trauma) and sitting loosely around the anal canal. Simple placation without division of the muscle can be combined with formal reconstruction of the perineal body via levatorplasty.

Anterior Repair with Levatorplasty

This is the operation of choice for patients with anterior injury. The intersphincteric space is approached through a curvilinear incision close to the vaginal introitus and extending laterally around the anal margin. The skin flap is dissected toward the anal margin to expose the fibers of external sphincter. Once the external sphincter has been mobilized from the surrounding tissue, it is retracted caudally and dissection is continued in the rectovaginal septum. At times there is some bleeding, as this plane is quite vascular. Care must be taken not to enter into the rectum. The vagina is separated through its entire length from the anterior rectal wall. The levator muscle can then be identified in the base of the wound, running anteriorly and superiorly. Anterior levatorplasty is performed by suturing the two sides of the levator using two or three interrupted sutures of PDS 2/0 or prolene. The external sphincter is divided through scar tissue and an overlapping repair is performed as described earlier. After the levatorplasty and sphincter repair, the semicircular incision now becomes longitudinal. The skin is closed using an absorbable or nonabsorbable suture. A small defect is left in the wound to facilitate drainage of collection **(Figs. 5A to G)**.

Postanal Repair

Postanal repair was developed by Parks in 1975. Parks had discovered that the anorectal angle was obtuse in patients with idiopathic fecal incontinence and puborectalis muscle was responsible for maintaining this angle. Therefore this operation was designed to restore the anorectal angle. A curved incision is made approximately 5 cm posterior to the anal margin. The skin flap is dissected and elevated toward the anal margin. The internal sphincter is encountered as the dissection proceeds the anal canal and the intersphincteric plane is identified. Now the dissection is continued in the intersphincteric plane until the puborectalis muscle is reached. Waldeyer's fascia is identified and divided, the supralevator space is entered, and the levator muscles are identified. The dissection is developed laterally on top of the levator ani using combination of sharp and blunt dissection. Approximation of the iliococcygeus muscle on either side is taken, followed by second row of sutures incorporating the pubococcygeus. The puborectalis limbs are approximated and external anal sphincter is plicated. All the sutures are taken interrupted before being tied. Posterior plication of the puborectalis theoretically restores the anorectal angle and the anal canal **(Table 3)**.

Dynamic graciloplasty: Dynamic graciloplasty combines transposition of the gracilis muscle with electrical stimulation via an implantable pulse generator. The gracilis muscle is preferred because it is the most superficial in the medial aspect of the thigh and has a proximal neurovascular bundle and can be tunneled under the skin in the proximal thigh and wrapped around the anal canal. The operation is best carried out with the patient in the Lloyd Davis position. Three incisions are given in order to mobilize and divide the distal tendon of gracilis. The muscle is mobilized as its neurovascular bundle lies at the junction of proximal and middle thirds. A tunnel is developed on either

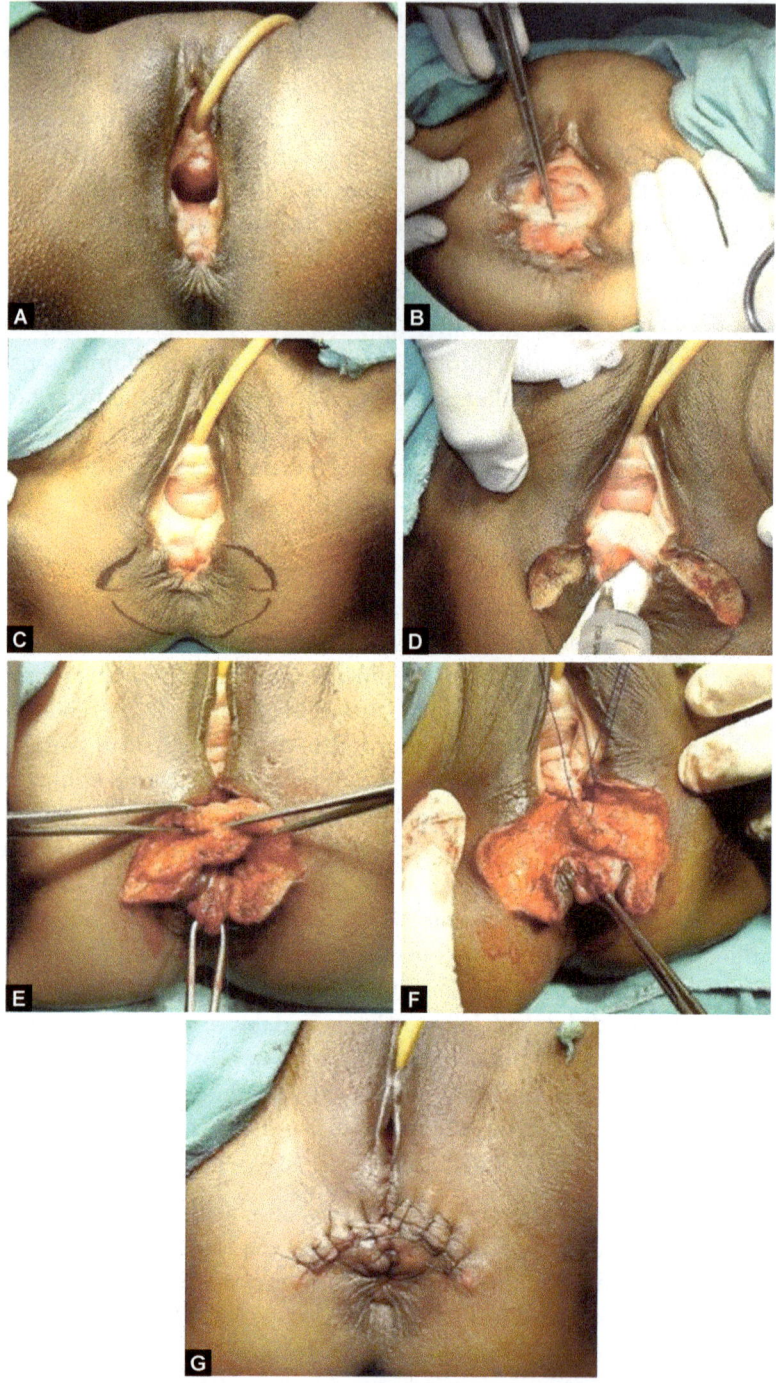

Figs. 5A to G: Overlapping sphincteroplasty with anterior levatorplasty. (A) Grade III obstetric perineal injury; (B) Loss of perineal body; (C) Marking of external anal sphincter; (D) Injection of 2% xylocaine with adrenaline; (E) Overlapping of external sphincter; (F) Repair of external sphincter with prolene suture; (G) Final shape after skin closure.

TABLE 3: Result of post anal repair.

Authors	No. of patients	Good/Excellent result (%)
Browning et al. (1983),[25]	140	86
Henry et al. (1985),[26]	129	70
Yoshioka et al. (1985),[27]	116	57

TABLE 4: Result of dynamic graciloplasty.

Authors	No. of patients	Success %	Follow-up period (months)
Geerdes et al. (1996),[28]	67	52	32
DMP trial (1999),[29]	75	53	24
DGTSG trial (2000),[30]	83	45	12

(DMP: dynamic muscle plasty; DGTSG: dynamic graciloplasty therapy study group)

side of the anal canal and the tendon of the gracilis muscle is passed around the anal canal to encircle it. The wrap configuration may be of different kind (alpha, gamma or epsilon). An incision is made over the contralateral ischial tuberosity and the gracilis tendon is sutured with nonabsorbable sutures (Prolene/Nylon) **(Table 4)**.

None of the skeletal muscles used to augment sphincter has the property of the EAS, which has resting tone and preponderance of slow twitch fibers (80% type I fibers-fatigue resistant). Gracilis muscle has only 43% type I muscle fibers. Chronic low-frequency stimulation induces a transformation from fast twitch to slow twitch muscle fibers. The first electrical stimulation of a transposed gracilis muscle was reported by Dikson and Nixon in 1968. There are two techniques for muscle stimulation. In the procedure devised by Williams et al., the electrodes are placed directly over the nerves to gracilis. After identifying the nerve with the help of nerve locator, the stimulator and the electrodes are attached. The stimulator lies in a pocket overlying the lower ribs. The lead is tunneled subcutaneously via a small incision in the suprainguinal region and the electrode is brought down to the appropriate nerve. The electrode plate is sutured over the main nerve bundle in a longitudinal fashion. The alternative technique is insertion of the electrode into the gracilis muscle adjacent to the supplying nerve. The connection to the stimulator is assessed using external temporary programmer. The gracilis muscle is then transposed around the anal canal as described earlier.

Postoperatively the patients are nursed with legs banded loosely together. Electrical stimulation of the muscle commences at day 10, provided the wound is healed. The stimulator is programmed using a standard training protocol. Once the muscle is trained the patient can be admitted for the closure of covering stoma. The stimulator can be stitched on or off by passing a magnet over it.

A successful functional outcome for graciloplasty, dynamic and adynamic, is consistently reported to be about 70%.[31]

In many respects gluteus maximus muscle is in ideal position to augment anal sphincter function. It involves formation of a defunctioning stoma as a preliminary procedure. The surgery is performed in prone jack-knife position. Two mirror image cutaneous incisions are made on each side from the border of the mid sacrum toward acetabulum. The sacrococcygeal origin of the muscle is detached with its aponeurosis. A 5 cm wide strip of muscle is divided parallel with the fascia up to the point where the neurovascular pedicle enters the deep surface. Blunt dissection of the muscle is continued until it is sufficiently mobilized to allow transposition around the anal orifice. Two lateral incisions are made parallel to the anal margin 2 cm from the anal orifice. The detached halves of the gluteus maximus muscles are then wrapped around the anal canal.

Artificial Anal Sphincter

Artificial anal implants have been used for urinary incontinence for many years. The device has undergone many modifications. The prosthesis currently in use is a modification of an artificial urinary sphincter AMS800 (American Medical system). The device is composed of a silicon elastomer which has three components: (1) an inflatable cuff, which wraps around the anus; (2) a pressure regulating balloon; and (3) a control pump **(Figs. 6A and B)**. The patient controls the device via pump in the scrotum or labia. Squeezing the pump 9–12 times forces the fluid from the cuff into the reservoir balloon, which is implanted in the space of Retzius. This deflates the cuff and opens the anal canal, allowing the passage of stool. The cuff then automatically slowly reinflates and occludes the anal canal providing continence until defecation is desired again. First result of implantation was reported by Christensen and Lorentzen in 1987. In the ABS group of multicenter

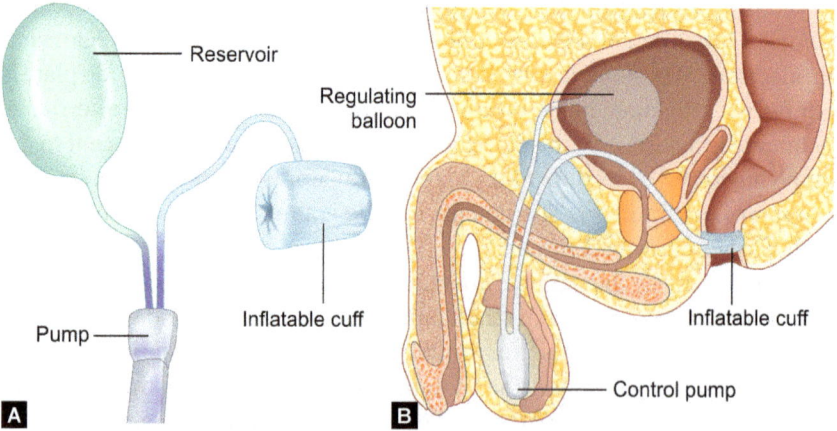

Figs. 6A and B: Artificial bowel sphincter. (A) Device; (B) Placement of device.

TABLE 5: Artificial bowel sphincter and success rate.

Authors (year)	No. of patients	Successful outcome (%)
Christiansen (1992),[35]	12	50
Lehur (1996),[36]	14	70
Vaizey (1998),[37]	7	71

TABLE 6: Artificial anal sphincter and complication.

Authors (year)	No. of patients	Infection	Erosion	Failure	Explanation
Lehur et al. (1996),[36]	24	1	3	3	8
Malouf et al. (2000),[38]	18	7	2	2	12
Vaizey et al. (1998),[37]	6	6	1	10	1
Dodi et al. (2000),[39]	8	2	1	0	2
Ortiz et al. (2002),[40]	22	3	5	2	9

clinical trial including 112 patients in 19 centers in US, Canada and Europe-1 year device function rate was 67%. The infection rate was 25%. Forty-six percent of the implanted patients required revision surgery. **Tables 5 and 6** describe long term outcomes and complications of artificial anal sphincter respectively.

Secca Procedure

This procedure involves delivering temperature-controlled radiofrequency energy (465 kHz, 2-5 W) to the anorectal junction with a goal of remodeling, scarring, and causing contraction of the collagen tissues in anal region. In a 5-year follow-up of 19 patients, sustained improvements in FI symptoms and FIQOL were reported when compared to baseline. In a review of 10 Secca studies comprising 220 patients, FI improved in 55-80% of patients, complications occurred in 20% of patients. Manometry and endoanal ultrasound tests did not reveal any changes. Most studies included small numbers of patients. There are no randomized controlled trials, but it has been FDA-approved since 2002 for patients who have failed conservative therapy for FI.[32,33]

Magnetic Anal Sphincter

The magnetic anal sphincter (MAS) comprises a series of interlinked titanium beads with internal magnetic cores that form a flexible ring, encircling the EAS and creating a barrier. During defecation, the beads separate, allowing stool to pass. Once the stool is passed, the inner core of magnet brings the ring in the normal position. Results of multicentric study was performed at four clinical sites in Europe and the United States, included patients (A total of 35 patients) with severe fecal incontinence for ≥6 months who had previously failed conservative therapy and were implanted with a magnetic anal sphincter

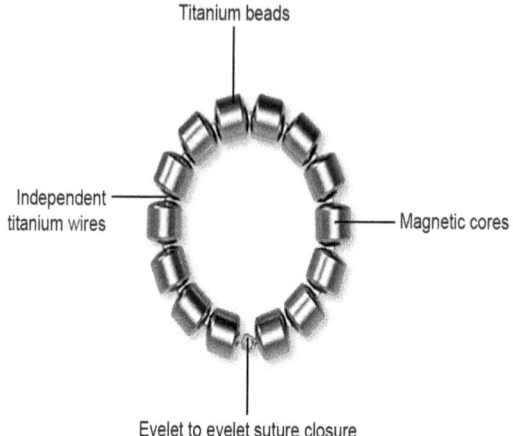

Fig. 7: Magnetic anal sphincter.

device, showed, the long-term overall outcomes at a median follow-up of 5 years were, therapeutic success rates were reported as 63% at 1 year, 66% at 3 years, and 53% at 5 years. The device was explanted in seven patients because of major adverse events. In total, 30 adverse events ranging from pain to device erosion were reported in 20 patients. The authors state that the majority (73%) of these were minor events and require little to no intervention and occurred during the first year after implantation **(Fig. 7)**.[34]

CONCLUSION

Fecal incontinence is a devastating problem as it affects the quality of life. There are many etiopathological factors leading to FI. History and thorough clinical examination is important to plan investigations and subsequent treatment. Investigations are required only in a small percentage of patients in therapeutic decision making. Majority of patients respond to nonsurgical treatments—medical, biofeedback and sacral nerve stimulation (SNS). Surgery is useful in select group of patients specifically those with sphincter injury. Sphincteroplasty with or without levatorplasty is procedure of choice, when there is anatomical defect and rest of the sphincter is normal. Colostomy may be last resort in selected patient.

REFERENCES

1. Nelson RL. Epidemiology of fecal incontinence. Gastroenterology. 2004;126 (1 Suppl 1):S3-7.
2. Faltin DL, Sangalli MR, Curtin F, Morabia A, Weil A. Prevalence of anal incontinence and other anorectal symptoms in women. Int Urogynecol J Pelvic Floor Dysfunct. 2001;12(2):117-21.
3. Rey E, Choung RS, Schleck CD, Zinsmeister AR, Locke GR 3rd, Talley NJ. Onset and risk factors for fecal incontinence in a US community. Am J Gastroenterol. 2010;105(2): 412-9.

4. Bharucha AE, Zinsmeister AR, Locke GR, Seide BM, McKeon K, Schleck CD, et al. Risk factors for fecal incontinence: a population-based study in women. Am J Gastroenterol. 2006;101(6):1305-12.
5. Bharucha AE, Fletcher JG, Melton LJ 3rd, Zinsmeister AR. Obstetric trauma, pelvic floor injury and fecal incontinence: a population-based case-control study. Am J Gastroenterol. 2012;107(6):902-11.
6. Rao SS. Current and emerging treatment options for fecal incontinence. J Clin Gastroenterol. 2014;48(9):752-64.
7. Sultan AH, Kamm MA, Hudson CN, Thomas JM, Bartram CI. Anal-sphincter disruption during vaginal delivery. N Engl J Med. 1993;329(26):1905-11.
8. Rogers RG, Leeman L, Borders A. Does cesarean delivery protect against pelvic floor dysfunction at 6 months postpartum? Female Pelvic Med Reconstr Surg. 2012; 18:S73.
9. Desai GJ, Junnare KK. Obstetric anal sphincter injures and outcome of primary repair. Int J Repord Contracept Obstet Gynecol. 2016;5(10):3568-71.
10. Gundabattula SR, Surampudi K. Risk factors for obstetric anal sphincter injuries (OASI) at a tertiary centre in south India. Int Urogynecol J. 2018; 29(3):391-6.
11. Falk PM, Blatchford GJ, Cali RL, Christensen MA, Thorson AG. Transanal ultrasound and manometry in the evaluation of fecal incontinence. Dis Colon Rectum. 1994;37(5):468-72.
12. Rao SS, Patel RS. How useful are manometric tests of anorectal function in the management of defecation disorders? Am J Gastroenterol. 1997;92(3):469-75.
13. Rockwood TH, Church JM, Fleshman JW, Kane RL, Mavrantonis C, Thorson AG, et al. Patient and surgeon ranking of the severity of symptoms associated with fecal incontinence: the fecal incontinence severity index. Dis Colon Rectum. 1999;42(12):1525-32.
14. Jorge JM, Wexner SD. Etiology and management of fecal incontinence. Dis Colon Rectum. 1993;36(1):77-97.
15. Goetz LH, Lowry AC. Overlapping sphincteroplasty: is it the standard of care? Clin Colon Rectal Surg. 2005;18(1):22-31.
16. Gregorcyk SG. The current status of the Acticon˙ Neosphincter. Clin Colon Rectal Surg. 2005; 18(1):32-7.
17. Karoui S, Leroi AM, Koning E, Menard JF, Michot F, Denis P. Results of sphincteroplasty in 86 patients with anal incontinence. Dis Colon Rectum. 2000;43(6):813-20.
18. Manning PC, Pratt JH. Fecal incontinence caused by lacerations of perineum. Arch Surg. 1964;88:569-76.
19. Fang DT, Nivatvongs S, Vermeulen FD, Herman FN, Goldberg SM, Rothenberger DA. Overlapping sphincteroplasty for acquired anal incontinence. Dis Colon Rectum. 1984;27(11):720-2.
20. Halverson AL, Hull TL. Long-term outcome of overlapping anal sphincter repair. Dis Colon Rectum. 2002;45(3):345-8.
21. Bravo Gutierrez A, Madoff RD, Lowry AC, Parker SC, Buie WD, Baxter NN. Long-term results of anterior sphincteroplasty. Dis Colon Rectum. 2004;47(5):727-32.
22. Barisic GI, Krivokapic ZV, Markovic VA, Popovic MA. Outcome of overlapping anal sphincter repair after 3 months and after a mean of 80 months. Int J Colorectal Dis. 2006;21(1):52-6.
23. Maslekar S, Gardiner AB, Duthie GS. Anterior anal sphincter repair for fecal incontinence: good long-term results are possible. J Am Coll Surg. 2007;204:40-6.
24. Chase S, Mittal R, Jesudason MR, Nayak S, Perakath B. Anal sphincter repair for fecal incontinence: experience from a tertiary care centre. Indian J Gastroenterol. 2010;29(4):162-5.
25. Browning GG, Parks AG. Postanal repair for neuropathic faecal incontinence: correlation of clinical result and anal canal pressures. Br J Surg. 1983;70(2):101-4.

26. Henry MM, Simson JN. Results of postanal repair: a retrospec-tive study. Br J Surg. 1985;72(Suppl):S17-9
27. Yoshioka K, Keighley MR. Critical assessment of the quality of continence after postanal repair for faecal incontinence. Br J Surg. 1989;76(10):1054-7.
28. Geerdes BP, Heineman E, Konsten J, Soeters PB, Baeten CG. Dynamic graciloplasty. Complications and management. Dis Colon Rectum. 1996;39(8):912-7.
29. Madoff RD, Rosen HR, Baeten CG, LaFontaine LJ, Cavina E, Devesa M, et al. Safety and efficacy of dynamic muscle plasty for anal incontinence (lessons from a prospective, multicenter trial). Gastroenterology. 1999;116:549-56
30. Baeten CG, Bailey HR, Bakka A, Belliveau P, Berg E, Buie WD, et al. Safety and efficacy of dynamic graciloplasty for fecal incontinence: report of a prospective, multicenter trial. Dynamic Graciloplasty Therapy Study Group. Dis Colon Rectum. 2000;43(6):743-51.
31. Hassan MZ, Rathnayaka MM, Deen KI. Modified dynamic gracilis neosphincter for fecal incontinence: an analysis of functional outcome at a single institution. World J Surg. 2010; 34(7):1641-7.
32. FDA. Summary of Safety and Probable Benefit (SSPB). [online] Available from http://www.accessdata.fda.gov/cdrh_docs/pdf13/H130006b.pdf. [Last Accessed December, 2020].
33. Frascio M, Mandolfino F, Imperatore M, Stabilini C, Fornaro R, Gianetta E, et al. The SECCA procedure for faecal incontinence: a review. Colorectal Dis. 2014;16:167-72.
34. Sugrue J, Lehur PA, Madoff RD, McNevin S, Buntzen S, Laurberg S, et al. Long-term experience of magnetic anal sphincter augmentation in patients with fecal incontinence. Dis Colon Rectum. 2017;60(1):87-95.
35. Christiansen J, Sparsø B. Treatment of anal incontinence by an implantable prosthetic anal sphincter. Ann Surg. 1992;215(4):383-6.
36. Lehur PA, Michot F, Denis P, Grise P, Leborgne J, Teniere P, et al. Results of artificial sphincter in severe anal incontinence. Report of 14 consecutive implantations. Dis Colon Rectum. 1996;39:1352-5.
37. Vaizey CJ, Kamm MA, Gold DM, Bartram CI, Halligan S, Nicholls RJ. Clinical, physiological, and radiological study of a new purpose-designed artificial bowel sphincter. Lancet. 1998;352:105-9.
38. Malouf AJ, Vaizey CJ, Kamm MA, Nicholls RJ. Reassessing artificial bowel sphincters. Lancet. 2000;355:2219-20.
39. Dodi G, Melega E, Masin A, Infantino A, Cavallari F, Lise M. Artificial bowel sphincter (ABS) for severe faecal incontinence (a clinical and manometric study). Int J Colorect Dis. 2000;2:207-11.
40. Ortiz H, Armendariz P, DeMiguel M, Ruiz MD, Alos R, Roig JV. Complications and functional outcome following artificial anal sphincter implantation. Br J Surg. 2002;89:877-81.

Targeted Therapy in Gastrointestinal Malignancy

Rahul, Mansi Sharma, Richa Sinha

INTRODUCTION

Surgery forms the backbone of treatment of most gastrointestinal (GI) malignancies, especially in curative settings. Chemotherapy or radiotherapy has defined roles used to further improve survival both perioperatively and in palliative scenario. The basic mechanism of all chemotherapeutic agents is to disrupt the cell cycle at different stages and inhibit cell division. The principles of radiation also remain the same. It damages nucleic acids in the target organ and prevents cell division. However, both of them affect cancerous as well as healthy replicating cells. The response to treatment remains unpredictable. In a similar pathology, a subset of patients shows complete clinical and pathological response, while another subset presents with progressive disease. The wide range of response may be subjected to finer differences at molecular level. This entails the need for personalized therapy. Recently, there has been a paradigm shift in the treatment of cancer. Molecular targeted agents have revolutionized the management of certain GI malignancies, leading to clinically meaningful improvement in patient outcome.

DEFINITION

Targeted cancer therapy or molecular therapy includes molecules that are meant to act selectively on the cancer cells preventing their growth and dissemination. The mode of action being specific for malignant cells, they are expected to be effective at low doses with less side effects as compared to chemotherapy and radiotherapy. However, this ultimate goal of the molecular therapy is an area of active research. A molecule in medical science refers to the genes and proteins. They form the basic units of cells in the body and are responsible for all the activities of the cells including metabolism, cell division, and cell death. Target therapy involves identification of targets—faulty molecule (gene/protein) in a malignancy and specifically blocking it to halt the progression of the disease. Such targets are termed as biomarkers. They also help in risk assessment, screening and at times in reaching to diagnosis. Moreover, the biomarkers can predict the efficacy of a drug, monitor the response, and prognosticate the disease behavior.

CELL PATHWAYS

The drugs available for cancer are directed toward halting the uncontrolled cell division. Hence, it becomes prudent to understand the cell signaling pathways or transduction pathways in order to design molecular therapy. The cells can release substances (hormones or growth factors which are mainly proteins) that affect the activity of other cells. These substances bind to the receptors present on the cell surface, which in turn brings about a metabolic change, like release of another protein inside the cell or phosphorylation of an intracellular component of the receptor. The changes are reflected in the activity of the nucleic acids and gene expression. These cellular pathways are responsible for cell division and growth.

CLASSES OF TARGETED THERAPY

Three main categories of target therapy have been described.

1. *Monoclonal antibodies*[1]: They are proteins designed in a way to attach to a specific substance (often protein) on the surface of cancer cells, thus blocking the signals for cell division. They are large Y-shaped molecules and usually cannot penetrate the cell membrane. The monoclonal antibodies are developed by injecting animals (usually mice) with a specific antigen. The spleen cells of the animals are collected and fused with myeloma cells which can replicate indefinitely. They are called hybridoma cells. Antibodies produced by them are checked for their activity against the antigen. The cells producing antibodies with desirable properties are isolated and used for monoclonal antibody production **(Fig. 1)**. The monoclonal antibodies produced by animals can produce undesirable reactions in humans such as rashes, joint swelling, anaphylaxis, and even death. One strategy to avoid such adverse effects is to chimerize the antigen-binding portion of the mouse antibody with other parts of the human antibody.[2] Another method to further reduce the chances of reaction is to humanize the antibody. Principle of genetic engineering is used to replace more than 90% of the molecule with human portions. This is called as humanized monoclonal antibody. They are well-tolerated and produce minimal reaction episodes. Most antibodies should be infused only after premedication with antiallergic drugs **(Fig. 2)**.

    Monoclonal antibodies have two names: a proprietary name owned by the manufacturer and a nonproprietary name assigned by World Health Organization (WHO). The nonproprietary names of all antibodies end in "-mab." The other suffices have been enumerated below.
    - Humanized monoclonal antibody: -zumab (example—trastuzumab)
    - Chimeric monoclonal antibody: -ximab (example—rituximab)
    - Mouse monoclonal antibody: - momab
    - Human monoclonal antibody: - mumab

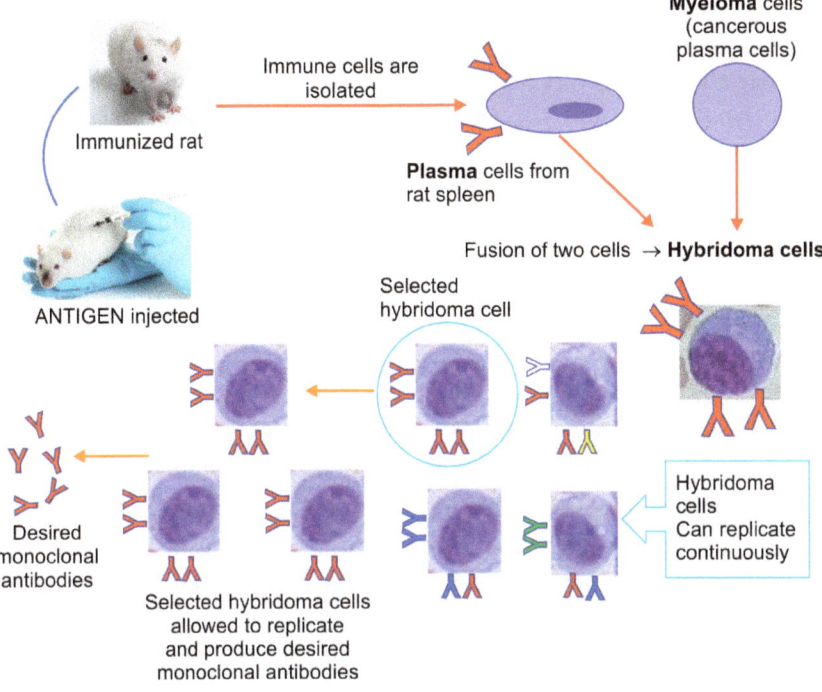

Fig. 1: Production of monoclonal antibodies.

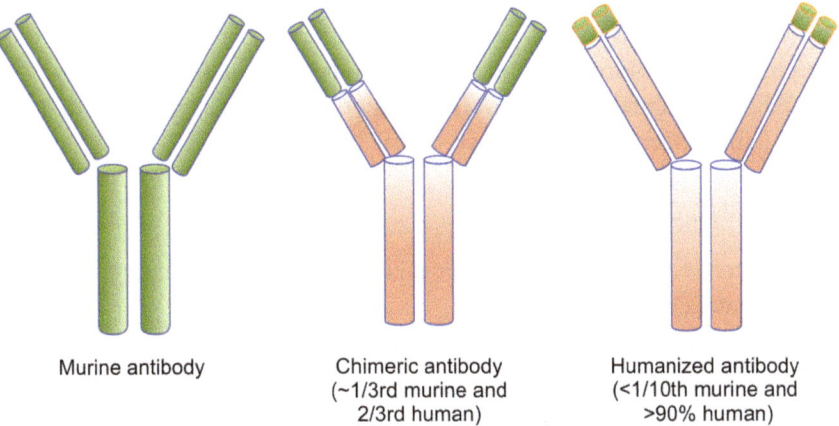

Fig. 2: Monoclonal antibodies—chimeric and humanized antibodies.

These antibodies can also be attached to specific substances that can kill cells. They are called as conjugated monoclonal antibodies. They can be:
– Radiolabeled (conjugated to radioactive particles)
– Chemolabeled (attached to chemotoxic agents)
– Immunotoxins (tagged with cell toxins)

Currently, the use of conjugated or tagged antibodies in cancer therapy is an area of active research.

2. *Small molecule inhibitors*: Small molecule inhibitors are manufactured in laboratories using chemicals, unlike antibodies which are bioengineered. They are relatively less costly and usually come as oral preparations. They are small in size and can enter the cells easily. They are detoxified by the liver and can produce drug interactions. The half-life is small and hence need to be administered on a daily basis, unlike antibodies which need to be given weekly or monthly. These molecules act by inhibiting "kinases," proteins which are responsible for transferring phosphate groups inside the cells. Tyrosine kinase is an important target for most of the molecule inhibitors available currently. Many growth receptors have an internal tyrosine kinase domain. It gets activated on binding of a growth factor and initiates a cascade of events resulting in gene expression and cell division. The names of small molecule inhibitors usually end in "ib" (example—imatinib). The drugs that inhibit the immune system end in "imus" (example—everolimus).

3. *Vaccines*: The immune system does not get activated against cancer cells as it does against an infective agent. Reasons being, immunity is suppressed by tumor growth. Moreover, cancer cells are not readily recognized as foreign substance by the plasma cells. Vaccines act as biological response modifiers. Two types of vaccines are known: prophylactic and therapeutic. Most of them in use presently are for cancer prevention. They target infections that are known to promote the development of malignancy. Hepatitis B virus (HBV) vaccine is very effective in preventing HBV infection. This in turn prevents chronic hepatitis, which is a proven risk factor for the development of hepatocellular carcinoma (HCC). Therapeutic use of vaccines in order to fight cancer cells is still a part of research protocol.

TARGETING CANCER CELLS

The cancer cells possess some typical characteristics that distinguish them from normal cells:

- Sustained growth signals and insensitivity to inhibitory signals
- Ability to evade programmed cell death and replicate indefinitely
- Angiogenesis to maintain sustained blood supply
- Ability to invade tissue and disseminate/metastasize as well evade immune system

These characteristics form the target for the molecular therapy. The most commonly employed targets include blocking the growth factor receptors or their effective enzymes (kinases). Other strategy to control the growth of cancers is by inhibiting the angiogenesis. Tumor cells evade apoptosis through p53 gene mutation. This produces growth factors that activate an enzyme called, PI3K. Inhibition of this kinase can prevent tumor growth.

Targeting Growth Factors and Their Receptors

Epidermal Growth Factor Receptor

Epidermal growth factor receptor (EGFR) is a cell surface receptor present in many organs such as intestine, skin, kidneys, and breast. It has an external domain which binds to specific ligands from the epidermal growth factor (EGF) family. This activates the intracellular tyrosine kinase domain, thus initiating the downstream signals of rat sarcoma (Ras)/mitogen-activated protein kinase (MAPK/MEK)/rapidly accelerated fibrosarcoma (Raf)/protein kinase B (Akt)/ mechanistic target of rapamycin (mTOR) pathway. This eventually results in DNA synthesis and cell division. Four types of EGFR have been described in literature: HER-1 (also known as EGFR), HER-2, HER-3, and HER-4. At present, HER-1 and HER-2 form the targets of molecular therapy **(Figs. 3A and B)**.

Targeting EGFR (HER-1)[3,4]

Overexpression of HER-1 has been shown in nearly one-third of GI cancers. It is associated with aggressive histology and poor prognosis. The receptor can be blocked at the extracellular domain by monoclonal antibodies (cetuximab/panitumumab) or at the intracellular tyrosine kinase domain by TKIs (tyrosine kinase inhibitors, example—erlotinib/gefitinib). The efficacy of TKIs is limited in GI malignancy.

Targeting HER-2

HER-2 overexpression has been associated with poor survival in GI malignancies. A recombinant monoclonal antibody, trastuzumab selectively blocks the extracellular domain of HER-2. It has also shown antibody-dependent cellular toxicity in few studies.[5] A dual TKI, lapatinib, has been developed, which inhibits both HER-2 and EGFR. It is being evaluated for its efficacy in GI cancers.[6]

Angiogenesis Inhibitors

Vascular endothelial growth factor (VEGF) is a protein that binds to vascular endothelial growth factor receptor (VEGFR) on the cell surface and stimulates angiogenesis (endothelial proliferation). Uncontrolled neovascularization is an important step in tumor growth and dissemination in majority of the solid tumors. This makes the VEGF pathway a vital target for molecular therapy.

Expression of VEGF is associated with poor prognosis (increased tumor vascularity and early metastasis). Alike EGFR pathways, VEGF pathway can be blocked at various levels[7]:
- Neutralizing antibodies to VEGF (bevacizumab)
- Antibodies that bind to the extracellular part of the receptor (ramucirumab)
- TKIs to inhibit the intracellular domains (sunitinib/sorafenib/cediranib/apatinib)

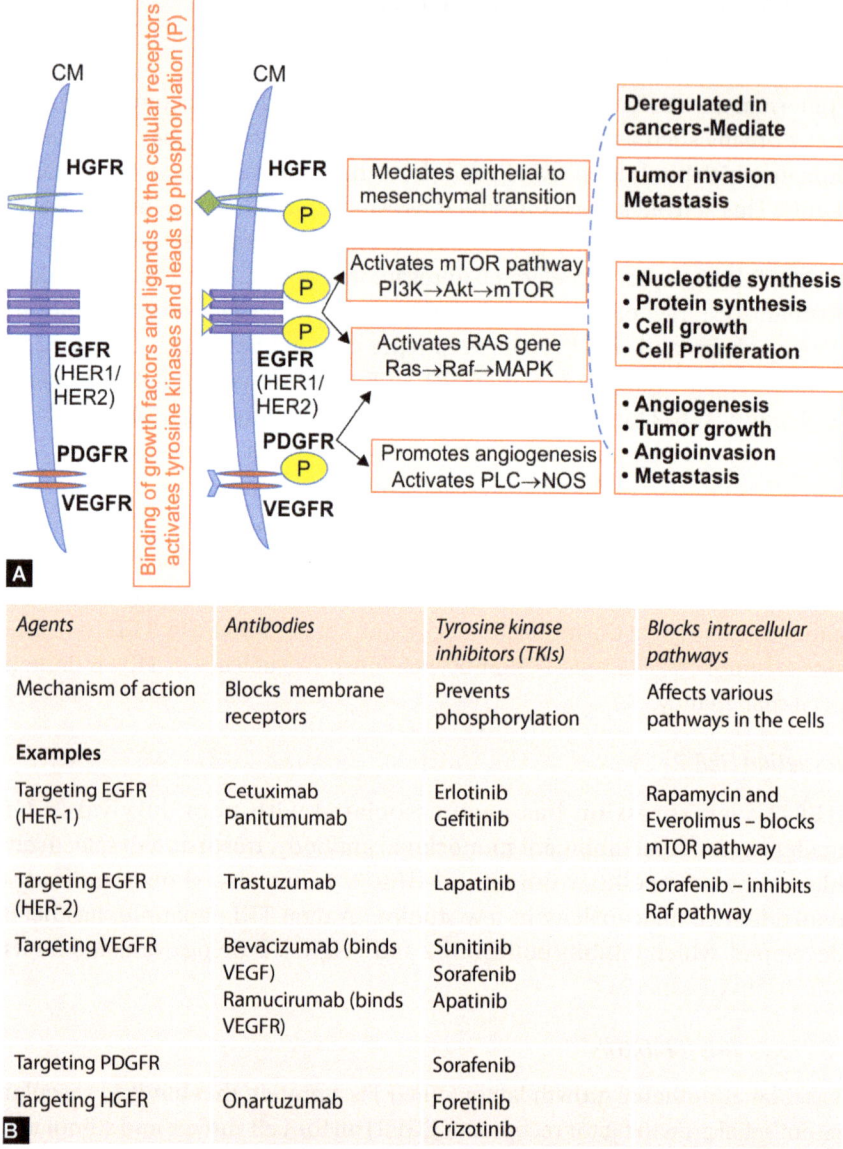

Figs. 3A and B: (A) Schematic diagram of signaling pathways crucial for cell proliferation and role in carcinogenesis when deregulated; (B) Molecular targets in cell pathway with mechanism of action. (Akt: protein kinase B; CM: cell membrane; EGFR: epidermal growth factor receptor; HGFR: hepatocyte growth factor receptor; HER: human epidermal growth factor receptor; MAPK: mitogen activated protein kinase; mTOR: mechanistic target of rapamycin; NOS: nitric oxide synthase; PDGFR: platelet derived growth factor receptor; PI3K: phosphoinositide 3-kinase; PLC: phospholipase C; Raf: rapidly accelerated fibrosarcoma; Ras: rat sarcoma; VEGFR: vasculoendothelial growth factor receptor)

Most of the VEGFR TKIs are multitargeted. Sorafenib also blocks the platelet-derived growth factor receptor (PDGFR) and other cell division pathways such as RAF/mitogen-activated protein kinase (MAPK/MEK)/extracellular-signal-regulated kinases (ERK) signaling pathways.[8]

Other Targeted Agents

PI3K-Akt-mTOR Pathway

The mTOR is activated by PI3K through Akt. It mediates signals responsible for cell division, cellular metabolism, and vasculogenesis. Its activity is triggered by receptors such as EGFRs and VEGFRs, and inhibited by intracellular factors [phosphatase and tensin homolog (PTEN)]. In a study by Yu et al., activated Akt was detected in >80% of the advanced gastric tumors in comparison to upregulation of just 30% of the upstream receptors.[9] Theoretically, targeting mTOR pathway should be more effective. Everolimus has been evaluated in a few trials.

Targeting Hepatocyte Growth Factor/MET[10]

The hepatocyte growth factor (HGF) binds to hepatocyte growth factor receptor (HGFR)/MET receptor and mediates the epithelial-to-mesenchymal transition (EMT). This transition is an important step during embryogenesis, as well as during tumor invasion and metastasis. Overexpression of MET has been documented in various tumors, but the prognostic value remains unclear. The agents developed to target this pathway include:
- Onartuzumab (anti-MET antibody) and rilotumumab (anti-HGF antibody)
- Foretinib and crizotinib (MET TKIs)

Targeting Gene Fusion

Developing techniques in gene sequencing have unveiled a variety of gene fusions which can promote cell division across different tumors. Chromosomal translocation of the NTRK gene family is associated with a variety of advanced solid tumors in children and adults. Larotrectinib is a potent inhibitor of tropomyosin receptor kinase (TRK). The final data from three randomised trials has led to a tissue agnostic approval for this drug to treat adult and pediatric patients with solid tumors that have a NTRK gene fusion and who have progressive systemic disease following treatment.[11]

Targeting Matrix Metalloproteins

The matrix metalloproteins (MMPs) are zinc-dependent endopeptidases that act to disintegrate the extracellular matrix. They are vital for tissue remodeling: angiogenesis, tissue repair, and morphogenesis. Unregulated expression of the

MMPs has been observed in several solid tumors and is linked with the potential to disseminate. Two drugs under evaluation are marimastat and prinostat.[12]

Challenges with Targeted Therapies

Targeted therapy has an array of limitations associated with it:

- *Compliance*: Though the side effects are low with these drugs, the compliance remains an issue. Factors that are responsible include: long duration of treatment, lack of motivation, cost of treatment associated with monoclonal antibodies, and complex regimens. New patient assist devices for drug delivery have the potential to improve compliance.[13]
- *Drug resistance*: Resistance tends to develop with all the drugs with time. The mechanism may include development of new mutations or presence of different mechanisms of tumor growth in the same person.
- *Determining optimal dose*: Dose determination with chemotherapeutic agents is easy as they produce side effects. Hence, upper safe limit can be calculated. Targeted therapy causes minimal side effects. No criterion exists to declare the dose as high. Many tumors do not shrink in size. Hence, the radiological response is also difficult to assess, though functional changes in the tumor based on nuclear scans can be helpful.
- Cost of the therapy and shortage of drugs remain an issue, especially when monoclonal antibodies are used.

ESOPHAGEAL CANCER

Worldwide, the most common variant of esophageal malignancy is squamous cell carcinoma (SCC). It is common in Asia and Africa, especially among low socioeconomic group of people. In the West, incidence of SCC is decreasing. Esophageal adenocarcinoma (EAC) is becoming commoner. The change has been attributed to greater incidence of reflux due to obesity and consumption of alcohol. Adenocarcinoma tends to arise from the metaplastic columnar epithelium in the lower esophagus (Barrett's esophagus). Molecular analysis often shows aneuploidy and p53 mutation in the area of metaplasia; long before frank neoplasia develops. Overexpression of HER2/neu gene has been documented in around 15% esophageal cancers. Wang et al. compared the genetic profile of SCC and EAC. Higher prevalence of HER2 and EGFR amplification, TGF-β signaling activation, and RAS/MEK/MAPK pathway activation was noted in EAC.[14] Adenocarcinoma esophagus is characterized by genomic instability and gross heterogeneity between patients. A systematic review including 12,749 patients documented increased incidence of serosal invasion, lymphatic and distant metastasis in association with HER2 positivity, which translated into poor survival as well.[15] Another systematic review by Chua et al.,[16] included 49 studies. More than two-thirds of them reported decreased overall survival (OS) with HER2 overexpression.

The mainstay of management of esophageal cancers at present remains multimodality therapy (surgery, chemotherapy, and radiotherapy). No molecular therapy has been approved by Food and Drug Administration (FDA) for clinical use in esophageal cancer, except for anti-HER2 drug, trastuzumab. It has been approved as a first-line therapy in HER2 positive advanced or metastatic EAC.[17] The OS has been shown to improve with the addition of trastuzumab to chemotherapy in metastatic setting. However, other HER2 targeted drugs have not yet shown a survival benefit, and studies are ongoing, especially in the adjuvant and neoadjuvant setting.[18,19] Other agents such as pertuzumab and afatinib are under evaluation in phase II and phase III clinical trials as a second-line therapy following trastuzumab-based regime.[20]

Nearly 17% of gastroesophageal cancer and esophageal malignancy have microsatellite instability (MSI). Immunotherapy with checkpoint inhibitors has shown promise in MSI-H tumors, including GE adenocarcinoma. The KEYNOTE-059 trial demonstrated survival benefit with anti-PD-1 monoclonal antibody pembrolizumab. It has been approved by FDA for use in programmed cell death-ligand 1 (PD-L1)-positive (>1%) advanced gastric cancer (AGC) or gastroesophageal junction (GEJ) adenocarcinoma.[21,22] A phase III study is currently underway to evaluate the benefit of combining pembrolizumab with first-line chemotherapy in neoadjuvant as well as adjuvant settings. Studies on genetic profiling and targeted therapy in esophageal cancers have demonstrated promising results, but needs further validation.

GASTRIC CANCER

Gastric cancer is the third most common cause of cancer-related death globally.[23] Over few decades, the incidence of gastric cancer has shown a decreasing trend in developed countries. This can be attributed to improved hygiene, good nutrition, and effective anti-*Helicobacter pylori* treatment. However, recently American cancer registry has documented a rise in noncardia malignancy among young white population (25–39 years).[24] Moreover, >50% new cases are registered in developing countries. This malignancy is a result of amalgamation of various factors: environmental and accumulation of genetic alterations.

Complete resection of the tumor remains the only chance for long-term survival. Sufficient data is available to establish the role of additional perioperative chemotherapy and adjuvant chemotherapy in improving the recurrence free and OS.[25,26] However, it is only in Japan that these tumors are diagnosed early and are amenable to cure with multimodality approach. This is possible due to intensive screening protocol in the country. In rest of the world, the patients often present in an advanced stage as the initial symptoms are nonspecific. This renders the disease inoperable at the offset. Conventional treatments (radiotherapy and chemotherapy) have shown a modest control on the disease progression in various studies. The overall median survival ranges from 6 to 11 months.[27] Combination chemotherapy [comprising 5-fluorouracil (or capecitabine) with a platinum compound (cisplatin) and/or docetaxel/epirubicin] is frequently used as the first-line regimen for AGC. This is often associated with considerable toxicities.[28] Use of radiotherapy in AGC is reserved for intractable pain or bleeding.

Lack of an effective treatment of AGC entails further research in understanding the molecular basis of carcinogenesis and development of targeted agents. In comparison to other solid tumors, gastric cancer follows a more complicated molecular and genetic pathway. However, clinical trials have shown that an addition of molecular-targeted therapy to the standard chemotherapy has favorable outcomes in patients with AGC. A phase III ToGA (Trastuzumab for Gastric Cancer) trial from South Korea[29] demonstrated significant benefit in OS with addition of trastuzumab to chemotherapy. Based on this practice changing study, trastuzumab was approved to be used as the first-line treatment in HER2-positive AGC and gastroesophageal cancer. In a recent study by Satoh et al.,[30] lapatinib in combination with paclitaxel as a second-line treatment of AGC produced a better overall response in comparison to paclitaxel alone, though the survival difference was not statistically significant (11 vs. 9 months). Ramucirumab (anti-VEGFR-2) is the first biological agent that has shown survival benefits as a single agent in advanced gastric or GEJ adenocarcinoma which has progressed post-first-line chemotherapy.[31] In AGC overexpressing HER2, addition of trastuzumab to platinum-based chemotherapy has become standard of care as front-line therapy. Trastuzumab deruxtecan (DS-8201) is an antibody-drug conjugate consisting of an anti-HER2 (human epidermal growth factor receptor 2) antibody, a cleavable tetrapeptide-based linker, and a cytotoxic topoisomerase I inhibitor. The drug has shown improved response rates as well as overall survival as compared to chemotherapy in patients with advanced HER2-positive gastric or gastroesophageal junction adenocarcinoma that had progressed after at least two previous therapies, including trastuzumab. Ramucirumab with paclitaxel for unselected population and pembrolizumab for MSI-H tumors are approved as second-line therapy in the West. In disease refractory to described regimens, apatinib, nivolumab, ramucirumab, and TAS-102 have demonstrated some benefit as single-agent therapy in terms of OS compared to placebo alone. Pembrolizumab is approved as a third-line agent in tumors expressing PD-L1. Drugs targeting the other pathways of cell division like PI3K/mTOR and HGF/MET are under phase I/II trial.

On the contrary, a Cochrane review analysis (2015) on the various targeted therapy alone or in combination with conventional chemotherapy failed to demonstrate a clear survival benefit in AGC. Even the subgroup analysis in the review could not establish the advantage of a particular agent (anti-VEGF/EGFR) as the first-line treatment. Possible benefits of targeted agents in HER2-positive AGC did not translate into better OS. Little information is available on any benefit in the quality of life with the use of these agents. There is definite evidence of increased adverse events in combination therapy. Majority of the studies were Phase II trials with limited number of patients with inconsistent outcomes. The level of evidence at present to support molecular therapy in AGC is modest. It needs further validation with well-constructed trials including large number of patients with predefined outcome measures.[32]

COLORECTAL AND SMALL BOWEL MALIGNANCY

Growing knowledge on genetic and protein changes at cellular level in colorectal cancer (CRC), have led to the significant development in the field of molecular therapy. Stage 1 and 2 disease is treated by surgery alone. Some stage 2 and all stage 3 disease are managed with surgery and chemotherapy/chemoradiotherapy. Currently, molecular targeted agents are recommended only in the treatment of stage 4 CRC or metastatic CRC. They can be used alone or in combination with other chemotherapeutic agents.

Use of EGFR inhibitor (panitumumab or cetuximab) is preferred in the management of left-sided tumors with wild-type KRAS or NRAS genes. Activating mutations in KRAS (mainly Exon-2) are detected in approximately 40% of metastatic colorectal cancers (mCRCs). In 2015, American Society of Clinical Oncology (ASCO) recommended that all patients eligible for anti-EGFR therapy should be tested for mutations in both KRAS and NRAS exon2. Presence of additional BRAF mutations, which is common in right colon and transverse colon cancer, may limit the effectiveness of EGFR inhibitors. Universal mismatch repair (MMR) or MSI testing is recommended in all colon cancers. They form an important guide to therapy decisions. Patients with stage II MSI-H tumors carry a good prognosis. The 5-fluorouracil-based chemotherapy would not be beneficial in these patients. Advanced tumors with dMMR (deficient MMR) and MSI-H (MSI-High) are likely to benefit from PD-1 inhibitors (nivolumab and pembrolizumab). In Checkmate 142 trial, nivolumab was found to provide durable disease control in patients with dMMR/MSI-H tumors who were pretreated for metastatic CRC (31% objective response and 3-month disease control in >69%). The benefit in these patients were observed regardless of BRAF/KRAS mutation or PD-L1 expression.[33,34]

The efficacy of EGFR inhibitors have been evaluated in well-conducted trials. Cetuximab in combination with FOLFIRI and FOLFOX-4 was assessed as first chemotherapy in mCRC in phase 3 CRYSTAL[35] and OPUS[36] study, respectively **(Table 1)**. The patients with wild-type KRAS demonstrated a significant improvement in response rates (57 vs. <40%) and progression free survival (PFS). The OS was also significantly more in CRYSTAL study in the cetuximab arm (24.9 vs. 21 months). The OS in OPUS study was also better with the addition of cetuximab (22.8 vs. 18.5 months), though the difference was not statistically significant. In contrast, two other studies, COIN trial[37] and NORDIC VII trial,[38] which evaluated cetuximab in addition to FOLFOX or

TABLE 1: Clinical Trials on Targeted Therapy in Advanced Colorectal Carcinoma (KRAS wild-type).

Serial no	Study	Year	Drugs/Therapy	Patients	PFS (months)	Median OS (months)
1	CRYSTAL trial[35]	2009	FOLFIRI + Cetuximab vs. FOLFIRI	172 vs. 176	9.9 vs. 8.7*	24.9 vs. 21*
2	OPUS trial[36]	2011	FOLFOX-4 + Cetuximab vs. FOLFOX	82 vs. 97	8.3 vs. 7.2*	22.8 vs. 18.5
3	COIN Trial[37]	2011	FOLFOX/ CapeOX + Cetuximab	362 vs. 367	8.6 vs. 8.6	17 vs. 17.9
4	NORDIC VII trial[38]	2012	FLOX + Cetuximab vs. FLOX	97 vs. 97	7.9 vs. 8.7	20.1 vs. 22
5	PRIME trial[39]	2010	FOLFOX-4 + Panitumumab vs. FOLFOX-4	325 vs. 331	9.6 vs. 8*	23.9 vs. 19.7
6	PEAK trial[40]	2014	Panitumumab vs. Bevacizumab with FOLFOX	142 vs. 143	10.9 vs. 10.1	34.2 vs. 24.3*
7	FIRE-3 trial[41]	2014	Cetuximab vs. Bevacizumab with FOLFIRI	297 vs. 295	10 vs. 10.3	28.7 vs. 25*
8	CALGB/ SWOG 80405 trial[42]	2014	Cetuximab vs. Bevacizumab with FOLFOX or FOLFIRI	578 vs. 559	10.4 vs. 10.8	29.9 vs. 29

(OS: overall survival; PFS: progression free survival)
*Clinically significant

CapeOX) as a first line of management in mCRC, did not show any difference in the PFS and OS.[39]

Three other randomized control trials (PEAK, FIRE-3, and CALGB/SWOG 80405) compared anti-EGFR agent with bevacizumab-containing chemotherapy regimen as first line of management in KRAS wild-type mCRC patients (*see* **Table 1**). The phase II PEAK study[40] used panitumumab in addition to FOLFOX and FIRE-3[41] used cetuximab in addition to FOLFIRI. Although the PFS and response rates were similar, the OS was better in anti-EGFR arm as compared to bevacizumab arm in both the studies (34.2 vs. 24.3 months and 28.4 vs. 25 months, respectively). The CALGB/SWOG 80405 study[42] compared cetuximab and bevacizumab along with cytotoxic chemotherapy (FOLFOX or FOLFIRI). Though the response rate was significantly higher in the cetuximab arm (65.6 vs. 57.2%, $P = 0.02$), the authors could not demonstrate a significant difference in PFS or OS. Although anti-EGFR-based regimen as a first-line therapy has a favorable trend in comparison to anti-VEGF-based regimen, the treatment strategy in RAS wild-type mCRC remains controversial. In patients with mutated KRAS, the efficacy of bevacizumab or cetuximab in addition to chemotoxic drugs could not demonstrate any substantial survival benefit.[41,43]

The efficacy of cetuximab and panitumumab alone or in combination has been evaluated as second-line therapy for mCRC in various trials. The results are variable with minimal improvement in OS in some studies. Recently, new agents have been evaluated for the use in mCRC [tyrosine kinase inhibitors—gefitinib/erlotinib and monoclonal antibody against insulin-like growth factor (IGF) receptor—ganitumab] with no demonstrable benefit.[44,45] However, a recently published randomized BEACON trial which included 665 patients with *BRAF* V600E-mutated mCRC with progressive disease on one or two previous regimens, demonstrated substantial benefit with combination therapy. The triple therapy including encorafenib, cetuximab, and binimetinib resulted in significantly longer OS (9 vs. 5.4 months) and better response rate than standard therapy.[46]

Small intestinal malignancy has molecular characteristics which resemble both CRC and gastric adenocarcinoma. The use of targeted therapy in small bowel adenocarcinoma (SBA) is limited to case reports. At present, the principles of CRC are followed for this entity. Further studies are desirable to establish unique molecular signatures of SBA.

HEPATOCELLULAR CARCINOMA

Hepatocellular carcinoma is the most common primary liver malignancy. It usually develops in diseased cirrhotic liver. The most common risk factors are chronic infection with HBV and hepatitis C virus (HCV). Other factors include regular alcohol consumption, obesity syndrome leading to nonalcoholic steatohepatitis (NASH), and various toxins. The lack of standard screening protocols and absence of symptoms in the early HCC leads to late presentation in majority of patients. This abrogates the application of any curative strategy (resection, transplantation, or ablation of the tumor). Poor hepatic reserve in these patients and chemorefractory nature of HCC due to overexpression of multidrug resistant genes such as MDRI precludes the routine use of systemic chemotoxic drugs.[47] This makes the application of targeted therapy prudent in advanced HCC (Child Pugh A and B).

Predominant mechanisms described in pathogenesis of HCC include cirrhosis (tissue damage) and oncogene or tumor suppressor gene mutations. Both affect the cell signaling pathways. Liver has an inherent property to regenerate. Adult hepatocytes are able to upregulate the production of the growth factors transiently in chronic parenchymal damage. In the setting of altered cell signaling, the growth becomes uninhibited. The signaling pathways associated with HCC include VEGFR, EGFR, and mTOR. Hepatocellular carcinoma is a vascular tumor and VEGF is the prime mediator for

TABLE 2: Clinical trials on targeted therapy in advanced hepatocellular carcinoma.

Serial no.	Study	Year	Drugs/Therapy	Patients	PFS (months)	Median OS (months)
1	Abou- Alfa et al.[50]	2006	Sorafenib	137	–	9.2
2.	SHARP[51] trial	2008	Sorafenib vs. Placebo	602 (299 vs. 303)	5.5 vs. 2.8	10.7 vs. 7.9
3	START trial[53]	2015	Sorafenib + TACE	50	13	3 years OS 86%
4	Abou- Alfa et al.[56]	2010	Sorafenib + Doxorubicin vs. Doxorubicin	96	6.4 vs. 2.8	13.7 vs. 6.5

(OS: overall survival; PFS: progression free survival; TACE: transarterial chemoembolization)

angiogenesis.[48] Drugs targeting VEGFR pathway (sorafenib and bevacizumab) are primarily investigated for advanced HCC **(Table 2)**.

Sorafenib is an oral multikinase inhibitor. It inhibits VEGFR-2, VEGFR-3, and PDGFR.[49] It inhibits neovascularization as well as induces tumor cell apoptosis. Abou-Alfa et al. in his study on 137 patients with advanced HCC demonstrated high pretreatment levels of pERK (phosphorylated extracellular regulated kinase) correlated with better response to sorafenib.[50] Two subsequent trials established the role of sorafenib in advanced HCC. The Sorafenib Hepatocellular Carcinoma Assessment Randomized Protocol (SHARP) trial compared the effect of sorafenib against a placebo in advanced HCC. The study was stopped prematurely as the survival benefit of sorafenib was much better than placebo.[51] Another study from Asia demonstrated better survival with sorafenib in advanced HCC.[52] In both the studies, majority of the patients were Child A or early Child B. The benefit of sorafenib in patients with severely deranged liver function is not clear. The recommended daily dose is 800 mg. Median duration of administration is 6 months. Common side effects include diarrhea, hand foot disease, weight loss, and anorexia.[53] Other drugs which have been evaluated for use in advanced HCC are bevacizumab, sunitinib, ABT-869 (antityrosine kinase), and rapamycin (mTOR inhibitor). The study groups are too small to establish a definite role of these agents alone or in combination. In recently published randomized trials, nivolumab and lenvatinib demonstrated better OS (though not statistically significant) and safety profile as compared to sorafenib when used as first-line therapy in advanced HCC.[54-56]

GASTROINTESTINAL CARCINOID TUMORS

Carcinoids are derived from the neuroendocrine (NE) cells. The substances (hormones) secreted by the tumor, and responsible for the symptoms include serotonin, corticotrophin, histamine, neurotensin, and dopamine. Localized tumors are amenable to surgical resection and cure. Metastatic disease in liver with symptoms can also be managed effectively by surgery. Chemotherapy has limited success rate in the management of carcinoids. In symptomatic patients, not suitable for surgical intervention, somatostatin analogs (octreotide, lanreotide, and pasireotide) are used to block the hormonal receptors and relieve symptoms. Radiolabeled (Indium-111/Yttrium-90 labeled) analogs and peptide receptor nucleotide therapy (PRRT) using Lu-177-Dotatate have produced encouraging symptomatic and radiologic response with few renal and hematological toxicities.[57]

The genetic changes in sporadic carcinoids are complex. The pattern of gain or loss of nucleic acids on the chromosomes is difficult to understand. However, all these mutations lead to the alteration in cell signaling pathways. Promising novel-targeted therapy in the carcinoids includes:

- VEGF inhibitors (bevacizumab) multikinase inhibitors (sunitinib and sorafenib)
- mTOR inhibitors (everolimus)

In a study by Yao et al. (2008) on advanced symptomatic carcinoids on octreotide therapy, addition of bevacizumab was associated with a PFS of 95% at 18 weeks in comparison to 68% in interferon group.[58] The mTOR inhibitor, everolimus, has been approved by FDA for use in metastatic carcinoids. Few trials (RADIANT-4) have shown good response rate with everolimus in addition to the somatostatin analogs.[59] Further understanding of the signaling pathways and development of new novel agents remains an area for research.

GASTROINTESTINAL STROMAL TUMORS

Gastrointestinal stromal tumor (GIST) is the most frequently (18% of all) occurring sarcoma in humans. It comprises 1% of all intestinal neoplasm. Historically, GISTs projected a poor prognosis. More than 50% of the tumors used to recur even after complete resection. The median survival in metastatic disease remained ~9 months as it is constitutionally resistant to chemoradiotherapy.[60] The discovery of gain of function mutation in the tyrosine kinase KIT gene by Hirota et al. was a path changer in the management of GISTs.[61] This association was validated in subsequent studies. Nearly three-fourths of the GISTs harbor a KIT mutation, most commonly in the juxtamembrane domain (Exon 11). Other infrequent mutations occur in extracellular domains (Exon 9 and rarely Exon 8) or the kinase domains (Exon 13 and 17). Of the KIT negative tumors, ~10% possess PDGFRA mutation. It also induces cell proliferation by activation of tyrosine kinase receptors. PDGFRA and KIT mutations do not occur in synchrony in GISTs. The tumors which are KIT and PDGFRA negative are termed as wild-type GISTs (WT-GIST). The common mutations detected in such tumors include BRAF and succinate dehydrogenase (SDH) mutations, which induce cell growth independent of KIT.

Targeting Tyrosine Kinase Pathway in GISTs (Table 3)

The unique characteristics of the non-WT-GISTs as described make them highly susceptible to TKIs. Presently, GISTs form an excellent example of application of targeted therapy in malignancy, both in perioperative and metastatic setting. The disease control in metastatic KIT-positive GISTs is exemplary with the use of imatinib (400 mg/800 mg daily). It has become the first line of treatment in metastatic GISTs. Currently, median OS reported in various studies ranges from 3 to 5 years as opposed to 9 months in the past, with nearly 20% 10-year survival.[62-65] Although majority respond well to imatinib, 50% develop resistance and present with progression of disease at 2 years. The recommendations for the management of resistance include: dose escalation of imatinib from 400 mg/day to 800 mg/day and use of other rescue TKIs (sunitinib, regorafenib and ripretinib).[66,67]

Imatinib as an adjuvant to surgical resection is an established practice. The trial published by American College of Surgeons in 2009 demonstrated significant improvement in recurrence free survival (RFS) (98 vs. 83% at 1 year) following 1 year of adjuvant, imatinib. A recent study by Joensuu et al. demonstrated greater benefit with 3 years of adjuvant therapy as compared to 1 year of treatment (RFS 66 vs. 48% and OS 92% vs. 81.7% at 5 years).[68,69] In borderline resectable or locally advanced tumors, neoadjuvant imatinib has shown promising results. RTOG (Radiation Therapy Oncology Group) 0132 trial[70] was the first of its kind to demonstrate the feasibility of neoadjuvant treatment (600 mg/day for 8-12 weeks) with imatinib. The response was assessed by RECIST criteria. The R0 resection in the patients was as high as 68%. Tirumani et al.[71] later reported that maximum benefit with neoadjuvant imatinib could be achieved between 28 and 34 weeks. The success of preoperative targeted therapy has helped in achieving R0 resection, application for minimal invasive techniques for curative resection, and organ preservation. The research is ongoing for the optimal dose and timing of surgery.

PANCREATIC CARCINOMA

The prognosis of pancreatic cancer remains poor, both because of late presentation and aggressive nature of the disease. Identification of specific molecular markers can help in early diagnosis in high-risk population as well as act as a guide to targeted therapy. 12 core signaling pathways have been linked to the development of pancreatic cancer, but none could be linked to a specific genetic mutation. Instead, it has been associated with post-transcriptional genetic changes involving micro-RNAs and RNA-binding proteins (RBP), essential for survival and growth of pancreatic cancer cells. HuR is an RBP, which has been found to downregulate or upregulate mRNA expressions which promote tumorigenesis. It increases the protein levels of angiogenic factors such as VEGF. Though high expression of HuR is associated

TABLE 3: Clinical trials on targeted therapy in gastrointestinal stromal tumors.

Serial no	Study	Year	Drugs/Therapy	Patients	PFS/RFS	OS	Conclusion
1.	SWOG S0033 trial[63]	2008	Imatinib in metastatic GISTs (400 mg vs. 800 mg/day)	746	2 years PFS (41 vs. 46%)	2 years OS (76 vs. 72%)	Initial dose should be 400 mg with escalation on disease progression
2.	Meta-analysis[64]	2010	Imatinib in metastatic GIST (400 mg vs. 800 mg/day)	1640	1.58 vs. 1.95 years (PFS)	4.08 vs. 4.05 years	Toxicity is dose dependent, so 400 mg should remain the standard starting dose. Only exception may be KIT exon 9 mutations
3.	Demetri et al.[67]	2006	Sunitinib vs. Placebo in metastatic GIST (second-line)	312	PFS—24.1 vs. 6 weeks ($p <0.001$)	Significantly better in sunitinib ($p <0.007$)	Significant disease control and better survival with sunitinib on failure with imatinib therapy
4.	ACOSOG Z9001 trial[68]	2014	Imatinib (400 mg for 1 year) vs. placebo as adjuvant	713	1 year RFS 98 vs. 83% ($p <0.001$)	1 year OS (99 vs. 99%)	Imatinib as adjuvant for one year in KIT exon 11 mutation has a longer RFS and is safe.
5.	SSG XVIII/AIO trial[69]	2012	Imatinib as adjuvant (1 year Vs 3 years 400 mg/day)	400	RFS at 5 years—48 vs. 66%	OS at 5 years—82 vs. 92%	Imatinib as adjuvant therapy should be continued for 3 years

(OS: overall survival; PFS: progression free survival; RFS: recurrence free survival) with worse pathologic prognosis (higher stage at diagnosis), it correlates with powerful response to gemcitabine therapy.[72,73] EGFR overexpression has been documented in 9–65% of the pancreatic tumors in various series. IGFR-1 receptor has also been associated with pancreatic malignancy and resistance to anti-EGFR therapy. Hence, combination therapy to block EGFR and IGF appears a viable option. New drugs targeting stem cells and DNA repair mechanisms (olaparib, a polyadenosine diphosphate-ribose polymerase inhibitor) in familial pancreatic cancer are being investigated.[74]

BILIARY TRACT CANCER

Biliary tract cancers, especially gallbladder carcinoma (GBC), are an aggressive disease and carry poor prognosis. Advanced stage portends an average survival of <6 months. Poor knowledge about the molecular pathogenesis of the malignancy has held the development of effective molecular therapy. Somatic mutations of KRAS (20%), p53 (44%), and PIK3CA are frequently reported in cholangiocarcinoma. Activating mutations in PIK3CA (13%) and hedgehog pathway (>70%) are being documented in patients with GBC. Hence, the therapeutic target potentials remain the RAS/RAF pathway and PI3K/AKT/MTOR pathway. Oral TKI, erlotinib, has been reported to show some benefit in advanced biliary tract cancer. Out of 42 patients in the series, 57% received erlotinib (150 mg/day). Partial response was seen in three and stable disease was present in seven at the end of 6 months.[75] Bevacizumab in combination with erlotinib has been investigated in advanced cholangiocarcinoma. It could achieve partial response in 12% and stable disease in >50% patients with median OS of 9.9 months.[76] EGFR inhibitors (cetuximab or panitumumab) alone or in combination with the chemotherapy have failed to demonstrate any survival benefit. Hedgehog pathway modifiers have shown decrease in tumor load in mouse models.[77] It needs further validation in humans and forms an important target in GBC. A recent addition to the armamentarium in the management of advanced cholangiocarcinoma are two targeted drugs: pemigatinib for FGFR2 fusions or rearrangements and Ivosidenib for IDH1 mutations.[78,79]

CONCLUSION

Personalized treatment is the most promising aspect of cure for malignancies. It is directed toward providing the best treatment in accordance with signs, symptoms, performance status, tumor morphology, and the molecular characteristics. Newer techniques that enable complete DNA sequencing can help in identification of the specific mutations. Every tumor though looking similar have unique molecular signature. Predicting the markers with accuracy can help to optimize therapy in both perioperative and metastatic setting. Presently, the targeted therapy is mainly used as salvage therapy in advanced diseases as far as the GI tumors are concerned, except for GISTs. Establishing the optimum dose and duration of therapy is an area of active research. Trend is toward companion diagnostics, i.e., identification of the patients who are likely to benefit maximum from a particular drug without serious adverse events. Ongoing research and trials in the field is expected to design regimens which will be effective as well as safe for use.

REFERENCES

1. Gerber DE. Targeted therapies: a new generation of cancer treatments. Am Fam Physician. 2008;77(3):311-9.
2. Naraev BG, Strosberg JR, Halfdanarson TR. Current status and perspectives of targeted therapy in well differentiated neuroendocrine tumors. Oncology. 2012;83(3):117-27.
3. Ilson DH, Kelsen D, Shah M, Schwartz G, Levine DA, Boyd J, et al. A phase 2 trial of erlotinib in patients with previously treated squamous cell and adenocarcinoma of the esophagus. Cancer. 2011;117(7):1409-14.
4. Kim JG. Molecular targeted therapy for advanced gastric cancer. Korean J Intern Med. 2013;28(2):149-55.
5. Spector NL, Blackwell KL. Understanding the mechanisms behind trastuzumab therapy for human epidermal growth factor receptor 2-positive breast cancer. J Clin Oncol. 2009;27(34):5838-47.
6. Iqbal S, Goldman B, Fenoglio-Preiser CM, Lenz HJ, Zhang W, Danenberg KD, et al. Southwest Oncology Group study S0413:a phase II trial of lapatinib (GW572016) as first-line therapy in patients with advanced or metastatic gastric cancer. Ann Oncol. 2011;22(12):2610-5.
7. Lieto E, Ferraraccio F, Orditura M, Castellano P, La Mura A, Pinto M, et al. Expression of vascular endothelial growth factor (VEGF) and epidermal growth factor receptor (EGFR) is an independent prognostic indicator of worse outcome in gastric cancer patients. Ann Surg Oncol. 2008;15(1):69-79.
8. Wilhelm SM, Adnane L, Newell P, Villanueva A, Llovet JM, Lynch M, et al. Preclinical overview of sorafenib, a multikinase inhibitor that targets both Raf and VEGF and PDGF receptor tyrosine kinase signaling. Mol Cancer Ther. 2008;7(10):3129-40.
9. Yu G, Wang J, Chen Y, Wang X, Pan J, Li G, et al. Overexpression of phosphorylated mammalian target of rapamycin predicts lymph node metastasis and prognosis of Chinese patients with gastric cancer. Clin Cancer Res. 2009;15(5):1821-9.
10. Graziano F, Galluccio N, Lorenzini P, Ruzzo A, Canestrari E, D'Emidio S, et al. Genetic activation of the MET pathway and prognosis of patients with high-risk, radically resected gastric cancer. J Clin Oncol. 2011;29(36):4789-95.
11. Ricciuti B, Genova C, Crino L, Libra M, Leonardi GC. Antitumor activity of Larotrectinib in tumor harboring NTRK gene fusions: a short review. Onco Targets Ther. 2019;12:1371-9.
12. Bramhall SR, Hallissey MT, Whiting J, Scholefield J, Tierney G, Stuart RC, et al. Marimastat as maintenance therapy for patients with advanced gastric cancer: a randomised trial. Br J Cancer. 2002;86(12):1864-70.
13. National Institute for Health and Clinical Excellence. Medicines adherence: involving patients in decisions about prescribed medicines and supporting adherence. NICE guideline (CG76). 2009.
14. Wang K, Johnson A, Ali SM, Klempner SJ, Bekaii-Saab T, Vacirca JL, et al. Comprehensive genomic profiling of advanced esophageal squamous cell carcinomas and esophageal adenocarcinomas reveals similarities and differences. Oncologist. 2015;20(10):1132-9.
15. Jørgensen JT, Hersom M. HER2 as a prognostic marker in gastric cancer—a systematic analysis of data from the literature. J Cancer. 2012;3:137-44.
16. Chua TC, Merrett ND. Clinicopathologic factors associated with HER2-positive gastric cancer and its impact on survival outcomes—a systematic review. Int J Cancer. 2012;130(12):2845-56.

17. Nagaraja V, Eslick GD. HER2 expression in gastric and oesophageal cancer: a meta-analytic review. J Gastrointest Oncol. 2015;6(2):143-54.
18. Thuss-Patience PC, Shah MA, Ohtsu A, Van Cutsem E, Ajani JA, Castro H, et al. Trastuzumab emtansine versus taxane use for previously treated HER2-positive locally advanced or metastatic gastric or gastro-oesophageal junction adenocarcinoma (GATSBY): an international randomised, open-label, adaptive, phase 2/3 study. Lancet Oncol. 2017;18(5):640-53.
19. Hecht JR, Bang YJ, Qin SK, Chung HC, Xu JM, Park JO, et al. Lapatinib in combination with capecitabine plus oxaliplatin in human epidermal growth factor receptor 2-positive advanced or metastatic gastric, esophageal, or gastroesophageal adenocarcinoma: TRIO-013/LOGiC—a randomized phase III trial. J Clin Oncol. 2016;34(5):443-51.
20. Tabernero J, Hof PM, Shen L, Ohtsu A, Shah MA, Cheng K, et al. 616OPertuzumab (P)+ trastuzumab (H)+ chemotherapy (CT) for HER2-positive metastatic gastric or gastrooesophageal junction cancer (mGC/GEJC): final analysis of a Phase III study (JACOB). Ann Oncol. 2017;28(5):v209-68.
21. Fuchs CS, Doi T, Jang RWJ, Muro K, Satoh T, Machado M, et al. KEYNOTE-059 cohort 1: efficacy and safety of pembrolizumab (pembro) monotherapy in patients with previously treated advanced gastric cancer. J Clin Oncol. 2017;35(15):4003-3.
22. Wainberg ZA, Jalal S, Muro K, Yoon HH, Garrido M, Golan T, et al. LBA28_PRKEYNOTE-059 Update: efficacy and safety of pembrolizumab alone or in combination with chemotherapy in patients with advanced gastric or gastroesophageal (G/GEJ) cancer. Ann Oncol. 2017;28(5):mdx440.020
23. Ferlay J, Soerjomataram I, Dikshit R, Eser S, Mathers C, Rebelo M, et al. Cancer incidence and mortality worldwide: sources, methods and major patterns in GLOBOCAN 2012. Int J Cancer. 2015;136(5):E359-86.
24. Anderson WF, Camargo MC, Fraumeni JF, Correa P, Rosenberg PS, Rabkin CS. Age-specific trends in incidence of noncardia gastric cancer in US adults. JAMA. 2010;303(17):1723-28.
25. Waddell T, Verheij M, Allum W, Cunningham D, Cervantes A, Arnold D, et al. Gastric cancer: ESMO-ESSO-ESTRO Clinical Practice Guidelines for diagnosis, treatment and follow-up. Ann Oncol. 2013;24(6):57-63.
26. Cunningham D, Allum WH, Stenning SP, Thompson JN, Van de Velde CJH, Nicolson M, et al. Perioperative chemotherapy versus surgery alone for resectable gastroesophageal cancer. N Engl J Med. 2006;355(1):11-20.
27. Wagner AD, Unverzagt S, Grothe W, Kleber G, Grothey A, Haerting J, et al. Chemotherapy for advanced gastric cancer. Cochrane Database Syst Rev. 2010;(3):CD004064.
28. Price TJ, Shapiro JD, Segelov E, Karapetis CS, Pavlakis N, Van Cutsem E, et al. Management of advanced gastric cancer. Expert Rev Gastroenterol Hepatol. 2012;6(2):199-208.
29. Bang YJ, Cutsem E, Feyereislova A, Chung HC, Shen L, Sawaki A, et al. Trastuzumab in combination with chemotherapy versus chemotherapy alone for treatment of HER2-positive advanced gastric or gastro-oesophageal junction cancer (ToGA): a phase 3, open-label, randomised controlled trial. Lancet. 2010;376(9742):687-97.
30. Satoh T, Doi T, Ohtsu A, Sun GP, Doi T, Xu JM, et al. Lapatinib plus paclitaxel versus paclitaxel alone in the second-line treatment of HER2-amplified advanced gastric cancer in Asian populations: TyTAN - A randomized, phase III study. J Clin Oncol. 2014;32(19):2039-49.
31. Fuchs CS, Tomasek J, Yong CJ, Dumitru F, Passalacqua R, Goswami C, et al. Ramucirumab monotherapy for previously treated advanced gastric or gastro-oesophageal junction adenocarcinoma (REGARD): an international, randomised, multicentre, placebo-controlled, phase 3 trial. Lancet. 2014;383(9911):P31-9.
32. Song H, Zhu J, Lu D. Molecular-targeted first-line therapy for advanced gastric cancer. Cochrane Database Syst Rev. 2016;7(7):CD011461.
33. Benedix F, Kube R, Meyer F, Schmidt U, Gastinger I, Lippert H, et al. Colon/Rectum Carcinomas (Primary Tumor) Study Group. Comparison of 17,641 patients with

right- and left-sided colon cancer: differences in epidemiology, perioperative course, histology, and survival. Dis Colon Rectum. 2010;53(1):57-64.
34. Overman MJ, McDermott R, Leach JL, Lonardi S, Lenz HJ, Morse MA, et al. Nivolumab in patients with metastatic DNA mismatch repair-deficient or microsatellite instability-high colorectal cancer (CheckMate 142): an open-label, multicentre, phase 2 study. Lancet Oncol. 2017;18(9):1182-91.
35. Van Cutsem E, Köhne CH, Hitre E, Zaluski J, Chien CRC, Makhson A, et al. Cetuximab and chemotherapy as initial treatment for metastatic colorectal cancer. NEJM. 2009;360(14):1408-17.
36. Bokemeyer C, Bondarenko I, Hartmann JT, de Braud F, Schuch G, Zubel A, et al. Efficacy according to biomarker status of cetuximab plus FOLFOX-4 as first-line treatment for metastatic colorectal cancer: the OPUS study. Ann Oncol. 2011;22(7):1535-46.
37. Maughan TS, Adams RA, Smith CG, Meade AM, Seymour MT, Wilson RH, et al. Addition of cetuximab to oxaliplatin-based first-line combination chemotherapy for treatment of advanced colorectal cancer: results of the randomised phase 3 MRC COIN trial. Lancet. 2011;377(9783):2103-14.
38. Tveit KM, Guren T, Glimelius B, Pfeiffer P, Sorbye H, Pyrhonen S, et al. Phase III trial of cetuximab with continuous or intermittent fluorouracil, leucovorin, and oxaliplatin (Nordic FLOX) versus FLOX alone in first-line treatment of metastatic colorectal cancer: the NORDIC VII study. J Clin Oncol. 2012;30(15):1755-62.
39. Douillard JY, Siena S, Classidy J, Tabernero J, Burkes R, Barugel M, et al. Randomized phase III trial of panitumumab with infusional fluorouracil, leucovorin and oxaliplatin (FOLFOX4) versus FOLFOX 4 as first line treatment in patient with previously untreated metastatic colorectal cancer: the PRIME study. J Clin Oncol. 2010;28(31):4697-705.
40. Schwartzberg LS, Rivera F, Karthaus M, Fasola G, Canon JL, Hecht JR, et al. PEAK: a randomized, multicenter phase II study of panitumumab plus modified fluorouracil, leucovorin, and oxaliplatin (mFOLFOX6) or bevacizumab plus mFOLFOX6 in patients with previously untreated, unresectable, wild-type KRAS exon 2 metastatic colorectal cancer. J Clin Oncol. 2014;32(21):2240-7.
41. Heinemann V, von Weikersthal LF, Decker T, Kiani A, Vehling-Kaiser U, Al-Batran SE, et al. FOLFIRI plus cetuximab versus FOLFIRI plus bevacizumab as first-line treatment for patients with metastatic colorectal cancer (FIRE-3): a randomised, open-label, phase 3 trial. Lancet Oncol. 2014;15(10):1065-75.
42. Venook AP, Niedzwiecki D, Lenz HJ, Innocenti F, Mahoney MR, O'Neil BH, et al. Cancer and Leukemia Group B (Alliance), SWOG, and ECOG. CALGB/SWOG 80405: Phase III trial of irinotecan/5- FU/leucovorin (FOLFIRI) or oxaliplatin/5-FU/leucovorin (mFOLFOX6) with bevacizumab (BV) or cetuximab (CET) for patients (pts) with KRAS wild-type (wt) untreated metastatic adenocarcinoma of the colon or rectum (MCRC). J Clin Oncol. 2014;32(15):LBA3.
43. Venook AP, Niedzwiecki D, Lenz HJ, Innocenti F, Fruth B, Meyerhardt JA, et al. Effect of first-line chemotherapy combined with cetuximab or bevacizumab on overall survival in patients with KRAS wildtype advanced or metastatic colorectal cancer: a randomized clinical trial. JAMA. 2017;317(23):2392-401.
44. Santoro A, Comandone A, Rimassa L, Granetti C, Lorusso V, Oliva C, et al. A phase II randomized multicenter trial of gefitinib plus FOLFIRI and FOLFIRI alone in patients with metastatic colorectal cancer. Ann Oncol. 2008;19(11):1888-93.
45. Cohn AL, Tabernero J, Maurel J, Nowara E, Sastre J, Chuah BYS, et al. A randomized, placebo-controlled phase 2 study of ganitumab or conatumumab in combination with FOLFIRI for second-line treatment of mutant KRAS metastatic colorectal cancer. Ann Oncol. 2013;24(7):1777-85.
46. Kopetz S, Grothey A, Yaeger R, Van Cutsem E, Desai J, Yoshino T, et al. Encorafenib, binimetinib, and cetuximab in BRAF V600E-mutated colorectal cancer. N Engl J Med. 2019;381(17):1632-43.
47. Huang M, Liu G. The study of innate drug resistance of human hepatocellular carcinoma Bel cell line. Cancer Letters. 1998;135(1):97-105.

48. Moon WS, Rhyu KH, Kang MJ, Lee DG, Yu HC, Yeum JH, et al. Overexpression of VEGF and angiopoietin 2: a key to high vascularity of hepatocellular carcinoma? Mod Pathol. 2003;16(6):552-7.
49. Hopfner M, Schuppan D, Scherubl H. Growth factor receptors and related signaling pathways as targets for novel treatment strategies of hepatocellular cancer. World J Gastroenterol. 2008;14(1):1-14.
50. Abou-Alfa GK, Schwartz L, Ricci S, Amadori D, Santoro A, Figer A, et al. Phase II study of sorafenib in patients with advanced hepatocellular carcinoma. Journal of Clinical Oncology. 2006;24(26):4293-300.
51. Llovet JM, Ricci S, Mazzaferro V, Hilgard P, Gane E, Blanc JF, et al. Sorafenib in advanced hepatocellular carcinoma. N Engl J Med. 2008;359(4):378-90.
52. Cheng L, Kang YK, Chen Z, Tsao CJ, Qin S, Kim JS, et al. Efficacy and safety of sorafenib in patients in the Asia-Pacific region with advanced hepatocellular carcinoma: a phase III randomised, doubleblind, placebo-controlled trial. Lancet Oncol. 2009;10(1):25-34.
53. Chao Y, Chung YH, Han G, Yoon JH, Yang J, Wang J, et al. The combination of transcatheter arterial chemoembolization and sorafenib is well tolerated and effective in Asian patients with hepatocellular carcinoma: final results of the START trial. Int J Cancer. 2015;136(6):1458-67.
54. Yau T, Park JW, Finn RS, Cheng AL, Mathurin P, Edeline J, et al. Checkmate 459: A Randomized, Multi-Center Phase 3 Study of Nivolumab (NIVO) vs Sorafenib (SOR) as First-Line (1L) treatment in patients (pts) with unresectable hepatocellular carcinoma. Ann Oncol. 2019;30(5):851-934.
55. Kudo M, Finn RS, Qin S, Han KH, Ikeda K, Piscaglia F, et al. Lenvatinib versus sorafenib in first-line treatment of patients with unresectable hepatocellular carcinoma: a randomised Phase 3 non-inferiority trial. Lancet. 2018;391(10126):1163-73.
56. Abou-Alfa GK, Johnson P, Knox JJ, Capanu M, Davidenko I, Lacava J, et al. Doxorubicin plus Sorafenib vs doxorubicin alone in patients with advanced hepatocellular carcinoma A randomized trial. JAMA. 2010;304(19):2154-60.
57. Anthony LB, Waltering EA, Espenan GD, Cronin MD, Maloney TJ, McCarthy KE. Indium-111-penteriotide prolongs survival in gastroenteropancreatic malignancies. Semin Nucl Med. 2002;32(2):123-32.
58. Yao JC, Phan A, Hoff PM, Chen HX, Charnsangavej C, Yeung SCJ, et al. Targeting vascular endothelial growth factor in advanced carcinoid tumor: a random assignment phase II study of depot octreotide with Bevacizumab and pegylated interferon alpha-2b. J Clin Oncol. 2008;26(8):1316-23.
59. Yao JC, Phan AT, Chang DZ, Wolff RA, Hess K, Gupta S, et al. Efficacy of RAD001 (Everolimus) and octreotide LAR in advanced low to intermediate grade neuroendocrine tumors: results of a phase II study. J Clin Oncol. 2008;26(26):4311-8.
60. DeMatteo RP, Lewis JJ, Leung D, Mudan SS, Woodruff JM, Brennan MF, et al. Two hundred gastrointestinal stromal tumors: recurrence patterns and prognostic factors for survival. Ann Surg. 2000;231(1):51-8.
61. Hirota S, Isozaki K, Moriyama Y, Hashimoto K, Nishida T, Ishiguro S, et al. Gain-of-function mutations of c-kit in human gastrointestinal stromal tumors. Science. 1998; 279(5350):577-80.
62. Joensuu H, Hohenberger P, Corless CL. Gastrointestinal stromal tumour. Lancet. 2013;382:973-83.
63. Blanke CD, Rankin C, Demetri GD, Ryan CW, von Mehren M, Benjamin RS, et al. Phase III randomized, intergroup trial assessing imatinib mesylate at two dose levels in patients with unresectable or metastatic gastrointestinal stromal tumors expressing the kit receptor tyrosine kinase: S0033. J Clin Oncol. 2008;26(4):626-32.
64. Gastrointestinal Stromal Tumor Meta-Analysis Group. Comparison of two doses of imatinib for the treatment of unresectable or metastatic gastrointestinal stromal tumors: a meta-analysis of 1,640 patients. J Clin Oncol. 2010;28:1247-53.

65. Casali PG, Zalcberg J, Cesne AL, Reichardt P, Blay JY, Lindner LH, et al. Ten-year progression-free and overall survival in patients with unresectable or metastatic GI stromal tumors: Long-term analysis of the European organisation for research and treatment of cancer, Italian sarcoma group, and Australasian gastrointestinal trials group intergroup phase III randomized trial on imatinib at two dose levels. J Clin Oncol. 2017;35(17):1713-20.
66. Antonescu CR, Besmer P, Guo T, Arkun K, Hom G, Koryotowski B, et al. Acquired resistance to imatinib in gastrointestinal stromal tumor occurs through secondary gene mutation. Clin Cancer Res. Jun 1, 2005;11(11):4182–90.
67. Demetri GD, van Oosterom AT, Garrett CR, Blackstein ME, Shah MH, Verweij J, et al. Efficacy and safety of Sunitinib in patients with advanced gastrointestinal stromal tumour after failure of Imatinib: a randomised controlled trial. Lancet. 2006;368: 1329-38.
68. Corless CL, Ballman KV, Antonescu CR, Kolesnikova V, Maki RG, Pisters PWT, et al. Pathologic and molecular features correlate with long-term outcome after adjuvant therapy of resected primary GI stromal tumor: the ACOSOG Z9001 trial. J Clin Oncol. 2014;32(15):1563-70.
69. Joensuu H, Eriksson M, Sundby Hall K, Hartmann JT, Pink D, Schütte J, et al. One vs three years of adjuvant imatinib for operable gastrointestinal stromal tumor: a randomized trial. JAMA. 2012;307(12):1265-72.
70. Eisenberg BL, Harris J, Blanke CD, Demetri GD, Heinrich MC, Watson JC, et al. Phase II trial of neoadjuvant/adjuvant imatinib mesylate (IM) for advanced primary and metastatic/recurrent operable gastrointestinal stromal tumor (GIST): early results of RTOG 0132/ ACRIN 6665. J Surg Oncol. 2009;99(1):42-7.
71. Tirumani SH, Shinagare AB, Jagannathan JP, Krajewski KM, Ramaiya NH, Raut CP. Radiologic assessment of earliest, best, and plateau response of gastrointestinal stromal tumors to neoadjuvant imatinib prior to successful surgical resection. Eur J Surg Oncol. 2014;40(4):420-8.
72. Jones S, Zhang X, Parsons DW, Lin JCH, Leary RJ, Angenendt P, et al. COre signaling pathways in human pancreatic cancers revealed by global genomic analyses. Science. 2008;321(5924)1801-6.
73. Richards NG, Rittenhouse DW, Freydin B, Cozzitorto JA, Grenda D, Rui H, et al. HuR status is a powerful marker for prognosis and response to gemcitabine-based chemotherapy for resected pancreatic ductal adenocarcinoma patients. Ann Surg. 2010;252(3);499-505.
74. Golan T, Hammel P, Reni M, Van Cutsem E, Macarulla T, Hall MJ, et al. Maintenance olaparib for germline BRCA-mutated metastatic pancreatic cancer. N Engl J Med. 2019;381:317-27.
75. Philip PA, Mahoney MR, Allmer C, Thomas J, Pitot HC, Kim G, et al. Phase II study of erlotinib in patients with advanced biliary cancer. J Clin Oncol Off J Am Soc Clin Oncol. 2006;24(19):3069-74.
76. Lubner SJ, Mahoney MR, Kolesar JL, Loconte NK, Kim GP, Pitot HC, et al. Report of a multicenter phase II trial testing a combination of biweekly bevacizumab and daily erlotinib in patients with unresectable biliary cancer: a phase II consortium study. J Clin Oncol. 2010;28(21):3491-7.
77. Riedlinger D, Bahra M, Boas-Knoop S, Lippert S, Bradtmöller M, Guse K, et al. Hedgehog pathway as a potential treatment target in human cholangiocarcinoma. J Hepatobiliary Pancreat Sci. 2014;21(8):607-15.
78. Abou-Alfa GK, Sahai V, Hollebecque A et al. Pemigatinib for previously treated, locally advanced or metastatic cholangiocarcinoma: a multicentre, open-label, phase 2 study. Lancet Oncol. 2020;21(5):671-84.
79. Abou-Alfa GK, Macarulla T, Javle MM et al. Ivosidenib in IDH1-mutant, chemotherapy-refractory cholangiocarcinoma (ClarIDHy): a multicentre, randomised, double-blind, placebo-controlled, phase 3 study. Lancet Oncol. 2020;21(6):796-807.

CHAPTER 6

Recent Advances in Endoscopy

Jayanta Samanta, Akash Singh, Virendra Singh

INTRODUCTION

The role of endoscopy in the practice of gastroenterology and gastrointestinal (GI) surgery cannot be overstated. Over the years, its use has transformed from an initial diagnostic tool to one of the key therapeutic modalities for patient care.[1] With the advent of newer technologies, the art of endoscopy has advanced from basic tissue harvesting to early detection of disease conditions and hence advocate better management options. Moreover, the armamentarium of therapeutic endoscopy has exponentially expanded in recent years to even obviate surgery in various cases and thus, catapulted its popularity to become the touchstone for gastroenterology practice.

Technological advancement is a part and parcel of our daily life and the world of endoscopy has advanced with the advent of high-resolution endoscopes, newer devices such as capsule endoscopy, ability for endoscopic microscopic assessment, and various accessories. In fact, procedures such as endoscopic retrograde cholangiopancreatography, endoscopic ultrasound (EUS), and "third space" endoscopy have surely brought a paradigm shift in the management options for patients with GI diseases. A brief overview of the recent advances in the field of GI endoscopy will be highlighted in this review.

ADVANCES IN ENDOSCOPIC IMAGING

Flexible endoscopes, pioneered by Hirchowitz et al.[2] in 1957, used the fiber optic technology which transmitted light using the principle of total internal reflection through optic bundles and created an image at the tip using a lens. From the use of charged couple devices (CCDs), the world of image acquisition technology in the field of gastroenterology has come a long way to the current era of image-enhanced endoscopy with landmark technologies such as magnification endoscopy, autofluorescence imaging (AFI), electronic chromoendoscopy techniques such as narrow-band imaging (NBI), i-scan, or flexible spectral imaging color enhancement (FICE) and confocal laser endomicroscopy (CLE). The cutting edge technology allows endoscopist to view the minutest of details and clinch the culprit lesion. In today's era of early cancer detection, these technologies have given comprehensive tools to create the effect of in vivo histological prediction, the concept of "optical biopsy."[3]

High-resolution, High-magnification Endoscopy

A high-magnification capability in an endoscope enables the power of optical zoom to get a closer image of the target keeping the resolution intact. This is in stark contrast to an electronic magnification, wherein the image is merely brought closer at the cost of loss of pixels and hence image quality is hampered after a certain extent. This electronic magnification or digital zoom is usually to the tune of 1.5–2 times. While standard scopes have optical zoom of 30–35, high-magnification ("zoom") endoscopes can magnify up to 150 times. All the currently available manufacturers have zoom endoscopes with both optical and digital zoom.[4]

Majority of the studies have clubbed this high-resolution magnification technology with other image-enhanced technologies such as NBI, i-scan, FICE, or the conventional chromoendoscopy and promote enhanced image viewing experience and lesion detection rates for the endoscopist.

Virtual Chromoendoscopy

Virtual chromoendoscopy uses enhanced tissue architecture visualization by optical filtering or software-driven image processing. Various available technologies are narrow-band imaging (NBI, Olympus Corporation), multiband imaging with FICE (Fujinon, Japan), and i-scan (Pentax, Japan). Majority of the studies experimenting image enhancement systems have been with the use of NBI.

Narrow-band Imaging

Narrow-band imaging system primarily aims at targeting the mucosal vasculature and henceforth highlights the alterations therein during pathologic settings. The shorter blue wavelength (i.e., 415 nm), corresponding to the main peak absorption spectrum of hemoglobin, enhances the superficial mucosal capillaries as brown and the longer green wavelength (i.e., 540 nm) corresponding to a secondary hemoglobin absorption peak displays the deeper mucosal and submucosal vessels as cyan.[5] NBI can be used for the diagnosis of a variety of conditions such as Barrett's esophagus, gastric metaplasia, *Helicobacter pylori* infection, celiac disease, and also classifying colorectal tumors using NBI International Colorectal Endoscopic (NICE) Classification[6] based on color, microvascular architecture and surface pattern of lesions, and a host of other conditions. The technology of NBI has shown promise as far as better mucosal detail description is concerned and adequate training in this technology holds the key to its better utilization **(Figs. 1A and B)**.

Optical Biopsy

The correlation of endoscopic findings and the pathological picture is often a tricky affair and in spite of techniques aiding for targeted biopsies, the

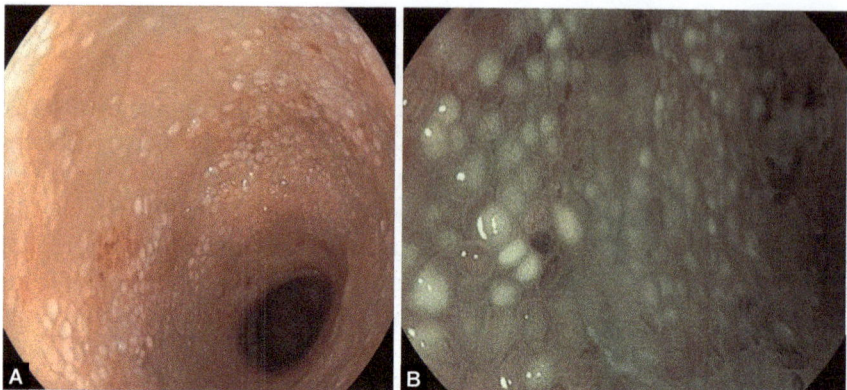

Figs. 1A and B: Terminal ileum in a case of primary intestinal lymphangiectasia: (A) White light image; (B) narrow-band imaging (NBI) image showing the enlarged whitish villi.

exact representative tissue for a corroborative histology keeps eluding the endoscopist and frustrating the pathologist. Hence, the concept of so called "optical biopsy" or "virtual biopsy." It encompasses three technologies, namely CLE, endocytoscopy (EC), and optical coherence tomography (OCT). The most widely studied is CLE.

Confocal Laser Endomicroscopy

Confocal laser endomicroscopy is a technique of high-resolution image acquisition of the mucosal layers of the GI tract. The current CLE devices are based on tissue fluorescence wherein exogenous fluorescence contrast agents such as fluorescein (most commonly used) (Pharmalab, Lane Cove, New South Wales, Australia) are used.[7] The devices commercially available are the Pentax Endomicroscopy system integrated in to the conventional endoscopy (Pentax, Tokyo, Japan) and the probe-based Cellvizio Endomicroscopy system (Mauna Kea Technologies, Paris, France).

Various applications for CLE include Barrett's esophagus, early gastric cancer, colonic polyps, and for inflammatory bowel diseases (IBD). Yet another advancement is in the form of needle-based CLE (nCLE; AQ-Flex19; Mauna Kea), which can be inserted through a 19-gauge EUS-FNA needle, and have found utility in the diagnosis of pancreatic cysts.[8]

The spectrum of CLE is rapidly expanding and even molecular imaging is being done along with it. More than its use in the GI lumen, it has applicability for the unmet needs in the pancreatobiliary domain where lack of a histological "gold standard" further complicates the scenario.

Endocytoscopy

Another emerging technique for real time in vivo histology is endocytoscopy (Olympus, Tokyo, Japan) (EC). Using the concept of contact white-light microscopy, EC, unlike CLE, can characterize cellular structures of only the superficial epithelial layer, not the deeper layers, in a plane parallel to the mucosal surface. Limited studies exist in its evaluation for esophageal lesions[9] and colorectal lesions.[10] More and more data are being generated in favor of EC's role, although it is still in its infancy.

Video Capsule Endoscopy

Video capsule endoscopy (VCE) has come a long way in becoming an invaluable tool in the diagnostic armamentarium of small bowel diseases including bleed[11] celiac disease, inflammatory bowel disease, tuberculosis, lymphoma, and a host of other conditions **(Figs. 2A and B)**. VCE is not only limited to the small bowel, and dedicated colon capsule (Pillcam Colon 2-Given Imaging, Israel) and esophageal capsule (PillCam Eso) are available for the specific imaging of the respective areas.[12] Image-enhancement techniques have also been incorporated in the VCE with as wider 360-degree viewing capsule[13] and FICE in the Given Imaging workstation (Pillcam SB2)[14] for "better" visualization.

The major drawback of VCE is the lack of facilities to intervene or take biopsies in case a lesion is detected. Magnetic steerable capsule endoscopy is now being evaluated for their potential role in better image-capturing capacity.[15] Future lies in the development of its capability to both diagnose as well as administer therapy such as drug delivery systems.

ADVANCES IN ENDOSCOPIC RETROGRADE CHOLANGIOPANCREATOGRAPHY

Endoscopic retrograde cholangiopancreatography (ERCP) has been the standard-of-care therapeutic tool for management of pancreatobiliary diseases for quite some time now. Management of cholangiocarcinoma (CCA)

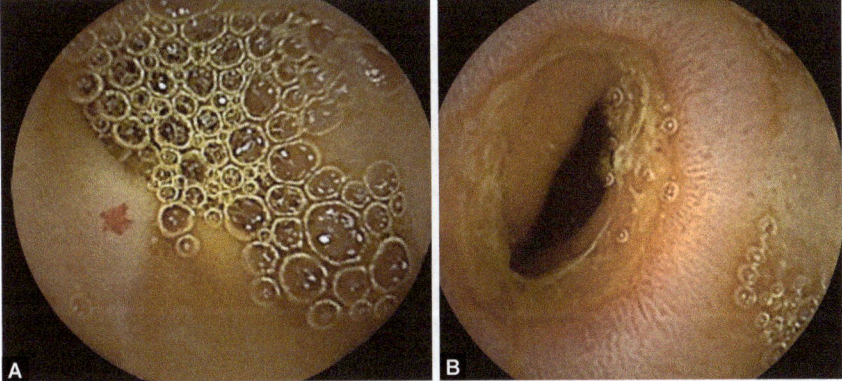

Figs. 2A and B: Video capsule endoscopy images of various conditions: (A) Telangiectasia in a case of occult gastrointestinal (GI) bleed; (B) Diaphragmatic disease in a case of pain abdomen with nonsteroidal anti-inflammatory drug (NSAID) abuse.

included biliary stenting which improved the quality of life but did not aid in improvement of survival. Hence, the newer concept of tumor ablative therapies such as photodynamic therapy (PDT) and radiofrequency ablation (RFA) which is believed to not only improve stent patency but also augment survival.

Endoscopic Retrograde Cholangiopancreatography-guided Photodynamic Therapy

Photodynamic therapy (PDT) is an ablative modality for the local control of tumor and entails the administration of photosensitizing agent that concentrates inside target cells and is activated by specific wavelength of light to generate reactive-oxygen species (ROS). ROS cause cellular damage and antiangiogenic pathways too get activated.[16] Recent meta-analysis hints toward improved survival in patients undergoing PDT with stenting compared to stenting alone.[17] Side effects include phototoxicity. More data are needed to define the ideal number of sessions required or need for bilateral versus unilateral treatment.

Endoscopic Retrograde Cholangiopancreatography-guided Radiofrequency Ablation

Radiofrequency ablation is another modality for management of perihilar CCA using electromagnetic wave frequencies in the range of 10^4 to 3×10^{12} Hz to create molecular friction and heat generation leading to coagulative necrosis and tissue destruction.[18] Recent meta-analysis showed better stent patency and survival benefit in patients with RFA and stenting.[19] RFA is a relatively well-tolerated procedure with rare adverse effect profile.

Hence, both PDT and RFA are now being used not only for palliation of unresectable CCA but also as neoadjuvant therapy for patients awaiting liver transplantation.

Cholangioscopy and Pancreatoscopy

Slim endoscopes and optical catheters are used to visualize the bile duct or the pancreatic duct directly and hence facilitate identification and management of intraductal lesions. The systems available are endoscope-based dual-operator systems, also known as "mother-daughter" (Olympus America, Center Valley, PA, and Pentax, Montvale, NJ) and a catheter-based system, known as "single-operator" cholangioscopy (SpyGlass DS Direct Visualization System, Boston Scientific Endoscopy, Marlboro, MA). Moreover, slim scopes (4.9–5.9 mm outer diameter) can be used for direct cholangioscopy. Fiberoptic cholangioscopes have a working channel of 1.2 mm allowing passage of forceps and lithotripsy fibers with up/down tip deflection,[20] for sampling and therapy. Pancreatoscopy is done with the same devices as that for cholangioscopy.

Cholangioscopy is commonly used for difficult bile duct stones and for evaluation of indeterminate strictures, with or without biopsy. NBI

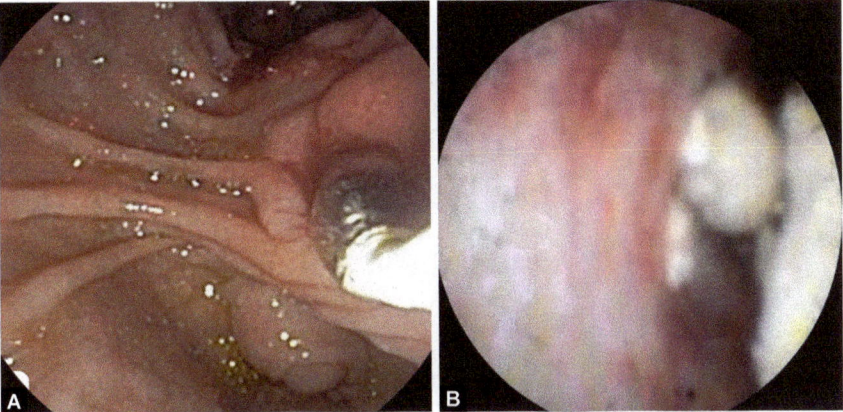

Figs. 3A and B: Pancreatoscopy using SpyGlass in a case of chronic pancreatitis: (A) Pancreatoscopy through minor papilla; (B) Pancreatic duct with intraductal stones.

cholangioscopy has been used in various biliary tract diseases such as biliary strictures, CCA, and biliary papillomatosis. Pancreatoscopy is used for pancreatic ductal stones and for neoplastic lesions such as intraductal papillary mucinous neoplasm (IPMN) **(Figs. 3A and B)**.

ADVANCES IN DIAGNOSTIC ENDOSCOPIC ULTRASOUND

Endoscopic ultrasound has come a long way into becoming one of the most valuable tool for investigation and plan management in a wide variety of GI diseases. Diagnostic accuracy of EUS-guided tissue acquisition reaches a sensitivity and specificity of 80% and 100%, respectively, but can be technically demanding and require multiple passes. Therefore, newer technologies are needed to not only reduce the need for sampling but also help in obtaining targeted tissue for accurately clinching the diagnosis.

Endoscopic Ultrasound-guided Elastography

Elastography is a real-time method for the assessment of tissue stiffness based on the internal force concept, wherein stiffer tissues pose lower strain and hence deform less on compression.[21] Two different modes are available—qualitative and quantitative. Qualitative elastography quantifies the degree of deformation after compression in the B-mode imaging and the strain is smaller in hard tissues than in soft tissues.[22] Hard tissue is dark blue and soft tissue is red with intermediate being green and medium in yellow **(Fig. 4)**. Quantitative elastography uses strain ratio and strain histogram for quantification of the hardness of the tissue and various cut-off points are taken to determine malignancy **(Table 1)**.

Endoscopic ultrasound-elastography has been used primarily for the assessment of solid pancreatic lesions and enlarged lymph nodes. Since the

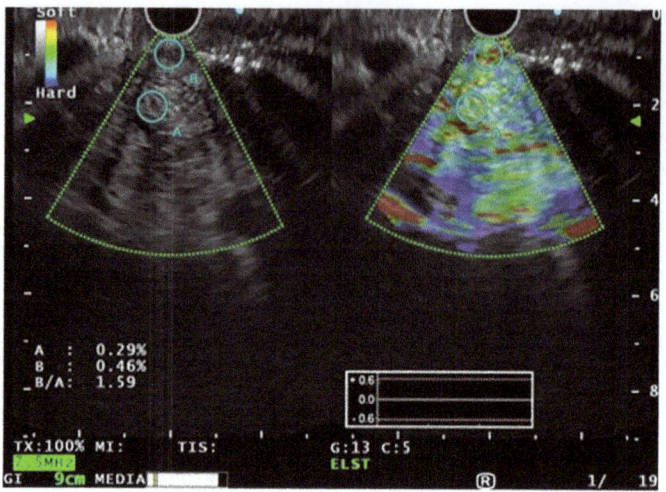

Fig. 4: Endoscopic ultrasound (EUS) elastography with strain ratio assessment.

TABLE 1: Endoscopic ultrasound (EUS) elastography: Qualitative and quantitative.		
Qualitative assessment		
Color and pattern	Hardness	Chance of malignancy
Heterogeneous red and green	Soft	No
Homogenous green	Soft	No
Heterogeneous green predominant	Intermediate	No
Heterogeneous blue	Hard	Yes
Homogeneous blue	Hard	Yes
Heterogeneous green and blue	Intermediate hard	Not definite
Quantitative assessment		
Parameter	Value	Chance of malignancy
Strain ratio	>10	yes
Strain histogram	<50	Yes

(Adapted from: Iglesias-Garcia J, Dominguez-Munoz JE. Endoscopic ultrasound image enhancement elastography. Gastrointest Endosc Clin N Am. 2012;22(2):333-48, x-xi.)

first study by Giovanni et al.,[23] describing EUS-elastography in pancreatic masses, multiple studies have assessed the role of this modality for its accuracy in predicting malignancy. Meta-analysis has shown that elastography could differentiate pancreatic malignancy from inflammatory masses with a sensitivity of 95% and specificity of 67-69%.[24] It has also been shown to be helpful to differentiate benign from malignant lymph node and hence its role in cancer staging.

Various other upcoming uses of this modality include transrectal elastography for prostate cancer, rectal cancer, IBD, and for evaluation of subepithelial masses and adrenal glands.

Contrast-enhanced Endoscopic Ultrasound

Evaluation of vascularity of solid lesions can help differentiate benign from malignant lesions. This concept is used in contrast-enhanced harmonic endoscopic ultrasound (CH-EUS). The CH-EUS uses the technology of signal generation by hitting gas-filled microbubbles (diameter 2–5 mm) of contrast agents with ultrasonic waves.[25] Second-generation contrast agents such as SonoVue (sulfur hexafluoride microbubbles; Bracco, Italy) and Sonazoid (perflurobutane microbubbles; GE Healthcare, USA) are commonly used.

Contrast-enhanced harmonic endoscopic ultrasound has wide applicability including solid pancreatic lesions such as pancreatic adenocarcinoma, mural nodule of IPMN, neuroendocrine tumor, inflammatory masses, and gastrointestinal stromal tumor (GIST). It can be used for tumor staging and nodal staging as well as for assessment of chemotherapeutic response.

Advances in Endoscopic Ultrasound-guided Tissue Acquisition

The art of EUS-guided tissue acquisition (EUS-TA) has evolved over the last 25 years since its first description. Multiple factors such as site of lesion, technique of sampling, needle-type, and expertise of the endosonographer influence the outcome in EUS-TA. Recent advancements in the field of needle design have enabled the art of EUS-guided biopsy sampling (EUS-FNB) with better tissue acquisition for a core biopsy. The ProCore FNB (EchoTip Procore; Cook Medical, USA) has additional beveled side cut of the distal needle shaft, while two other FNB needles have different needle tip design—Sharkcore (Medtronic, Minneapolis, MN, USA) and Franseen needle tip (Acquire; Boston Scientific, Natick, MA, USA) **(Figs. 5A to C)**.

The advent of EUS-FNB needles enables core tissue acquisition, need for less number of passes and may eventually obviate the need for rapid onsite cytological evaluation (ROSE), a facility entailing higher costs. Moreover, newer devices such as through the needle cytology brushes and forceps can help improve the diagnostic yield in pancreatic cystic lesions.

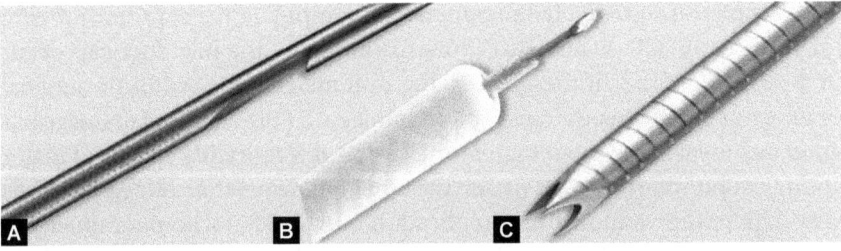

Figs. 5A to C: The different kinds of FNB needles: (A) EchoTip ProCore HD EUS needle (*Courtesy:* Cook Medical, Bloomington, IN); (B) SharkCore FNB needle (*Courtesy:* Medtronic, Minneapolis, MN); and (C) Acquire EUS-FNB device (*Courtesy:* Boston Scientific, Natick, MA).

Needle-based Confocal Laser Endomicroscopy

The technique of CLE provides the ability to produce real-time microscopic imaging of the lesion, the art of "optical biopsy." Of late, the development of needle-based CLE (nCLE) have been used predominantly for the characterization of pancreatic cysts,[26] although its use extends to solid pancreatic lesions as well as lymph nodes.

ADVANCES IN THERAPEUTIC ENDOSCOPIC ULTRASOUND

There has been remarkable progress in the field of pancreatobiliary endoscopy in the past few years with immense progress in the use of EUS as a therapeutic tool. The spectrum of therapeutic EUS has expanded from drainage of pancreatic fluid collections to EUS-guided bile duct and pancreatic duct access in cases of failed ERCP, gallbladder drainage, gastrojejunostomy (GJ), and EUS-guided cancer therapy including celiac plexus neurolysis (CPN).

Lumen-apposing Metal Stents

Lumen-apposing metal stents (LAMS) has opened the gates of therapeutic endoscopy to a wide array of interventional options. Earlier plastic stents were used to drain pancreatic fluid collections but with the advent of LAMS, not only can the fluid be drained but also provide a wide conduit (10-20 mm) allowing the endoscopist to pass regular endoscopes beyond the lumen of the GI tract for carrying out procedures such as necrosectomy (termed as direct endoscopic necrosectomy).[27] The various LAMS available in the market are the Hot Axios (Boston Scientific. Marlborough, MA, USA), NAGI, and SPAXUS stents (Taewoong Medical, South Korea).

The use of these LAMS provides high technical and clinical success with short procedure duration. Its use is not only restricted to drainage of pancreatic fluid collections, but also for EUS-guided choledochoduodenostomy, gallbladder drainage, and GJ as will be discussed in the subsequent text.

Endoscopic Ultrasound-guided Biliary Drainage

Endoscopic retrograde cholangiopancreatography is the standard-of-care for endoscopic biliary access. Failure to cannulate the bile duct can occur in 4-16% of cases.[28] In these cases, the options earlier used to be surgical drainage or percutaneous transhepatic drainage (PTBD). Surgical drainage has good technical success but high mortality (30-day mortality 15%) and major complications rate (39%). PTBD, on the other hand, is technically easy but has very high reintervention and complication rates (~80%) with poor quality of life due to external catheter. With the advent of endoscopic ultrasound-guided biliary drainage (EUS-BD), these shortcomings can be circumvented and can be used in suitable cases safely and effectively.

The indications for EUS-BD include failed ERCP, altered anatomy, inaccessible papilla due to tumor infiltration, and large ascites precluding PTBD.[29]

Technique

Endoscopic ultrasound-guided biliary drainage can be performed in multiple ways depending on the site of biliary obstruction, the accessibility of papilla, and the expertise and comfort of the interventionist.

The basic steps involve access into either the left hepatic ductal system or the common bile duct (CBD) with the help of, preferably, a 19G EUS-FNA needle. After puncturing the system, the position of the needle is confirmed by aspiration of bile, followed by injection of contrast to obtain a cholangiogram. Guide-wire is then negotiated through the needle into the ductal system. The tract is then dilated using graded diameter stiff catheter, balloon catheter, or cystotome. Once the access is secured and tract is dilated, then stenting is done.

There are four ways of EUS-BD, namely, hepaticogastrostomy (EUS-HGS) choledochoduodenostomy (EUS-CDS), EUS-guided antegrade stent (EUS-AS) placement, and EUS-guided rendezvous procedure (EUS-RV). EUS-HGS **(Figs. 6A to D)** entails placement of stent in the left ductal system with proximal

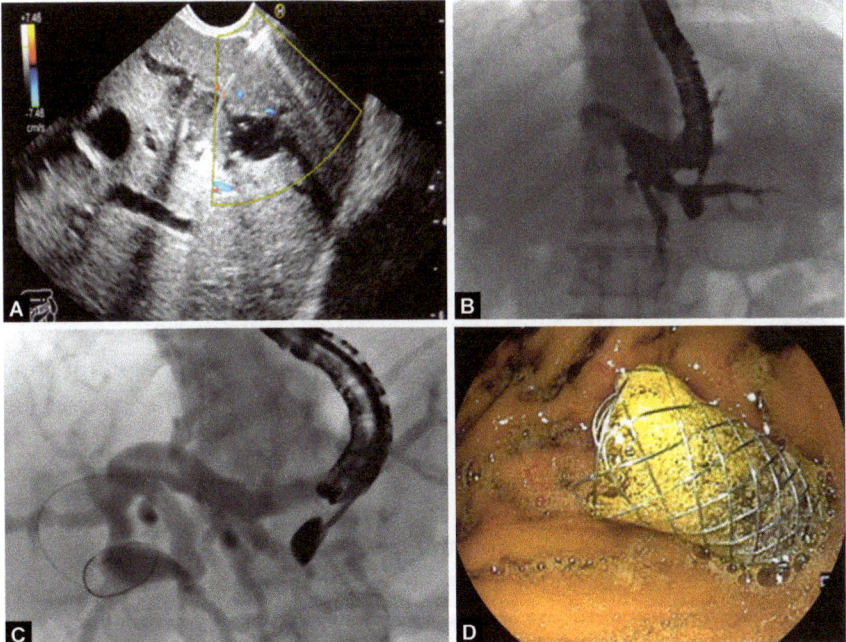

Figs. 6A to D: Endoscopic ultrasound (EUS)-hepaticogastrostomy: (A) EUS-guided puncture of the dilated left ductal system; (B) Contrast injection to confirm and obtain cholangiogram; (C) Guidewire negotiated up to the hilum; and (D) Intragastric part of the self expandable metallic stent (SEMS) seen.

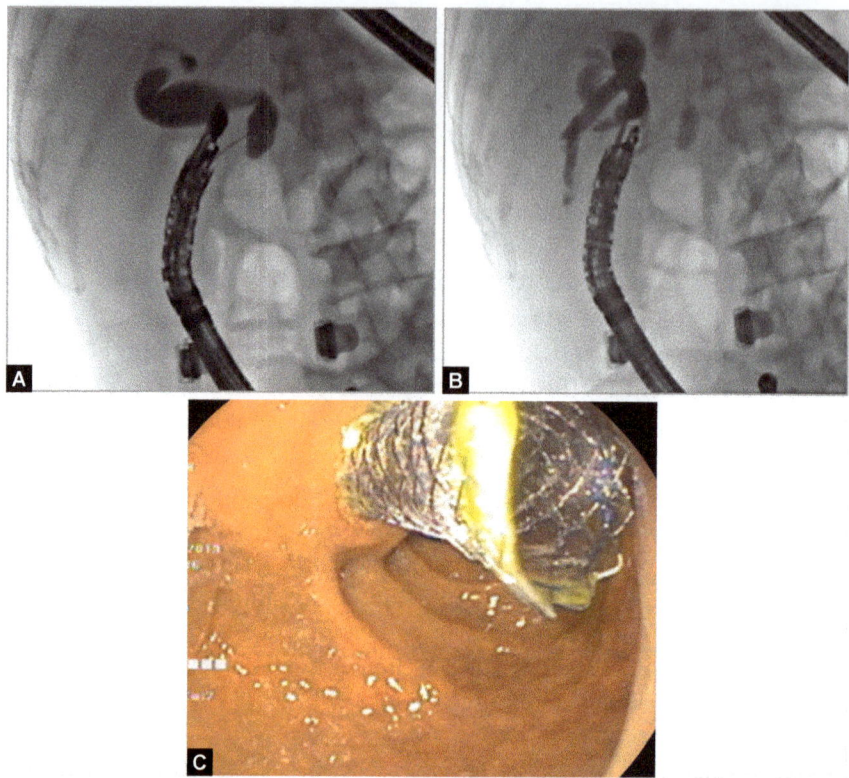

Figs. 7A to C: Endoscopic ultrasound (EUS) choledochoduodenostomy in pancreatic cancer with duodenal obstruction: (A) EUS-guided puncture of the CBD from D1 station; (B) Guidewire looped inside the CBD; and (C) Endoscopic image of the CDS stent in D1.

end in the stomach creating a permanent transgastric-transhepatic fistula. EUS-CDS **(Figs. 7A to C)** creates a transduodenal-CBD fistula for transmural drainage. EUS-AS helps in the placement of stent in the biliary system across the papilla akin to ERCP. EUS-RV is a technique to assist the conventional ERCP by negotiating the guide wire across the papilla and then complete the procedure using conventional ERCP. The various nuances of the four techniques and indications are detailed in **Table 2**. No definite consensus exists as to which technique or approach is best.

Published data suggest a cumulative success rate of EUS-BD to be 88–93%,[30] with complications rate of 13–20% cases. Complications include infection (cholangitis, cholecystitis, etc.), pneumoperitoneum, bile leak, bleeding, and stent migration. In fact, recent review showed that EUS-BD fared better than PTBD in terms of better clinical success, less adverse events, and lower rates of reinterventions.[31]

Overall, EUS-BD scores over both surgery and PTBD with good safety profile. Nevertheless, EUS-BD is a complex procedure and should be done by skilled endoscopists with good surgical and interventional radiology back-up.

TABLE 2: The various techniques of endoscopic ultrasound-guided biliary drainage (EUS-BD).

Technique	Indications	Route	Remarks	Advantages/Disadvantages
EUS-hepaticogastrostomy (EUS-HGS)	• Hilar or CBD obstruction with inaccessible papilla • Failure to access left ductal system through PTBD	Intrahepatic puncture	• Creation of permanent fistula—transgastric transhepatic • Metallic SEMS preferable	• Stable scope position • Technically challenging stent deployment
EUS-Choledochoduodenostomy (EUS-CDS)	• Lower or mid-CBD obstruction with inaccessible papilla	Extrahepatic route	• Creation of permanent fistula transduodenal • SEMS preferable	• Stable long loop scope position • Technically easier stent deployment
EUS-antegrade stent placement (EUS-AS)	• Lower CBD obstruction with inaccessible papilla	Intrahepatic route	• Placement of stent across papilla akin to ERCP	• Technically difficult guidewire negotiation • Temporary fistula across the transgastric puncture route
EUS-Rendezvous (EUS-RV)	Failed ERCP with accessible papilla	• Intrahepatic route • Extrahepatic route	Placement of guidewire across papilla for facilitation of conventional ERCP	• Intrahepatic route: Stable scope position but difficult guidewire manipulation • Extrahepatic route: Unstable scope position at D1-D2 junction but easier guidewire manipulation

(CBD: common bile duct; ERCP: endoscopic retrograde cholangiopancreatography; PTBD: percutaneous transhepatic drainage; SEMS: scanning electron microscopes)

Endoscopic Ultrasound-guided Pancreatic Duct Drainage

Similar to EUS-BD, EUS-guided pancreatic duct drainage (EUS-PD) can be performed with the technical steps similar to that of EUS-BD. Primarily, it is done in cases of chronic pancreatitis requiring stenting in whom ERCP has failed probably due to strictures or other causes. Other indication can be pancreatic trauma with duct disruption.

Access to the duct can be obtained at either the neck or body of the pancreas and pancreatic rendezvous is attempted. In cases where this cannot be done, transluminal drainage of the duct is carried out by creating a pancreaticogastrostomy or pancreaticoduodenostomy **(Figs. 8A to D)**. EUS-PD is technically more challenging and complications include pancreatitis, bleeding, pneumoperitoneum, and stent migration.

Endoscopic Ultrasound-guided Gallbladder Drainage

Cholecystitis is ideally managed by antibiotics and surgery. However, in high surgical risk candidates, patients can be managed either by the percutaneous route by placement of cholecystostomy tube or by ERCP-guided transpapillary

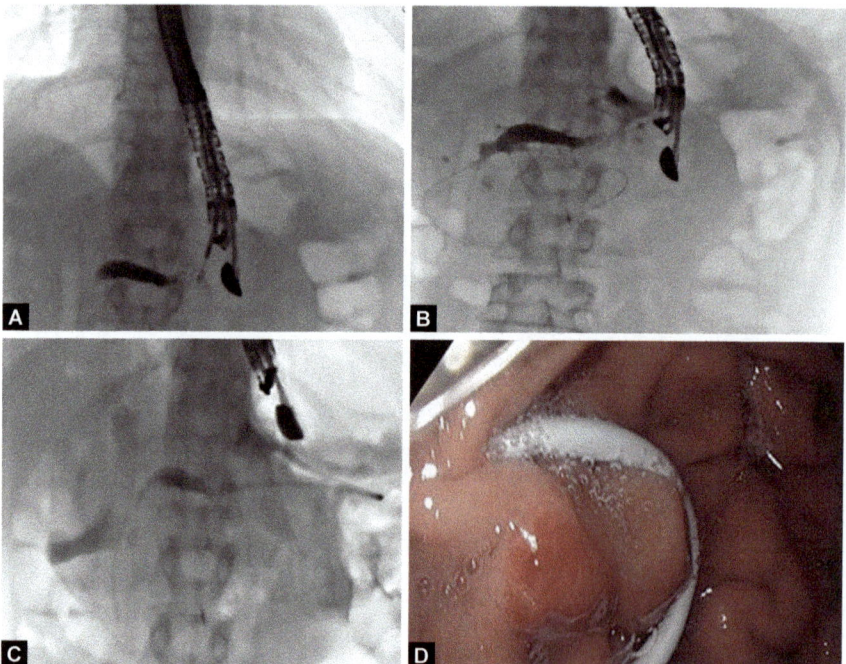

Figs. 8A to D: Endoscopic ultrasound (EUS)-guided pancreatic duct drainage (EUS-PD) in a case of groove pancreatitis: (A) EUS-guided pancreatic duct (PD) puncture; (B) Pancreatogram showing stricture in head with dilated PD, guidewire negotiated across stricture; (C) Long plastic stent placed and pancreatogastrostomy created; and (D) Endoscopic view of stent.

stent placement. However, the percutaneous route has the risk of an externally lying catheter, while the ERCP route has a technical success of only 81%. EUS-guided gallbladder drainage (EUS-GBD) has gained immense popularity since its first description in 2007.[32]

The access to the gallbladder is gained either through the prepyloric area or the first part of duodenum, usually with a 19G needle and drainage can be done either by placement of naso-gallbladder drains, plastic stents, or metallic stents. The technique has a technical and clinical success rates of nearly 100% with adverse events rate of 6–12%.[33] With the recent advent of "Hot LAMS," having electrocautery mounted tip, the steps of the procedure are reduced. Long-term data on outcome of EUS-GBD needs to be established.

Endoscopic Ultrasound-guided Gastrojejunostomy

Gastric outlet obstruction commonly occurs with advanced upper GI and pancreatobiliary malignancies and requires intervention. The available options are surgical GJ and endoscopic enteral stenting. Surgical GJ is fraught with prolonged recovery time and gastroparesis while enteral stenting may migrate or occlude with tumor overgrowth. EUS-guided GJ (EUS-GJ) has come up as an excellent option with the use of a LAMS with long-term patency.[34]

Endoscopic ultrasound-guided gastrojejunostomy can be done by four techniques, namely, water immersion, water-inflated balloon technique, EPASS balloon, and the free-hand technique. In order to reduce the steps of procedure, electrocautery-mounted LAMS ("Hot LAMS") are preferred (**Figs. 9A to E**).

Technical success reported is 92%.[35] Compared to enteral stenting, EUS-GJ had less reintervention rates,[36] similar clinical success compared to surgical GJ.[37] Thus, early data of this new technique of EUS-GJ is promising and long-term data needs to be established.

Endoscopic Ultrasound-guided Vascular Interventions

The advantage of obtaining high-resolution images of the mediastinal and abdominal vasculature enables EUS with Doppler facility as a modality for an accurate vascular access and possible therapy. It has been shown to be feasible for Dieulafoy's lesions, bleeding tumors, and pseudoaneurysms.

For gastric varices (GV), the standard-of-care is endoscopic glue (cyanoacrylate) injection with hemostasis rates of 58–100% and rebleeding rates of 0–40%.[38] EUS has multiple technical advantages over conventional endoscopic therapy in the management of GV. With EUS, (1) detection rate of GV increases and is more accurate because of the Doppler facility; (2) residual patency can be assessed as that can predict rebleed; (3) enables accurate delivery of the hemostatic agent into the lumen of the varix; (4) "feeder" vessel can be identified and targeted, if needed; (5) stainless steel coils can be injected and hence can reduce the need for glue injection reducing embolization risk.

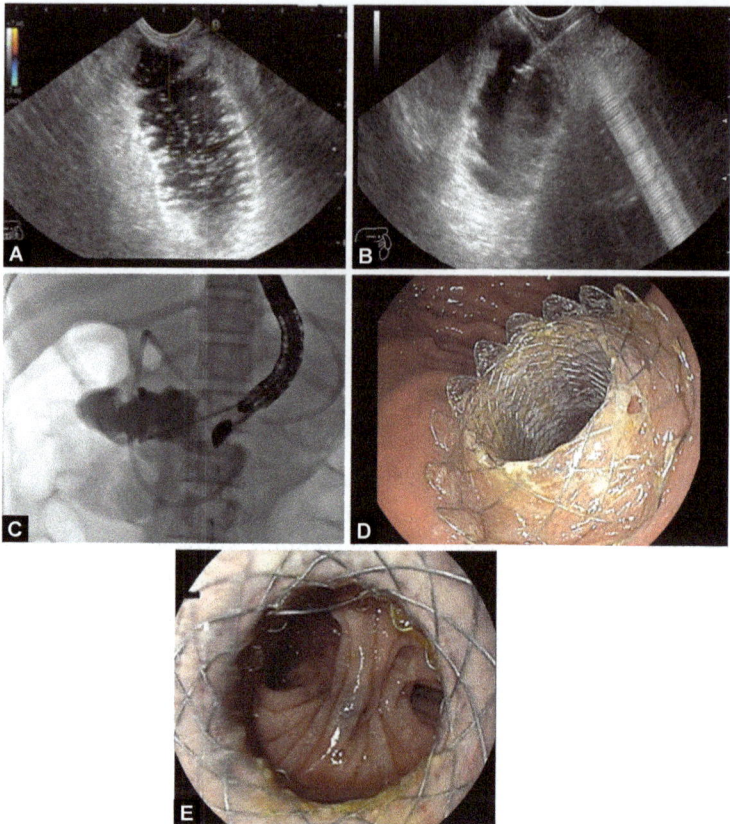

Figs. 9A to E: Endoscopic ultrasound (EUS)-gastrojejunostomy using Spaxus system by the free-hand technique: (A) Dilated jejunal loops filled with saline infused through nasojejunal (NJ) tube; (B) Dilated loop punctured with 19G needle; (C) Contrast injected and confirmed followed by tract dilation; (D) Lumen-apposing metal stents (LAMS) placed; and (E) Dilated with balloon, jejunal loops seen.

Combination of coil and glue can act synergistically having additive benefit with reduced adverse events and reported a rebleeding rate of only 3%.[27] **(Figs. 10A to D)**. Ectopic varices such as duodenal varices and rectal varices can also be managed with EUS-guided therapy.

Portal vein (PV) can be easily visualized on EUS and have been accessed and pressure measurement carried out. Huang et al. have done the first human study measuring portal pressure gradient.[39] PV access through EUS has led to an array of therapeutic possibilities such as sampling of PV thrombus in hepatocellular carcinoma (HCC), PV blood sampling for circulating tumor cells, and selective PV embolization.[40]

Endoscopic Ultrasound-guided Cancer Therapy

The management of pain in pancreatic cancer with the help of EUS-guided CPN is well established. The various other upcoming oncotherapies using EUS

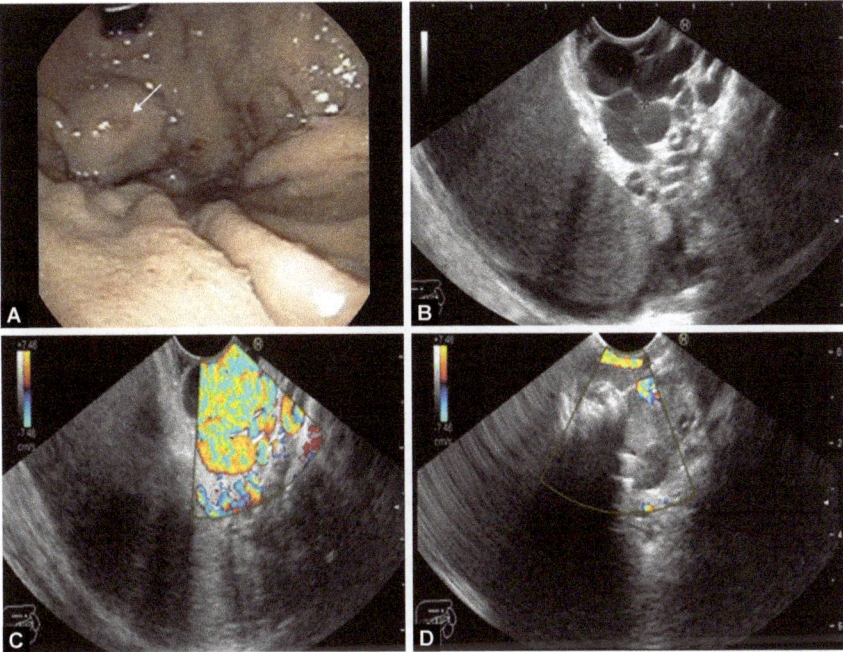

Figs. 10A to D: Endoscopic ultrasound (EUS)-guided gastric variceal coiling: (A) Endoscopic vision of gastric varices (GV) with red color signs (RCS); (B) EUS image of large GV; (C) Doppler flow demonstrated; and (D) EUS-guided coiling done.

interventions include assistance with radiotherapy such as fiducial marker placement and brachytherapy. Moreover, tumor ablative therapies such as alcohol, RFA, and PDT are being done using EUS guidance. Immunotherapy and gene therapy are also being explored using EUS-guidance for targeted delivery.[41]

THIRD SPACE ENDOSCOPY

The reach of endoscopist has extended from the first space (Lumen) to second space (peritoneal cavity) and now the third space (intramural or submucosal space). The art of submucosal endoscopy with the creation of a mucosal flap safety valve (SEMF) was first described by Sumiyama et al.[42] It entails injection of saline and dye in order to expand the potential submucosal space and enter with a flexible endoscopy for further management. Per oral endoscopic myotomy (POEM), for the management of achalasia cardia, using this principle was first demonstrated in animal by Pasricha et al. in 2007[43] followed by the first human study by Inoue et al. in 2010.[44] These two landmark studies paved the way for an ever-expanding field of submucosal endoscopy and increasing number of conditions and indications where this technique can be adopted.

The spectrum of "third space" endoscopy covers a host of various procedures for treating the various conditions as highlighted in **Flowchart 1**.

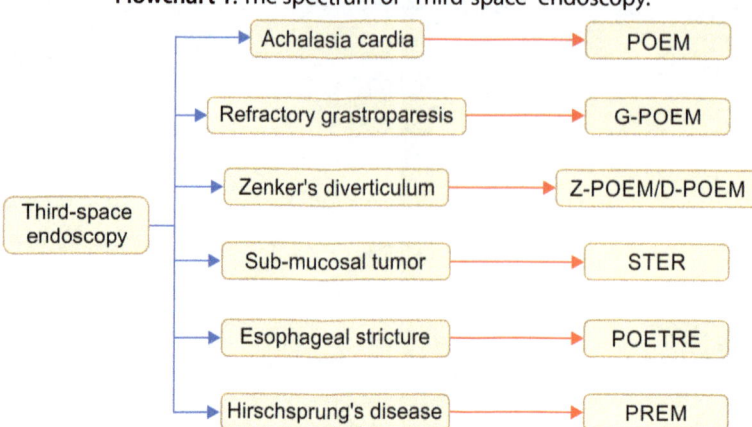

Flowchart 1: The spectrum of "Third-space" endoscopy.

(G-POEM: gastric per oral endoscopic myotomy; POEM: per oral endoscopic myotomy; POETRE: per oral endoscopic tunneling for restoration of the esophagus; PREM: per rectal endoscopic myotomy; STER: submucosal tunneling endoscopic resection; Z-POEM: per oral endoscopic myotomy for Zenker's diverticulum)

Equipment and Accessories

Few specialized accessories are needed for the procedure. The solution used for submucosal injection is either saline or hydroxyethyl starch with a dye, usually methylene blue or indigo carmine. Standard scope such as GIF-HQ190, Olympus with integrated water channel, electrosurgical unit, carbon dioxide insufflators with low flow tubes, and endoscopic flushing pumps are required. The various knives used are Triangle tip Knife J (KD-645L, Olympus, Japan), Hybrid Knife (201150-060, Erbe, Germany), Hook Knife (KD-620LR, Olympus, Japan), and IT-Knife 2 (KD-611L, Olympus, Japan) as per the operator's choice along with coagulation forceps (Coagrasper; FD-410/11, Olympus, Japan).

Per Oral Endoscopic Myotomy

Per oral endoscopic myotomy is used for the management of achalasia and other spastic esophageal motility disorders. Most of the data on "third space" entails POEM. The steps include: (1) formation of a submucosal bleb; (2) mucosal incision; (3) tunneling in the submucosal space; (4) myotomy including the lower esophageal sphincter, and (5) closure of the mucosal entry point **(Figs. 11A to E)**.

Per oral endoscopic myotomy is safe and effective with good clinical success at 5-year follow-up of 83%.[45] It is more effective than the pneumatic dilatation at 1-year Follow-up (92.2 vs. 70%) as shown in a recent randomized controlled trial (RCT).[46] It is equally effective for treatment naïve (87%) and treatment failure (76.3%) cases. With clear advantages over the conventional Heller's myotomy in terms of hospital stay, operating time, and blood loss, POEM would soon become the standard-of-care for achalasia and spastic motility disorders.

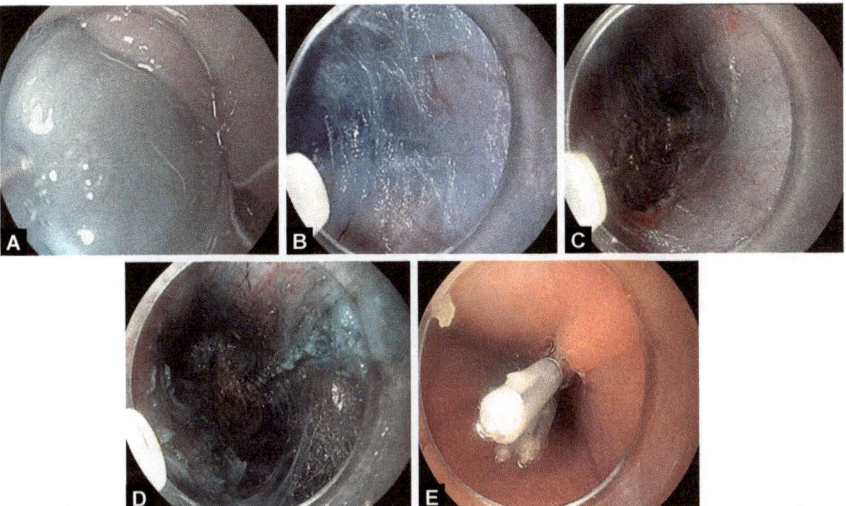

Figs. 11A to E: Per oral endoscopic myotomy (POEM): (A) Submucosal injection forming a bleb; (B) Submucosal dissection using Triangular Tip J Knife; (C) Myotomy done after dissection; (D) Complete full thickness myotomy done; and (E) Mucosal entry point closed with clips.

A common symptom that patient complains after POEM is that of reflux. To circumvent this problem, a newer addition to the technique of POEM is partial fundoplication, also termed as POEM+F. Described by Inoue et al.,[47] the procedure entails advancing the scope into the peritoneal cavity, at the end of myotomy, retracting the anterior gastric wall close to the gastroesophageal (GE) junction to create a partial wrap.

Beyond Per Oral Endoscopic Myotomy

Submucosal tunneling is being used beyond the standard POEM for a host of other procedures. For gastroparesis, pyloromyotomy can be done for the relief of symptoms, the procedure known as G-POEM. The clinical efficacy of this procedure was around 86%.[48]

Zenker's diverticulum and other types of esophageal diverticulum such as epiphrenic diverticulum can also be managed in the similar lines. The principle of therapy in symptomatic esophageal diverticular disease is to shed off the muscular bar/septum and the success depends on the completeness of this septostomy. Unlike the conventional endoscopic myotomy, submucosal tunneling and myotomy (Z-POEM or D-POEM) ensure a more complete and longer myotomy while avoiding the risk of perforation at the same time. A recent multicenter data of 75 patients of Z-POEM showed 97.3% technical success and 92% clinical success[49] **(Figs. 12A to D)**.

For Hirschsprung's disease, similar technique of submucosal tunneling and myotomy was first described by Bapaye et al. and was coined as PREM (per rectal endoscopic myotomy).[50] Submucosal tunneling and endoscopic

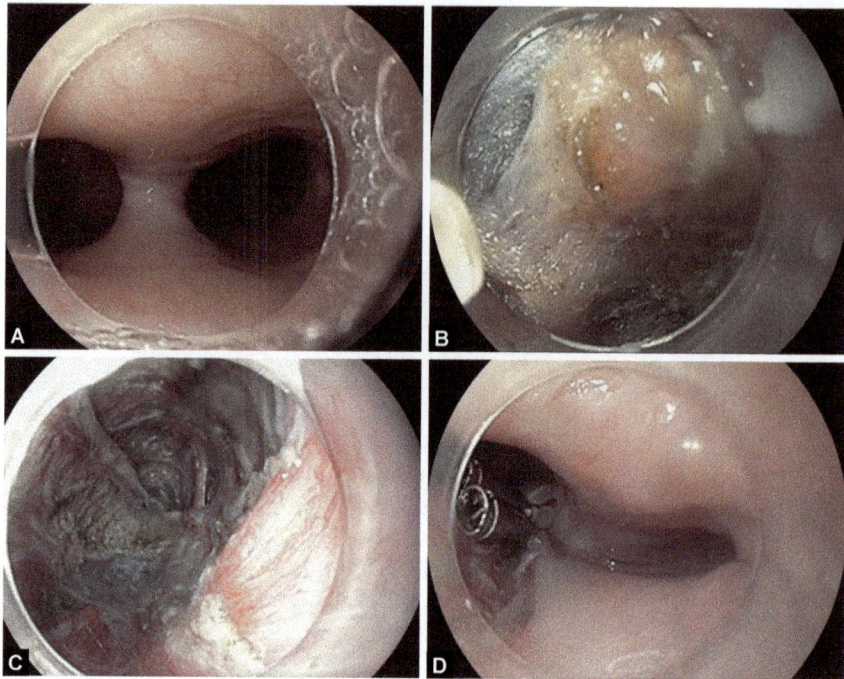

Figs. 12A to D: Z-POEM for Zenker's diverticulum: (A) Endoscopic view of the diverticulum; (B) Muscular septum noted after submucosal dissection; (C) Complete septostomy done; and (D) Mucosal entry point closed with clips.

resection (STER) is the technique of removal of submucosal tumors in the esophagus, stomach, and even rectum.

ENDOSCOPIC SUBMUCOSAL DISSECTION

Endoscopic submucosal dissection (ESD) is a well-established procedure used for "en bloc" resection of superficial malignancies of the GI tract. It entails the similar technique of submucosal dissection for removal of the lesion. The procedure is technically challenging and needs precise training. Various technical advancements have occurred over the ensuing years and a host of various kind of knives are available and are used depending on the location and type of lesion, the degree of fibrosis, and axis of the device with respect to the dissection plane.[51] Various countertraction techniques have been developed such as clip with line or snare, clip-flap, and Endolifter (Olympus). Newer methods such as magnetic countertraction and overtube with manipulatory arms are being evaluated. Indications for ESD include early esophageal carcinoma, gastric cancer, colorectal lateral spreading tumors—nongranular type (LST-NG), large depressed or protruded type tumors and carcinoma with shallow T1 submucosal invasion.

ENDOSCOPIC FULL THICKNESS RESECTION

Endoscopic full thickness resection (EFTR) is a recent modality for local excision of a GI malignancy using the similar principle of ESD. Unlike ESD, a full thickness resection is done, creating a deliberate rent in the GI wall, and then closing the defect using over the scope clip (OTSC) (Ovesco, Tubingen, Germany) or suturing (Overstitch Endoscopic suturing system, Apollo Endosurgery, Texas). GIST is a good indication for the conventional *exposed* EFTR with less risk of tumor cell dissemination and does not require lymphadenectomy. The technical difficulty of *exposed* EFTR is that after the full thickness perforation created, there is loss of intraluminal CO_2 into the peritoneal cavity.

In *nonexposed* EFTR, the lesion is inverted and sutured before excision. This principle has been used in the new full thickness resection device (FTRD). It is composite device consisting of an OTSC cap and a snare.[52] FTRD has shown technical success of 89% with R0 resection rate of 58-87%. Limitations include lesions larger than 25 mm cannot be resected and inadequate endoscopic view due to long attached cap.

ADVANCES IN MANAGEMENT OF GASTROINTESTINAL BLEED

Nonvariceal upper GI bleed is commonly managed using the conventional endoscopic techniques such as injection therapy, hemostatic clips, and bipolar (gold and silver) probes. Despite these measures, the rebleeding rates and mortality have remained same.[53]

The OTSC (Ovesco, Tubingen, Germany), also known as the "bear claw," is a nitinol clip originally designed for closure of fistulae and leaks, is currently being used for the management of bleeding ulcers, and works like variceal band ligation wherein the bleeding ulcer is sucked in the cap and the clip is applied. In a recent prospective RCT, it was found that OTSC fared better than conventional hemostatic clips for patients with recurrent peptic ulcer bleeding.[54] Other emerging therapies for the management of nonvariceal bleed include RFA for gastric antral vascular ectasia (GAVE), Endoclot, a new hemostatic powder and cryotherapy.

ADVANCES IN THE MANAGEMENT OF GASTROESOPHAGEAL REFLUX DISEASE

Gastroesophageal reflux disease (GERD) is a common condition and various endoscopic modalities have emerged besides medical therapy as 20-40% are refractory. The various endoscopic therapies are mentioned below.
- *Stretta* (Mederi Therapeutics, Greenwich, CT, USA) procedure delivers radiofrequency current at the lower esophageal sphincter (LES) causing LES fibrosis with improved tonicity and better antireflux barrier.

- *Transoral incisionless fundoplication* (TIF) is done using EsophyX® (Endo Gastric Solutions, Redmond, WA, USA) device creating a partial (270°) fundoplication for a length of 2–3 cm. Recent data suggest stable outcome at 3 years with healed esophagitis in 86% cases.
- *Medigus Ultrasonic Surgical Endostapler* (MUSE™; Medigus, Omer, Israel) has ultrasound transducer to locate the Z line and endostapler for partial anterior fundoplication.
- *GERDx™* (G-SURG GmbH, Seeon-Seebruck, Germany) is a full thickness endoscopic plication device with better maneuverability and polytetrafluoroethylene (PTFE) plate-reinforced suture. This device is being commonly used with good results.
- *ARMS* (antireflux mucosectomy) procedure uses the property of scar formation that occurs after endoscopic mucosal resection (EMR) or endoscopic submucosal dissection (ESD) and thus narrows the GE junction causing reduced reflux. Recent data suggest good outcome at 1 year with discontinuation of proton-pump inhibitor (PPI) in 55% of patients.[55]

ADVANCES IN ENDOSCOPIC BARIATRIC AND METABOLIC THERAPIES

Endoscopic bariatric metabolic therapies (EBMTs) are a battery of techniques used for obesity treatment as well as glycemic control. It causes more weight loss than mere lifestyle modifications or medications.[56] They are not as good as bariatric surgery but definitely has better safety profile.

Intragastric balloons (IGBs) have been used very commonly for quite some time now. IGBs do have postremoval effects as 66–90% of the weight loss is maintained at 6 months after IGB removal. The various balloons used are: (1) Orbera Intragastric Balloon System (Orbera, Apollo Endosurgery, Austin, TX); (2) ReShape Dual Integrated Balloon System (ReShape medical, San Clemente, CA); (3) Obalon Balloon system (Obalon Therapeutics, Carlsbad, CA); and (4) Spatz3 Adjustable Balloon System (Spatz FGIA, Great Neck, NY). Common side effects include nausea, vomiting, abdominal pain, or need for early device removal.

The principle of aspiration therapy is used with *Aspire Assist System* (Aspire Bariatrics, Prussia, PA) wherein a part of the ingested chyme is aspirated through a gastrostomy tube akin to the conventional percutaneous gastrostomy tube (PEG). Study showed that 58.6% of patients achieved >10% weight loss compared to 22.1% in the control arm.[57]

Gastric plication and suturing can be done endoscopically and mimics the surgical suturing. Two techniques are used to alter the gastric anatomy, namely primary surgery obesity endoluminal (POSE) using incisionless operating platform (IOP, USGI Medical, San Clemente, CA) and endoscopic sleeve gastroplasty (ESG) using Overstitch (Apollo Endosurgery, Austin, TX).

Endoscopic sleeve gastroplasty is often referred to as the mimicker of surgical sleeve gastrectomy. The OverStitch system allows full-thickness plication by applying running sutures in a triangular fashion from anterior wall to greater curvature to posterior gastric wall with at least six stitch placements. A large multicenter data of 248 patients showed that at 24 months, 84.2% patients had >10% body weight loss.[58] Pooled body weight loss at 24 months in a meta-analysis was 17.2% with only 2.2% serious adverse events.[59] More long-term data is warranted.

Duodenal mucosal resurfacing (DMR) is a new kid on the block for the management of type 2 diabetes mellitus wherein the duodenal mucosa is circumferentially lifted with saline beyond the ampulla of Vater and then subjected to hydrothermal ablation using the Revita DMR (Fractyl, Lexington. MA). The mechanistic hypothesis is of postablative regeneration of normal duodenal mucosa after the destruction of the diseased one. The first multicenter large data recently published of 46 patients found that HbA_1c, fasting plasma glucose, and HOMA-IR improved and sustained at 12 months follow-up with only a modest weight loss.[60]

THE ADVENT OF ARTIFICIAL INTELLIGENCE

Artificial intelligence (AI) is nothing but computer programs designed to function like human intelligence or even better. The terms AI, machine learning (ML), and deep learning (DL) are close compatriots. DL involves artificial neural network (ANN) akin to the human brain and can process large amount of data. Deep neural network (DNN) models on the other hand uses several consecutive filters allowing the automatic detection of relevant features of input data.[61] Convoluted neural network (CNN) is a type of ANN with a connectivity pattern akin to our visual cortex and hence is an apt tool for endoscopic imaging. The current focus is on AI-assisted endoscopy. Most of the studies use one set of data to train in ML process and then test its performance with a second set. AI is being used for identifying malignant and premalignant lesions, inflammatory and other lesions such as IBD and celiac disease, GI bleeding, and for diagnosis of polyps and enhancing the accuracy of the endoscopist.

FUTURE IMAGE INNOVATIONS

The various technologies that are in the pipeline for image innovations include hypoxia imaging for neoplastic lesions and IBD, three-dimensional imaging for enhanced polyp detection, and finally robotic-assisted endoscopes (RAE) for maximizing mucosal viewing area and enhanced patient comfort. Self-propelled colonoscopes controlled by endoscopist remotely are being evaluated. Aer-O-Scope™ (GI view Ltd., Ramat Gan, Israel) is a 360° viewing colonoscope, others are Endotics Endoscopy System (Era Endoscopy, Peccioli, Italy) and Invendoscope™ (Invendo Medical, Kissing, Germany). Small bowel capsules can be directed by external magnet such as NaviCam (Anchon technologies, Wuhan, China).

CONCLUSION

The world of endoscopy is ever expanding with the advent of more and better technologies. Experience of decades of research is adding on to the use of similar technologies for more advanced procedures as has been witnessed in the field of therapeutic EUS. The reach of the endoscopist is no longer confined within the lumen and the expanse in various spaces highlights the fine line between the endoscopist and their surgical colleagues. A substantial number of procedures underline the expanding territory of an endoscopist which were once purely the domain of radiologist or surgeons. Nevertheless, amidst such exciting times in the endoscopy world, one must understand that advanced technology and techniques need to be mastered adequately and with patience and applied only in cases with the right indication.

REFERENCES

1. Sivak MV. Gastrointestinal endoscopy: past and future. Gut. 2006;55(8):1061-4.
2. Hirschowitz BI, Peters CW, Curtiss LE. Preliminary report on a long fiberscope for examination of stomach and duodenum. Med Bull (Ann Arbor). 1957;23(5):178-80.
3. Beg S, Ragunath K. Image-enhanced endoscopy technology in the gastrointestinal tract: what is available? Best Pract Res Clin Gastroenterol. 2015;29(4):627-38.
4. ASGE TECHNOLOGY COMMITTEE; Kwon RS, Adler DG, Chand B, Conway JD, Diehl DL, et al. High-resolution and high-magnification endoscopes. Gastrointestinal endoscopy. 2009;69(3 Pt 1):399-407.
5. ASGE TECHNOLOGY COMMITTEE; Song LM, Adler DG, Conway JD, Diehl DL, Farraye FA, et al. Narrow band imaging and multiband imaging. Gastrointestinal endoscopy. 2008;67(4):581-9.
6. Tanaka S, Sano Y. Aim to unify the narrow band imaging (NBI) magnifying classification for colorectal tumors: current status in Japan from a summary of the consensus symposium in the 79th Annual Meeting of the Japan Gastroenterological Endoscopy Society. Dig Endosc. 2011;23(Suppl 1):131-9.
7. Kiesslich R GP, Neurath MF, (Eds). Atlas of Endomicroscopy. Germany: Springer; 2008.
8. Konda VJ, Aslanian HR, Wallace MB, Siddiqui UD, Hart J, Waxman I. First assessment of needle-based confocal laser endomicroscopy during EUS-FNA procedures of the pancreas (with videos). Gastrointest Endosc. 2011;74(5):1049-60.
9. Kumagai Y, Kawada K, Yamazaki S, Iida M, Momma K, Odajima H, et al. Endocytoscopic observation for esophageal squamous cell carcinoma: can biopsy histology be omitted? Dis Esophagus. 2009;22(6):505-12.
10. Kudo SE, Wakamura K, Ikehara N, Mori Y, Inoue H, Hamatani S. Diagnosis of colorectal lesions with a novel endocytoscopic classification - a pilot study. Endoscopy. 2011;43(10):869-75.
11. Sealock RJ, Thrift AP, El-Serag HB, Sellin J. Long-term follow up of patients with obscure gastrointestinal bleeding examined with video capsule endoscopy. Medicine (Baltimore). 2018;97(29):e11429.
12. Parker CE, Spada C, McAlindon M, Davison C, Panter S. Capsule endoscopy--not just for the small bowel: a review. Expert Rev Gastroenterol Hepatol. 2015;9(1):79-89.

13. Tontini GE, Wiedbrauck F, Cavallaro F, Koulaouzidis A, Marino R, Pastorelli L, et al. Small-bowel capsule endoscopy with panoramic view: results of the first multicenter, observational study (with videos). Gastrointest Endosc. 2017;85(2):401-8.e2.
14. Imagawa H, Oka S, Tanaka S, Noda I, Higashiyama M, Sanomura Y, et al. Improved visibility of lesions of the small intestine via capsule endoscopy with computed virtual chromoendoscopy. Gastrointest Endosc. 2011;73(2):299-306.
15. Hale MF, Drew K, Sidhu R, McAlindon ME. Does magnetically assisted capsule endoscopy improve small bowel capsule endoscopy completion rate? A randomised controlled trial. Endosc Int Open. 2016;4(2):E215-21.
16. Henderson BW, Dougherty TJ. How does photodynamic therapy work? Photochem Photobiol. 1992;55(1):145-57.
17. Moole H, Tathireddy H, Dharmapuri S, Moole V, Boddireddy R, Yedama P, et al. Success of photodynamic therapy in palliating patients with nonresectable cholangiocarcinoma: A systematic review and meta-analysis. World J Gastroenterol. 2017;23(7):1278-88.
18. Ni Y, Mulier S, Miao Y, Michel L, Marchal G. A review of the general aspects of radiofrequency ablation. Abdom Imaging. 2005;30(4):381-400.
19. Sofi AA, Khan MA, Das A, Sachdev M, Khuder S, Nawras A, et al. Radiofrequency ablation combined with biliary stent placement versus stent placement alone for malignant biliary strictures: a systematic review and meta-analysis. Gastrointest Endosc. 2018;87(4):944-51.e1.
20. ASGE Technology Committee; Shah RJ, Adler DG, Conway JD, Diehl DL, Farraye FA, et al. Cholangiopancreatoscopy. Gastrointest Endosc. 2008;68(3):411-21.
21. Iglesias-Garcia J, Dominguez-Munoz JE. Endoscopic ultrasound image enhancement elastography. Gastrointest Endosc Clin N Am. 2012;22(2):333-48, x-xi.
22. Frey H. [Realtime elastography. A new ultrasound procedure for the reconstruction of tissue elasticity]. Radiologe. 2003;43(10):850-5.
23. Giovannini M, Hookey LC, Bories E, Pesenti C, Monges G, Delpero JR. Endoscopic ultrasound elastography: the first step towards virtual biopsy? Preliminary results in 49 patients. Endoscopy. 2006;38(4):344-8.
24. Pei Q, Zou X, Zhang X, Chen M, Guo Y, Luo H. Diagnostic value of EUS elastography in differentiation of benign and malignant solid pancreatic masses: a meta-analysis. Pancreatology. 2012;12(5):402-8.
25. Kitano M, Yamashita Y. New imaging techniques for endoscopic ultrasonography: Contrast-enhanced endoscopic ultrasonography. Gastrointest Endosc Clin N Am. 2017;27(4):569-83.
26. Napoleon B, Palazzo M, Lemaistre AI, Caillol F, Palazzo L, Aubert A, et al. Needle-based confocal laser endomicroscopy of pancreatic cystic lesions: a prospective multicenter validation study in patients with definite diagnosis. Endoscopy. 2019;51(9):825-35.
27. Wallace MB, Wang KK, Adler DG, Rastogi A. Recent Advances in Endoscopy. Gastroenterology. 2017;153(2):364-81.
28. Holt BA, Hawes R, Hasan M, Canipe A, Tharian B, Navaneethan U, et al. Biliary drainage: role of EUS guidance. Gastrointest Endosc. 2016;83(1):160-5.
29. Nussbaum JS, Kumta NA. Endoscopic ultrasound-guided biliary drainage. Gastrointest Endosc Clin N Am. 2019;29(2):277-91.
30. Moole H, Dharmapuri S, Duvvuri A, Dharmapuri S, Boddireddy R, Moole V, et al. Endoscopic versus percutaneous biliary drainage in palliation of advanced malignant hilar obstruction: A meta-analysis and systematic review. Can J Gastroenterol Hepatol. 2016;2016:4726078.
31. Sharaiha RZ, Khan MA, Kamal F, Tyberg A, Tombazzi CR, Ali B, et al. Efficacy and safety of EUS-guided biliary drainage in comparison with percutaneous biliary drainage when ERCP fails: a systematic review and meta-analysis. Gastrointest Endosc. 2017;85(5):904-14.

32. Baron TH, Topazian MD. Endoscopic transduodenal drainage of the gallbladder: implications for endoluminal treatment of gallbladder disease. Gastrointest Endosc. 2007;65(4):735-7.
33. Penas-Herrero I, de la Serna-Higuera C, Perez-Miranda M. Endoscopic ultrasound-guided gallbladder drainage for the management of acute cholecystitis (with video). J Hepatobiliary Pancreat Sci. 2015;22(1):35-43.
34. Amin S, Sethi A. Endoscopic ultrasound-guided gastrojejunostomy. Gastrointest Endosc Clin N Am. 2017;27(4):707-13.
35. Tyberg A, Perez-Miranda M, Sanchez-Ocana R, Penas I, de la Serna C, Shah J, et al. Endoscopic ultrasound-guided gastrojejunostomy with a lumen-apposing metal stent: a multicenter, international experience. Endosc Int Open. 2016;4(3):E276-81.
36. Chen YI, Itoi T, Baron TH, Nieto J, Haito-Chavez Y, Grimm IS, et al. EUS-guided gastroenterostomy is comparable to enteral stenting with fewer re-interventions in malignant gastric outlet obstruction. Surg Endosc. 2017;31(7):2946-52.
37. Khashab MA, Bukhari M, Baron TH, Nieto J, El Zein M, Chen YI, et al. International multicenter comparative trial of endoscopic ultrasonography-guided gastroenterostomy versus surgical gastrojejunostomy for the treatment of malignant gastric outlet obstruction. Endosc Int Open. 2017;5(4):E275-E81.
38. de Franchis R, Primignani M. Endoscopic treatments for portal hypertension. Semin Liver Dis. 1999;19(4):439-55.
39. Huang JY, Samarasena JB, Tsujino T, Lee J, Hu KQ, McLaren CE, et al. EUS-guided portal pressure gradient measurement with a simple novel device: a human pilot study. Gastrointest Endosc. 2017;85(5):996-1001.
40. ASGE Technology Committee; Trikudanathan G, Pannala R, Bhutani MS, Melson J, Navaneethan U, et al. EUS-guided portal vein interventions. Gastrointest Endosc. 2017;85(5):883-8.
41. Mukewar S, Muthusamy VR. Recent advances in therapeutic endosonography for cancer treatment. Gastrointest Endosc Clin N Am. 2017;27(4):657-80.
42. Sumiyama K, Gostout CJ, Rajan E, Bakken TA, Knipschield MA, Marler RJ. Submucosal endoscopy with mucosal flap safety valve. Gastrointest Endosc. 2007;65(4):688-94.
43. Pasricha PJ, Hawari R, Ahmed I, Chen J, Cotton PB, Hawes RH, et al. Submucosal endoscopic esophageal myotomy: a novel experimental approach for the treatment of achalasia. Endoscopy. 2007;39(9):761-4.
44. Inoue H, Minami H, Kobayashi Y, Sato Y, Kaga M, Suzuki M, et al. Peroral endoscopic myotomy (POEM) for esophageal achalasia. Endoscopy. 2010;42(4):265-71.
45. Teitelbaum EN, Dunst CM, Reavis KM, Sharata AM, Ward MA, DeMeester SR, et al. Clinical outcomes five years after POEM for treatment of primary esophageal motility disorders. Surg Endosc. 2018;32(1):421-7.
46. Ponds FA, Fockens P, Lei A, Neuhaus H, Beyna T, Kandler J, et al. Effect of peroral endoscopic myotomy vs pneumatic dilation on symptom severity and treatment outcomes among treatment-naive patients with achalasia: A randomized clinical trial. JAMA. 2019;322(2):134-44.
47. Inoue H, Ueno A, Shimamura Y, Manolakis A, Sharma A, Kono S, et al. Peroral endoscopic myotomy and fundoplication: a novel NOTES procedure. Endoscopy. 2019;51(2):161-4.
48. Khashab MA, Ngamruengphong S, Carr-Locke D, Bapaye A, Benias PC, Serouya S, et al. Gastric per-oral endoscopic myotomy for refractory gastroparesis: results from the first multicenter study on endoscopic pyloromyotomy (with video). Gastrointest Endosc. 2017;85(1):123-8.
49. Yang J, Novak S, Ujiki M, Hernandez O, Desai P, Benias P, et al. An international study on the use of peroral endoscopic myotomy in the management of Zenker's diverticulum. Gastrointest Endosc. 2020;91(1):163-8.

50. Bapaye A, Wagholikar G, Jog S, Kothurkar A, Purandare S, Dubale N, et al. Per rectal endoscopic myotomy for the treatment of adult Hirschsprung's disease: First human case (with video). Dig Endosc. 2016;28(6):680-4.
51. Mavrogenis G, Hochberger J, Deprez P, Shafazand M, Coumaros D, Yamamoto K. Technological review on endoscopic submucosal dissection: available equipment, recent developments and emerging techniques. Scand J Gastroenterol. 2017;52(4): 486-98.
52. Schmidt A, Beyna T, Schumacher B, Meining A, Richter-Schrag HJ, Messmann H, et al. Colonoscopic full-thickness resection using an over-the-scope device: a prospective multicentre study in various indications. Gut. 2018;67(7):1280-9.
53. Martinez-Alcala A, Monkemuller K. Emerging endoscopic treatments for nonvariceal upper gastrointestinal hemorrhage. Gastrointest Endosc Clin N Am. 2018;28(3):307-20.
54. Schmidt A, Golder S, Goetz M, Meining A, Lau J, von Delius S, et al. Over-the-scope clips are more effective than standard endoscopic therapy for patients with recurrent bleeding of peptic ulcers. Gastroenterology. 2018;155(3):674-86.e6.
55. Inoue H, Sumi K, Tatsuta T, Ikebuchi Y, Tuason J. 998 Clinical results of antireflux mucosectomy (ARMS) for refractory GERD. Gastrointest Endosc. 2017;85(5):AB120.
56. Sullivan S, Edmundowicz SA, Thompson CC. Endoscopic bariatric and metabolic therapies: New and emerging technologies. Gastroenterology. 2017;152(7):1791-801.
57. Thompson CC, Abu Dayyeh BK, Kushner R, Sullivan S, Schorr AB, Amaro A, et al. Percutaneous gastrostomy device for the treatment of class II and class III obesity: Results of a randomized controlled trial. Am J Gastroenterol. 2017;112(3):447-57.
58. Lopez-Nava G, Sharaiha RZ, Vargas EJ, Bazerbachi F, Manoel GN, Bautista-Castano I, et al. Endoscopic sleeve gastroplasty for obesity: a multicenter study of 248 patients with 24 months follow-up. Obes Surg. 2017;27(10):2649-55.
59. Hedjoudje A, Dayyeh BA, Cheskin LJ, Adam A, Neto MG, Badurdeen D, et al. Efficacy and safety of endoscopic sleeve gastroplasty: A systematic review and meta-analysis. Clin Gastroenterol Hepatol. 2020;18(5):1043-53.e4.
60. van Baar ACG, Holleman F, Crenier L, Haidry R, Magee C, Hopkins D, et al. Endoscopic duodenal mucosal resurfacing for the treatment of type 2 diabetes mellitus: one year results from the first international, open-label, prospective, multicentre study. Gut. 2020;69(2):295-303.
61. Le Berre C, Sandborn WJ, Aridhi S, Devignes MD, Fournier L, Smail-Tabbone M, et al. Application of artificial intelligence to gastroenterology and hepatology. Gastroenterology. 2020;158(1):76-94.e2.

Evaluation of Incidental Dilated Bile Duct

Supriya Sharma, Anu Behari

INTRODUCTION

The biliary system transports bile from hepatocytes, through intra- and extrahepatic ducts, sphincter of Oddi and ampulla of Vater into the duodenum where it facilitates absorption of lipids and excretion of certain toxic metabolites in the small bowel. In recent years, widespread use of high resolution imaging techniques to investigate causes of nonspecific abdominal symptoms has resulted in increasing reports of isolated bile duct (BD) dilatation in minimally symptomatic and non-jaundiced patients with normal or near normal liver function tests. Discovery of an unexplained BD dilatation poses a diagnostic and therapeutic dilemma. There are many possible causes of both obstructive and non-obstructive biliary dilation. However, there are few studies which examine the yield of diagnostic evaluation and outcome of common bile duct (CBD) dilation in asymptomatic patients or patients with no laboratory abnormalities. This chapter attempts to better understand the causes in this specific clinical scenario, identify predictors of disease, and suggest the most appropriate investigation algorithm.

CAUSES OF INCIDENTAL BILIARY DILATATION

Smith I et al. conducted a systematic review of published studies on patients with incidental dilatation of CBD.[1] An etiology was identified in only 33% of patients evaluated **(Box 1)**. The authors suggest that although significance of incidental dilated CBD as a predictor of underlying disease, particularly malignancy is unknown, and long-term outcomes have not been well elucidated, symptomatic patients or patients with abnormalities on liver function tests, especially elevated bilirubin, should undergo additional investigation to identify the cause.[1]

A logical approach to incidentally identified biliary dilatation would be to identify the level of biliary dilatation – hilar or lower end block and tailor the investigation best suited to pick up the most common etiologies which have been described at these levels. **Table 1** suggests the most common etiologies depending upon the level of biliary dilatation.

BOX 1: Causes for incidental biliary dilatation as reported in literature[1]

- CBD stone
- Chronic pancreatitis
- IPMN, pancreatic cancer
- Ampullary tumor
- Mucinous cystic neoplasm
- Pancreaticobiliary malignancy
- Chronic calcific pancreatitis
- Pancreatic cyst
- Benign biliary stricture
- Choledochal cyst
- Clonorchis sinensis infection
- Hepatobiliary ascariasis
- Papillary stenosis
- Primary sclerosing cholangitis
- Hepatic cyst
- Juxtapapillary diverticulum
- Anomalous pancreatobiliary maljunction
- Choledochal cyst
- Distal CBD cancer
- Distal CBD adenoma
- Cholangiocarcinoma
- Malignant lymphoma
- Plasma cell neoplasm
- Neuroendocrine tumor
- Cancer gallbladder
- Ampullary stenosis
- Tumor of papilla of Vater
- CBD mass/polyp
- Microlithiasis
- Extrahepatic portal vein obstruction producing portal biliopathy

RADIOLOGICAL EVALUATION OF THE BILE DUCT: PEARLS AND PITFALLS

Transabdominal ultrasonography (USG) is the most commonly used radiological tool for evaluating the hepatobiliary tree. For an accurate assessment, USG should be done after overnight fasting or fasting of at least 6 hours to permit adequate distension of the biliary system. To ensure uniformity in reporting, the bile duct should be measured at the porta where it is parallel to the portal vein posteriorly and is crossed by the right hepatic artery anteriorly. Measure height of duct rather than the width, from one inner wall to the other, in anteroposterior transverse sonograms of the bile duct obtained at this level **(Fig. 1)**. The height of the duct is measured as the bile duct is oval in shape and oblique in its course. Thus the same bile duct can have different measurements depending upon the site and dimension being measured. In addition the lumen of a low inserting cystic duct may be included in ductal measurement if this is taken at a site other than the porta **(Fig. 2)**.

There are controversies regarding the upper normal diameter of the CBD but it is conventionally accepted to be 7 mm.[1] A variety of factors can

TABLE 1: Commonly identified causes of biliary dilatation depending on level of obstruction

Anatomical location	Malignant	Benign
Hilar	Gallbladder cancer	
	Hilar cholangiocarcinoma	
Low/Mid CBD	Pancreatic cancer	Pancreatitis (acute/chronic)
	Periampullary cancer	Choledochal cyst
	Biliary type - Intraductal papillary mucinous tumor	Pancreatic pseudocyst
		Choledochal cyst, Anomalous pancreatobiliary junction
		Periampullary diverticulum
		Papillary stenosis
Either	Cholangiocarcinoma	Stones
	Metastases	Mirizzi's syndrome
	Lymphoma	Postoperative strictures
		Primary sclerosing cholangitis
		Other cholangiopathies e.g., Portal cavernomatous cholangiopathy
		Bile duct polyp
		Haemobilia
		Parasites

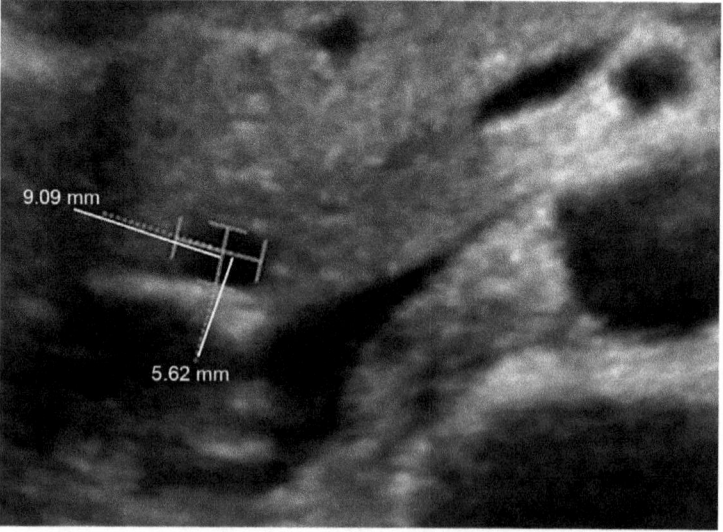

Fig. 1: Transverse view of pancreatic head with distal common bile duct (CBD) that is wider (9.1 mm) than taller (5.6 mm).

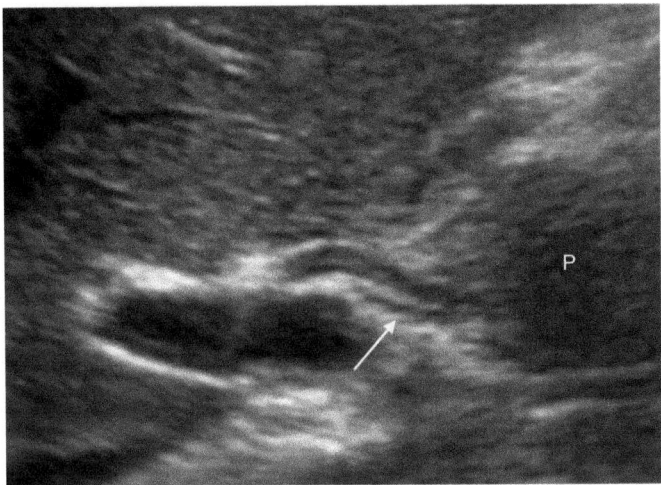

Fig. 2: Sagittal view of extrahepatic bile duct with low insertion of cystic duct (arrow) at level of pancreatic head (P). If one does not look at sagittal view and just takes measurement on transverse views, a low inserting CD lumen will falsely increase the measurement of the bile duct.

influence bile duct size such as imaging modality and age as discussed later. Besides USG, the other imaging modality used to report on bile duct size can be magnetic resonance cholangiopancreatography (MRCP), endoscopic retrograde cholangiopancreatography (ERCP) or percutaneous transhepatic cholangiography (PTC) and computed tomography (CT). There can be some discrepancy between the observed BD diameters between each of these modalities in the same patient.[2,3]

In transabdominal USG, BD may be difficult to visualize because of bowel gas, resulting in underestimation of duct size compared to other imaging techniques. On CT and MRCP imaging, bile duct wall is included in the measurement resulting in overestimation. Additionally measurements are made of the duct width rather than height on the axial images. This may cause inaccuracies as the bile duct has an oblique extrahepatic course.[4] The lumen of a low inserting cystic duct may be erroneously included in calculation in an axial image especially if measurements are not taken at porta. Finally, magnification and duct distension by contrast, used in ERCP and PTC, may overestimate duct size.

To determine the normal size of the extrahepatic BD and to evaluate the effect of aging on the duct diameter, 256 healthy subjects, and patients without hepatobiliary disease were examined using high-resolution real-time USG scanner.[5] The inner diameter of the widest point of the duct varied from 1 to 10 mm, and was found to be age-dependent (r = 0.60, P <0.001). The authors concluded that, based on visualization of the entire extrahepatic duct echographically, normal inner diameter of CBD can be up to 10 mm, and there is small increase of duct size with age. Other studies too have reported an increase in the CBD diameter in older patients, even if with consistent variability.[6,7] Based on autopsy observations, authors have identified loss of elastic fibers and fragmentation of the longitudinal smooth myocyte bands in elderly subjects with proximal compensatory dilatation.[8,9] There could also be an element of hypotonicity of the choledochus due to use of drugs such as calcium channel blockers and nitroglycerine in elderly subjects. However, recent prospective studies with more than 1,000 patients aged between 60 and 90 years and followed up for 4 years demonstrated only a small increase in the caliber of the CBD with increasing age (60 years old or less, mean diameter 3.6 mm ± 0.2 mm, vs. over 85 years old, mean diameter 4 mm ± 0.2 mm, p = 0.009).[10] The authors concluded that although the CBD did increase in size with aging, 98% of CBDs remained below 6-7 mm, the commonly accepted upper range of normal.

Autopsy study of 655 patients suggested that there is dilatation of the choledochus in man after cholecystectomy as has been previously noted in animals. After removal of gallbladder with its powers of absorption and distensibility, the entire secretory pressure of the liver is transmitted to the walls of the choledochus and the sphincter of Oddi resulting in dilatation.[11] But it is also known that following the removal of gallbladder in dogs the sphincter of Oddi loses most of its tone and intraductal pressure falls to a much lower level than when normal gallbladder is intact. Studies which looked at this more critically by measuring CBD before the cholecystectomy and repeatedly at defined time intervals postoperatively for 5 years found no change in BD diameter before and following cholecystectomy.[12] A prospective study with 234 patients also observed that the diameter of the CBD measured on sonograms increase only slightly if at all after cholecystectomy and concluded that most patients do not have significant compensatory dilatation of the duct after cholecystectomy.[13]

Probably the most pragmatic way to summarize would be to state that combination of cholecystectomy and advancing age does tend to be associated with slightly larger extrahepatic bile ducts. This phenomenon is most appreciated in the middle segment of the bile duct where it is not surrounded by liver or pancreas.

CHOLEDOCHOLITHIASIS AND CBD DILATATION

At time of cholecystectomy, it has been estimated that 5-20% of patients have choledocholithiasis with the incidence increasing with age.[14,15] Although most patients with choledocholithiasis are symptomatic, occasional patients are asymptomatic and pose diagnostic and therapeutic dilemmas. In asymptomatic patients, the diagnosis may be suspected because of abnormal liver blood tests, abnormalities seen on imaging studies obtained for unrelated reasons, or when an intraoperative cholangiogram obtained during cholecystectomy suggests the presence of a CBD stone. Since liver tests may be elevated due to a wide variety of etiologies, the positive predictive value of elevated liver tests is poor. On the other hand, the negative predictive value of normal liver tests is high. Thus, normal liver tests play a greater role in excluding choledocholithiasis than elevated liver tests play in diagnosing stones. The sensitivity of transabdominal USG for choledocholithiasis ranges from 20 to 90%.[16] Stone is suspected when an intraductal echogenic focus is identified on longitudinal or transverse planes with or without ductal dilatation. One has to always bear in mind stone mimickers like intraductal gas which produce linear and mobile shadows, blood and sludge which produce diffuse echoes, hydatid membranes and surgical clips which lie outside the duct lumen. Transabdominal ultrasound has poor sensitivity for stones in the distal CBD because the distal CBD is often obscured by bowel gas in the imaging field.[17] The sensitivity of ERCP for choledocholithiasis is estimated to be 80-93%, with a specificity of 99-100%.[18,19] However, ERCP is invasive, requires technical expertise, and is associated with complications such as pancreatitis, bleeding, and perforation. As a result, ERCP is now reserved for patients who are at high risk for having a CBD stone, particularly if there evidence of cholangitis, or who have had a stone demonstrated on other imaging modalities. **Table 2** describes the criteria laid down by American Society of Gastrointestinal Endoscopists to classify patients as being at high and intermediate risk for choledocholithiasis.

Patients categorized as having a high risk of choledocholithiasis can be directly subjected to therapeutic ERCP. However, for patients at intermediate risk for choledocholithiasis, endoscopic ultrasound (EUS) or MRCP to be done to confirm the presence of choledocholithiasis before a therapeutic ERCP.

MRCP is noninvasive and EUS is certainly less invasive than ERCP. Both tests are highly sensitive and specific for choledocholithiasis.[20] Stone is identified as an intraluminal signal void in 2 thin section orthogonal planes on MRCP **(Fig. 3)**.

One has to be aware of certain pitfalls while interpreting MRCP images in a suspected case of choledocholithiasis.

TABLE 2: Risk factors which suggest presence of choledocholithiasis according to American Society of Gastrointestinal Endoscopy

High risk for choledocholithiasis; >50% risk of CBD stones	CBD stone on abdominal ultrasound OR
	Clinical acute cholangitis OR
	Serum bilirubin greater than 4 mg/dL with suspicion of stone on USG OR
	A dilated common bile duct on USG (more than 6 mm in a patient with a gallbladder in situ) and a serum bilirubin of 1.8 to 4 mg/dL
Intermediate risk for choledocholithiasis; 10-50% risk of CBD stones	A dilated common bile duct on ultrasound (more than 6 mm in a patient with a gallbladder in situ) OR
	A serum bilirubin of 1.8 to 4 mg/dL OR
	Abnormal liver biochemical test other than bilirubin OR
	Clinical gallstone pancreatitis

A signal void apparent on MRI may actually be the result of flow artifact and not an intraductal calculus. Flow void refers to low signal seen in vessels that contain vigorously flowing blood/fluid and is generally synonymous with vascular patency. Flow voids generally appear in a dilated CBD at site of insertion of cystic duct where swirling of flow can occur. An MRI image may miss stones due to partial volume effect **(Figs. 4A and B)**. This is caused by loss of contrast between two adjacent tissues in an image due to insufficient resolution so that more than one tissue occupies the same pixel. To improve the sensitivity and specificity of MRI, one should study thin-collimation

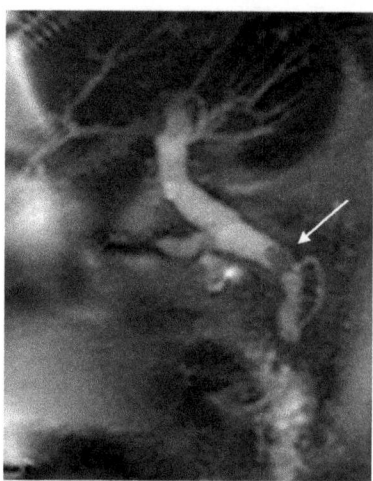

Fig. 3: Magnetic resonance cholangiopancreatography (MRCP) image showing (arrow) bile duct dilatation due to a stone.

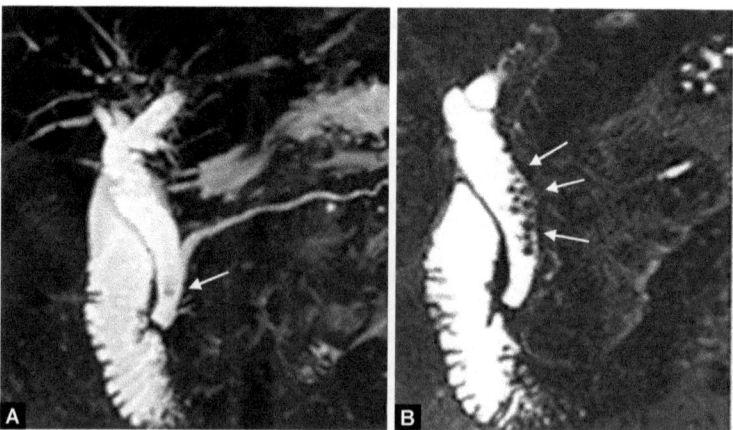

Figs. 4A and B: Errors due to partial volume effect on magnetic resonance cholangio-pancreatography (MRCP). Coronal maximum intensity projection reformat shows possible single filling defect (arrow) in dilated distal common bile duct (CBD). The thin section MRCP source image of the same patient in fact demonstrates multiple filling defects (arrows) in the CBD, in keeping with stones.

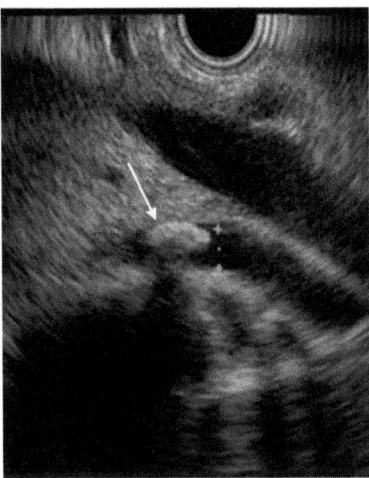

Fig. 5: Endoscopic ultrasound identifying (arrow) intraductal echogenic focus from a stone as the cause of biliary dilatation.

images which have a high spatial resolution and axial sections in addition to reformatted images for detecting small calculi. EUS provides excellent images of the CBD due to proximity of transducer in duodenum to the CBD which permits one to obtain high-resolution imaging without interference by overlying bowel gas. Intraductal stone appears as an intraductal echogenic focus with posterior acoustic shadowing (**Fig. 5**). EUS also offers opportunity to sample tissue/lesion thereby providing a histologic diagnosis. It also helps determine invasion and local staging of any malignant lesion.

Choosing between the two tests depends on various factors such as ease of availability, cost, patient-related factors, and the clinical suspicion for a small stone. Studies which have prospectively compared accuracy of EUS with MRCP in the diagnosis of choledocholithiasis have found the two to be comparable.[21,22] MRCP may be preferred for many patients as it is noninvasive. However, the sensitivity of MRCP may be lower than EUS for small stones <6 mm[23] and biliary sludge which are better picked up on EUS. Hence, EUS should be considered in patients in whom the suspicion for choledocholithiasis remains moderate to high despite a negative MRCP.

Intraoperative cholangiography (IOC) has an estimated sensitivity of 59–100% for diagnosing choledocholithiasis, with a specificity of 93–100% and has been suggested for patients with intermediate probability of having CBD stones if facilities for laparoscopic cholecystectomy and CBD exploration are available.[24] However, it is highly operator-dependent and may be technically unfeasible in patients with a severely inflamed gallbladder or with a short cystic duct.[25] Hence several surgeons do not routinely use IOC since asymptomatic common bile duct stones may pass spontaneously and/or have a low potential for causing complications, such that their identification may lead to unnecessary CBD exploration and/or conversion to open surgery.[26,27]

Another intraoperative approach for detecting choledocholithiasis is intraoperative ultrasonography. The reported sensitivity and specificity are over 90%, and it has been suggested that the routine use of intraoperative ultrasound followed by selective IOC and CBD exploration leads to the accurate diagnosis of choledocholithiasis, while reducing the need for routine IOC.[28] Compared with IOC, intraoperative ultrasound does not require entry into the bile duct. However, it is associated with a learning curve and is currently not as widely available.[29] The decision regarding intraoperative cholangiography or intraoperative ultrasonography depends upon patient selection and the surgeon's expertise and comfort with the techniques. CBD stones can also be picked up on contrast enhanced CT scans particularly when helical cholangiography protocol is used.[30] If a common bile duct stone is clearly visualized on CT, the finding is highly specific.

Chronic Pancreatitis and CBD Dilatation

EUS reveals features of chronic pancreatitis (CP) that are not appreciated with other imaging modalities. These include hyperechoic margins of the pancreatic duct, subtle lobularity of the parenchyma, small cystic changes in the parenchyma, and side branch duct ectasia. EUS should be the imaging modality of choice when evaluating biliary dilatation in suspected case of chronic pancreatitis avoiding need for further invasive investigations.

Mass Lesion and CBD Dilatation

When evaluating a dilated bile duct one wants to be absolutely certain of the absence of benign or malignant mass lesions anywhere from the porta till the ampulla of Vater. In this context it is helpful to have an idea of the level of biliary dilatation. Suspected small periampullary lesions can be elegantly assessed using EUS. Larger lesions can be assessed using contrast enhanced CT scans with multiplanar and cholangiography type reformats. Mass lesions suspected of producing hilar blocks are assessed using contrast enhanced MRI with coronal reconstructions.

Periampullary Diverticulum and CBD Dilatation

Duodenal diverticula have been reported in 2-5% of patients undergoing barium studies of the upper gastrointestinal tract, 7% of patients undergoing endoscopic retrograde cholangiopancreatography, and up to 20% in autopsy series.[31] But very few periampullary diverticula cause biliary indentation.[32] They may be associated with an increased risk of choledocholithiasis due to biliary stasis from extrinsic compression of CBD by diverticulum causing stasis-associated bacterial contamination with resultant deconjugation of bilirubin glucuronide and precipitation of bile salts and reflux through an incompetent sphincter of Oddi.[33] Lemmel's syndrome is a rare complication of periampullary duodenal diverticula, wherein there is obstruction of the intrapancreatic portion of the CBD by the periampullary diverticulum producing obstructive jaundice.[34] It can be suspected early on by the detection of a periampullary diverticulum and signs of distal bile obstruction. Pathogenesis varies from local compression to secondary sphincter of Oddi dysfunction or periampullary fibrosis.

Choledochal Cyst

Although the conventional terminology has been a choledochal cyst, but, because the anatomy may not always resemble a "cyst", the preferred nomenclature today is a congenital choledochal malformation (CCM). By definition, CCM refers to congenital bile duct dilatation affecting the extrahepatic bile duct with or without involvement of the intrahepatic bile duct. The configuration may be cystic wherein there is a distinct change in caliber both at the upper and lower end, or fusiform wherein the dilatation is mild and tapers gently. Although abdominal pain is the most frequent symptom in adult patients, non-specific symptoms are also reported and the cyst may be incidentally identified in patients undergoing radiologic evaluation for other clinical diagnosis.[35,36] Diagnosis of choledochal cyst and its classification is made on a cholangiography study, generally an MRCP. This is an important benign cause of biliary dilatation and may cause diagnostic confusion with secondary biliary dilatation from distal biliary obstruction due to stone or tumor. Demonstration of disproportionate central biliary dilatation, anomalous pancreaticobiliary junction, persistence of biliary dilatation even after endoscopic biliary stenting, a well distended gallbladder without stones and a long tortuous cystic duct and are some pointers toward a choledochal cyst (**Fig. 6**). These features become more relevant when attempting to differentiate a choledochal cyst from choledocholithiasis or early malignant BD obstruction, particularly in the asymptomatic patient.

It is also important to be aware of an anatomy wherein the biliary dilatation is minimal or absent but the patient presents with typical features of biliary obstruction or recurrent pancreatitis and a cholangiogram shows a long common channel which may contain sludge. This anatomy has been labeled as the forme fruste anatomy.[37,38] Forme fruste choledochal cyst (FFCC) is a known variant of a choledochal cyst that has minimal or no dilatation of the extrahepatic bile duct and is associated with pancreaticobiliary malunion (**Fig. 7**). Other subtle differences include higher incidences of dilatation of common pancreaticobiliary channel and presence of protein plugs or debris at the level of common channel in FFCC as compared to the classical choledochal cysts. Like choledochal cysts, the recommended treatment for symptomatic patients with FFCC is CBD excision and a bilioenteric anastomosis to achieve biliopancreatic disconnection.

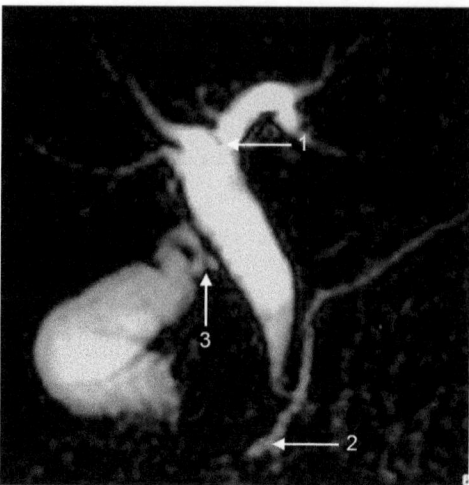

Fig. 6: Magnetic resonance cholangiopancreatography (MRCP) of cystic variant of choledochal cyst with typical features such as disproportionate central intrahepatic biliary dilatation (1), a long common pancreaticobiliary channel (2) and a long, tortuous, dilated cystic duct (3) which help differentiate from bile duct dilatation due to distal obstruction.

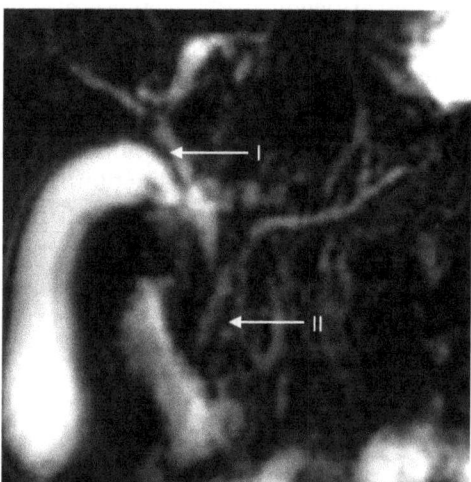

Fig. 7: Forme fruste variant of choledochal cyst with minimal dilatation of bile duct (I), long common pancreaticobiliary channel (II) in a patient with symptoms of jaundice or recurrent pancreatitis.

Biliary Stricture and CBD Dilatation

Biliary strictures can be benign resulting result from operative trauma or traumatic passage of BD stone or chronic pancreatitis or malignnat in nature. A benign stricture can be differentiated from a malignant one if it shows regular, symmetric, and short segment narrowing. Irregular, asymmetric, and long segment narrowing was more commonly found in malignant stricture.[39]

Other Causes of Bile Duct Dilatation

Rare causes of nonobstructive biliary dilatation are chronic opioid use and sphincter of Oddi dysfunction. In a recent study, opium addicts, symptomatic for abdominal pain were subjected to EUS. The authors observed CBD dilatation, especially in the extrahepatic tract, in all 15 patients and increased surface area of Vater's papilla in 12 of them, after a mean of 20 years of opium addiction.[40]

EVALUATION OF AN INCIDENTALLY DISCOVERED ASYMPTOMATIC OR MINIMALLY SYMPTOMATIC BILIARY DILATATION

Almost 95% of patients with biliary obstruction will have some form of biliary dilatation. There can be biliary obstruction without duct dilatation in some cases of choledocholithiasis, primary sclerosing cholangitis or postoperative structuring. But even in these patients if there is no demonstrable duct dilatation, there will be some clinical symptoms current or remote and/or biochemical abnormalities suggesting biliary obstruction and need for further evaluation by cholangiography. When opining on an USG report suggesting biliary dilatation (CBD diameter > 7 mm), it is important to bear in mind that bile duct dilatation beyond this level is not physiological and hence should be evaluated further.

Ultimately, the extent to which one investigates a patient with unexplained biliary dilatation depends on the presence of clinical symptoms and abnormal laboratory values, the probability of an underlying abnormality, and the appropriateness of further therapy if any abnormality is detected in the given patient. One has to be realistic in chasing the cause of biliary dilatation in an asymptomatic elderly patient with normal biochemistries who will not be a potential candidate for invasive intervention strategies because of comorbidities.

Although transabdominal USG provides a quick, noninvasive and a cheap method to evaluate the bile duct, it is operator-dependent and the image quality depends largely on the intervening tissues. When dealing with a patient with dilated bile duct demonstrated on initial USG, the first step is to determine the clinical probability that an underlying obstructive lesion is present. This decision is basic on the anatomical information about the level of obstruction (hilar block vs. distal obstruction) from the initial imaging study along with clinical and biochemical assessment. Presence of biliary tract symptoms, even if remote from the time of presentation and abnormalities on liver function tests greatly increase the diagnostic yield of further investigations.[41,42]

A bile duct dilatation reported on USG is generally verified and further investigated using either MRCP or EUS depending upon clinical suspicion, patient factors, and technical expertise.[43] MRCP is an excellent non-invasive modality for diagnosis of various pathologies causing CBD dilatation with its diagnostic results being comparable to ERCP.[44] Although advances in MR technology have improved the ability to image biliary abnormalities, the need for use of contrast and the inability to provide a histological diagnosis are its limitations.[45]

Endoscopic ultrasound, apart from providing important diagnostic information concerning the biliary anatomy, offers an opportunity to sample the tissue/lesion thereby providing a histologic diagnosis. It also helps determine invasion and local staging of any malignant lesion.[46] Scheiman et al., in a prospective study and cost analysis performed on a cohort of patients referred for ERCP, identified EUS as the preferred initial diagnostic test, compared to MRCP, for the evaluation of biliary system and identification of extrahepatic disease.[47]

Nonetheless the available literature is equivocal about the best way to approach patients with asymptomatic biliary dilatation as EUS is operator dependent while there are known pitfalls in interpreting MRI images. There is also lack of clarity about the role of EUS in patients where MRCP has not been able to pinpoint the etiology behind biliary dilatation when both modalities are optimally available. In clinical practice, we often encounter patients who have a dilated common bile duct (CBD) and thereafter undergo MRCP. The patients with a nondiagnostic MRCP pose a difficult diagnostic dilemma of either investigating further with modalities such as ERCP or assuring the patients that everything is normal and hence no further investigations are required. To answer this diagnostic dilemma, Rana et al. retrospectively evaluated patients who underwent EUS for unexplained dilatation of CBD on MRCP and subsequently underwent ERCP for confirmation of EUS findings or were followed-up for at least 1 year after EUS examination.[41] They found that EUS was able to establish diagnosis in 50% of patients with inconclusive MRCP. They found CBD stones in 15 (37.5%) with largest size of CBD stone being 9 mm, mass in CBD in 2 (5%), benign biliary stricture in 2 (5%), biliary stricture with underlying chronic pancreatitis in 1 (2.5%) patient. All the patients with abnormal LFT had a detectable CBD pathology whereas 20/30 (66.6%) patients with normal LFT had normal EUS findings. They concluded that EUS is a useful investigative modality for patients with unexplained CBD dilatation on MRCP. Other authors too have found utility of EUS in detecting a biliary pathology in presence of biliary dilatation and the yield increases in presence of symptoms or biochemical abnormalities.

RECENT ADVANCES IN BILIARY TRACT IMAGING

With advancement in technology, there has been renewed interest in not missing out early biliary tract neoplasia as a cause of incidental biliary dilatation. The various newer imaging modalities which have been explored in the setting of indeterminate biliary strictures are discussed here.

Intraductal Cholangioscopy in Evaluation of Dilated Bile Duct

In patients with indeterminate biliary strictures or filling defects, intraductal cholangioscopy permits direct inspection of the epithelium for subtle abnormalities or to obtain biopsies. Compared with conventional brush cytology or biopsy during ERCP, cholangioscopic visualization may enhance diagnosis by detecting "tumor vessels" (irregularly dilated and tortuous blood vessels) in the setting of malignancy. In addition, the presence of intraductal nodules or masses, infiltrative or ulcerated strictures, or papillary or villous mucosal projections may indicate malignancy and should prompt biopsies.[48]

Systems available for cholangiopancreatoscopy include endoscope-based systems, commonly referred to as "mother-daughter" systems and a catheter-based system (SpyGlass). Mother-daughter systems consist of a mother duodenoscope and a daughter cholangiopancreatoscope. The daughter scope is inserted through the accessory channel of the mother scope. Two endoscopists are required for mother-daughter systems. Daughter scopes range in diameter from 3.1-3.4 mm, with a working channel of 1.2 mm which permits passage of miniature biopsy forceps and intraductal lithotripsy fibers. The catheter-based system have a 0.77 mm optical probe that is passed through a 3.3 mm, 4-lumen catheter which also has a 2 mm working channel and two dedicated 0.6 mm irrigation channels. The tip of the catheter can be deflected in four directions. Spy glass can be operated by a single endoscopist. Complications specific to the performance of cholangioscopy include cholangitis, which is related to intraductal fluid irrigation and uncommonly, hemobilia and bile leaks attributable to intraductal lithotripsy.[49]

Intraductal Ultrasound in Evaluation of Dilated Bile Duct

The technical evolution of EUS has led to the development of small caliber intraductal ultrasound (IDUS) miniprobes (about 2 mm), which can be passed through standard endoscopes directly into the bile duct. The small caliber, flexibility, and excellent image quality produced by these catheters makes them ideal for evaluating cause of biliary obstruction and can also assist in local tumor staging.

In IDUS acoustic coupling is optimized by the tubular anatomy of the pancreatic and bile ducts, which are fluid filled and only slightly larger in caliber than the probe itself. In addition, the probes operate at higher frequencies (12-30 MHz) than standard EUS, which leads to higher image resolution and detailed examination of ductal and periductal tissues. However, the limited depth of penetration prevents examination of more distant sites. IDUS can help distinguish benign from malignant strictures based upon bile duct anatomy and unique sonographic imaging characteristics such as a hypoechoic mass, especially if infiltrating surrounding tissues, heterogeneity of the internal echo, notching or irregularity of the outer border, a papillary surface, disruption of the normal bile duct structure and suspicious lymph nodes (hypoechoic, round and smooth bordered).[50] Examination of more distant tissues is hindered by its limited depth of penetration. IDUS may also have limited value in evaluating lymph nodes, and unlike EUS, IDUS cannot be used to perform fine needle aspiration.

Three systems are available to perform IDUS:
- Electronic cylindrical phased array
- Combined probe (allows both radial and linear scanning)
- Mechanical radial sector scan system

Confocal Laser Endomicroscopy in Evaluation of Dilated Bile Duct

Confocal laser endomicroscopy (CLE) is an endoscopic technology for high-resolution assessment and "optical biopsies" of gastrointestinal mucosal histology at a cellular and subcellular level. CLE probe (pCLE) used for evaluation of biliary tract is very small (0.9 mm diameter) to fit through the biopsy channel of a cholangioscope. During cholangioscopy, the probe can be placed against the lesion or area of interest under direct visual control and guidance. The goal is to differentiate benign from malignant strictures. The available data on hepatobiliary CLE are promising. The hallmarks of neoplasia in the bile duct include epithelial structures characterized by glands or villi and increased vascularity. The reported sensitivity of CLE for diagnosing neoplasia is 83–98%, and the specificity is 67–100%.[51]

ADVANCES IN TISSUE SAMPLING TECHNIQUES AT ERCP AND ROLE OF BIOMARKERS

A biliary neoplasm typically appears as a stricture during ERCP. Some of the characteristics of malignant stricture are a length of more than 10 mm, a ragged contour, and the presence of a fixed filling defect and/or an abrupt transition from relatively normal to the stricture, so called shouldering, typically located above the stricture. Tissue diagnosis may be necessary when the cholangiographic images are not classical. Tissue sampling of suspected bile duct tumors can be obtained by cytologic brushings, biopsy forceps, bile aspiration, or a combination of all of these modalities. During cytological sampling, the expression of tumor markers by biliary neoplasms has been evaluated in several studies. Mutations in P53, k-ras and telomerase RNA in biliary samples have not shown consistent results. Assessing DNA proliferation by digital image analysis (DIA) and fluorescence in situ hybridization (FISH) have shown some promise in improving the specificity of cytology.[50] DIA quantifies the amount of cellular DNA by measuring the intensity of nuclei stained with a dye that binds to nuclear DNA. FISH uses fluorescently labeled DNA probe test to detect chromosomal abnormalities in cells. Adding DNA measurements as an adjunct to brush cytology in patients with biliary strictures has been suggested to increase diagnostic yield.[52]

A prospective study evaluating cholangiography, routine cytology, DIA and FISH of tissue samples, and intraductal ultrasound in 86 patients with indeterminate biliary strictures concluded that combination of DIA, FISH, and intraductal ultrasound increased the yield several-fold compared with routine cytology and histology alone.[50] Although exciting, all the above methods are limited by their restricted availability and essentially experimental status in the evaluation algorithms routinely applied during evaluation of an incidental dilatation of bile duct. Wider availability and more prospective data are needed before their indications and routine use become applicable in the setting of evaluation of an incidental bile duct dilatation.

CONCLUSION

It is important to have a clear and evidence-based approach to evaluation and management of an asymptomatic dilated biliary system. While those with sinister etiologies causing biliary obstruction should not be missed, it is also important that those who do not have a pathologic cause of biliary dilatation are not subjected to unnecessary invasive/semi-invasive evaluation. Presence of biliary tract symptoms and or abnormal LFTs can help identify the subset of patients with high pretest probability of an abnormality detected on further cross sectional imaging. CT scan is preferred when mass lesion is suspected and MRCP/EUS are recommended for biliary dilatation due to stone disease. It is good to keep in mind some of the rare causes of asymptomatic biliary dilatation. Finally, the truly asymptomatic patient with normal liver tests in whom bile duct dilatation is found incidentally and is not alarming can be followed closely with clinical and laboratory follow-up to help decide whether any additional imaging would be appropriate. Nonetheless, prospective studies with well-characterized patients and long-term follow-up are required to determine the ideal diagnostic algorithm for incidental CBD dilation incorporating the more recent advances in diagnostic imaging modalities.

REFERENCES

1. Smith I, Monkemuller K, Wilcox CM. Incidentally identified common bile duct dilatation. A systematic review of evaluation, causes, and outcome. J Clin Gastroenterol. 2015;49:810-5.
2. Coss A, Enns R. The investigation of unexplained biliary dilatation. Curr Gastroenterol Rep. 2009;11:155-9.
3. Wachsberg RH, Kim KH, Sundaram K. Sonographic versus ERCP measurements of the bile duct revisited: importance of the transverse diameter. AJR. 1998;170:669-74.
4. Jeon J, Song YS, Kyu TL, Lee KH, Bae MH, Lee JK. Clinical significance and long term outcome of incidentally found bile duct dilation. Dig Dis Sci. 2013;58:1-7.
5. Wu CC, Ho YH, Chen CY. Effect of aging on common bile duct diameter: a real-time ultrasonographic study. J Clin Ultrasound. 1984;12:473-8.
6. Bachar GN, Cohen M, Belenky A, Atar E, Gideon S. Effect of aging on the adult extrahepatic bile duct: a sonographic study. J Ultrasound Med. 2003;22:879-85.
7. Horrow MM. Ultrasound of the extrahepatic bile duct: issues of size. Ultrasound Q. 2010;26:67-74.

8. Nakada I. Changes in morphology of the distal common bile duct associated with aging. Gastroenterol JPN. 1981;16:54-63.
9. Kialian GP, Aznaurian AV. The age-related characteristics of the muscular layer of the common bile duct in man. Morfologiia. 1995;108:10-12.
10. Perret RS, Sloop GD, Borne JA. CBD measurements in elderly population. J Ultrasound Med. 2000;19:727-30.
11. Puestow CB, Morrison RB. The relationship of cholecystitis and cholecystectomy to dilatation of the choledochus. Ann Surg. 1935;101:599-602.
12. Majeed AW, Johnson AG. The preoperatively normal bile duct does not dilate after cholecystectomy: results of a five year study. Gut. 1999;45:741-3.
13. Feng B, Song Q. Does the common bile duct dilate after cholecystectomy? Sonographic evaluation in 234 patients. AJR. 1995;165:859-61.
14. Collins C, Maguire D, Ireland A, Fitzgerald E, O'Sullivan GC. A prospective study of common bile duct calculi in patients undergoing laparoscopic cholecystectomy: natural history of choledocholithiasis revisited. Ann Surg. 2004;239:28.
15. O'Neill CJ, Gillies DM, Gani JS. Choledocholithiasis: over diagnosed endoscopically and undertreated laparoscopically. ANZ J Surg. 2008;78:487.
16. Maple JT, Ben-Menachem T, Appalaneni V, Banerjee S, Cash BD, et al. ASGE Standards of Practice Committee. The role of endoscopy in the evaluation of suspected choledocholithiasis. Gastrointest Endosc. 2010;71:1.
17. Wermke W, Schulz HJ. Sonographic diagnosis of bile duct calculi. Results of a prospective study of 222 cases of choledocholithiasis. Ultraschall Med. 1987;8:116.
18. Prat F, Amouyal G, Amouyal P, Pelletier G, Fritsch J, Choury AD, et al. Prospective controlled study of endoscopic ultrasonography and endoscopic retrograde cholangiography in patients with suspected common-bile duct lithiasis. Lancet. 1996;347:75.
19. Gurusamy KS, Giljaca V, Takwoingi Y, Higgie D, Poropat G, Štimac D, et al. Endoscopic retrograde cholangiopancreatography versus intraoperative cholangiography for diagnosis of common bile duct stones. Cochrane Database Syst Rev. 2015;CD010339.
20. Giljaca V, Gurusamy KS, Takwoingi Y, Higgie D, Poropat G, Štimac D, et al. Endoscopic ultrasound versus magnetic resonance cholangiopancreatography for common bile duct stones. Cochrane Database Syst Rev. 2015;CD011549.
21. Verma D, Kapadia A, Eisen GM, Adler DG. EUS vs MRCP for detection of choledocholithiasis. Gastrointest Endosc. 2006;64:248.
22. Ledro-Cano D. Suspected choledocholithiasis: endoscopic ultrasound or magnetic resonance cholangio-pancreatography? A systematic review. Eur J Gastroenterol Hepatol. 2007;19:1007.
23. Zidi SH, Prat F, Le Guen O, Rondeau Y, Rocher L, Fritsch J, et al. Use of magnetic resonance cholangiography in the diagnosis of choledocholithiasis: prospective comparison with a reference imaging method. Gut. 1999;44:118.
24. Videhult P, Sandblom G, Rasmussen IC. How reliable is intraoperative cholangiography as a method for detecting common bile duct stones? A prospective population-based study on 1171 patients. Surg Endosc. 2009;23:304.
25. Massarweh NN, Devlin A, Elrod JA, Symons RG, Flum DR. Surgeon knowledge, behavior, and opinions regarding intraoperative cholangiography. J Am Coll Surg. 2008;207:821.
26. Snow LL, Weinstein LS, Hannon JK, Lane DR. Evaluation of operative cholangiography in 2043 patients undergoing laparoscopic cholecystectomy: a case for the selective operative cholangiogram. Surg Endosc. 2001;15:14.
27. Nickkholgh A, Soltaniyekta S, Kalbasi H. Routine versus selective intraoperative cholangiography during laparoscopic cholecystectomy: a survey of 2,130 patients undergoing laparoscopic cholecystectomy. Surg Endosc. 2006;20:868.

28. Machi J, Oishi AJ, Tajiri T, Murayama KM, Furumoto NL, Oishi RH. Routine laparoscopic ultrasound can significantly reduce the need for selective intraoperative cholangiography during cholecystectomy. Surg Endosc. 2007;21:270.
29. Machi J, Tateishi T, Oishi AJ, Furumoto NL, Oishi RH, Uchida S, et al. Laparoscopic ultrasonography versus operative cholangiography during laparoscopic cholecystectomy: review of the literature and a comparison with open intraoperative ultrasonography. J Am Coll Surg. 1999;188:360.
30. Tseng CW, Chen CC, Chen TS, Chang FY, Lin HC, Lee SD. Can computed tomography with coronal reconstruction improve the diagnosis of choledocholithiasis? J Gastroenterol Hepatol. 2008;23:1586.
31. Leivonen MK, Halttunen JA, Kivilaakso EO. Duodenal diverticulum at endoscopic retrograde cholangiopancreatography, analysis of 123 patients. Hepatogastroenterology. 1996;43(10):961.
32. Kim JE, Lee JK, Lee KT, Park DI, Hyun JG, Paik SW, et al. The clinical significance of common bile-duct dilatation in patients without biliary symptoms or causative lesions on ultrasonography. Endoscopy. 2001;33:495-500.
33. Bruno M, Ribaldone DG, Fasulo R, Gaia S, Marietti M, Risso A, et al. Is there a link between periampullary diverticula and biliopancreatic disease? An EUS approach to answer the question. Dig Liver Dis. 2018;50(9):925.
34. Khan BA, Khan SH, Sharma A. Lemmel's Syndrome: a rare cause of obstructive jaundice secondary to periampullary diverticulum. Eur J Case Rep Intern Med. 2017;4(6):000632.
35. Liu YB, Wang JW, Devkota KR, Ji ZL, Li JT, Wang XA, et al. Congenital choledochal cysts in adults: twenty-five-year experience. Chin Med J (Engl). 2007;120:1404-7.
36. Law R, Topazian M. Diagnosis and treatment of choledochoceles. Clin Gastroenterol Hepatol. 2014;12:196-203.
37. Lilly JR, Stellin GP, Karrer FM. Forme fruste choledochal cyst. J Pediatric Surg. 1985;20(4):449-51.
38. Shimotakahara A, Yamataka A, Kobayashi H, Okada Y, Yanai T, Lane GJ, et al. Forme fruste choledochal cyst: long-term follow-up with special reference to surgical technique. J Pediatr Surg. 2003;38(12):1833-6.
39. Suthar M, Purohit S, Bhargav V, Goyal P. Role of MRCP in Differentiation of Benign and Malignant Causes of Biliary Obstruction. J Clin Diagn Res. 2015;9(11):TC08-12.
40. Sharma SS, Ram S, Maharshi S, Shankar V, Katiyar P, Jhajharia A, et al. Pancreato-biliary Endoscopic Ultrasound in Opium Addicts Presenting with Abdominal Pain. Endosc Ultrasound. 2013;2:204-7.
41. Rana SS, Bhasin DK, Sharma V, Rao C, Gupta R, Singh K. Role of endoscopic ultrasound in evaluation of unexplained common bile duct dilatation on magnetic resonance cholangiopancreatography. Ann Gastroenterol. 2013;26:66-70.
42. Oppong KW, Mitra V, Scott J, Anderson K, Charnley RM, Bonnington S, et al. Endoscopic ultrasound in patients with normal liver blood tests and unexplained dilatation of common bile duct and or pancreatic duct. Scand J Gastroenterol. 2014;49:473-80.
43. Fernandez-Esparrach G, Gines A, Sanchez M, Pagés M, Pellisé M, Fernández-Cruz L, et al. Comparison of endoscopic ultrasonography and magnetic resonance cholangiopancreatography in the diagnosis of pancreatobiliary diseases: a prospective study. Am J Gastroenterol. 2007;102:1632-9.
44. Hekimoglu K, Ustundag Y, Dusak A, Erdem Z, Karademir B, Aydemir S, et al. MRCP vs. ERCP in the evaluation of biliary pathologies: review of current literature. J Dig Dis. 2008;9:162-9.
45. Holm AN, Gerke H. What should be done with a dilated bile duct? Curr Gastroenterol Rep. 2010;12:150-6.
46. Godfrey EM, Rushbrook SM, Carroll NR. Endoscopic ultrasound: a review of current diagnostic and therapeutic applications. Postgrad Med J. 2010;86:346-53.
47. Scheiman JM, Carlos RC, Barnett JL, Elta GH, Elta GH, Nostrant TT, Chey WD, et al. Can endoscopic ultrasound or magnetic resonance cholangiopancreatography replace

ERCP in patients with suspected biliary disease? A prospective trial and cost analysis. Am J Gastroenterol. 2001;96:2900-4.
48. Seo DW, Lee SK, Yoo KS, Kang GH, Kim MH, Suh DJ, et al. Cholangioscopic findings in bile duct tumors. Gastrointest Endosc. 2000;52:630.
49. Sethi A, Chen YK, Austin GL, Brown WR, Brauer BC, Fukami NN, et al. ERCP with cholangiopancreatoscopy may be associated with higher rates of complications than ERCP alone: a single-center experience. Gastrointest Endosc. 2011;73:251.
50. Levy MJ, Baron TH, Clayton AC, Enders FB, Gostout CJ, Halling KC, et al. Prospective evaluation of advanced molecular markers and imaging techniques in patients with indeterminate bile duct strictures. Am J Gastroenterol. 2008;103:1263.
51. Slivka A, Gan I, Jamidar P, Costamagna G, Cesaro P, Giovannini M, et al. Validation of the diagnostic accuracy of probe-based confocal laser endomicroscopy for the characterization of indeterminate biliary strictures: results of a prospective multicenter international study. Gastrointest Endosc. 2015;81:282.
52. Lindberg B, Enochsson L, Tribukait B, Arnelo U, Bergquist A. Diagnostic and prognostic implications of DNA ploidy and S-phase evaluation in the assessment of malignancy in biliary strictures. Endoscopy. 2006;38:561.

CHAPTER 8

Antibiotics in Abdominal Surgery: Current Guidelines and Practices

S Suresh Kumar, R Kalayarasan, Vikram Kate, N Ananthakrishnan

INTRODUCTION

Surgical site infection (SSI) is the most common health care associated infection among hospitalized patients and the most common nosocomial infection in surgical wards.[1] SSI rates considerably increase when the surgery is performed on the gastrointestinal tract ranging up to 30% compared to other general surgical procedures.[1,2] The reason for the higher rate of SSIs is that the GI tract harbors a high load of bacteria including anaerobic organisms from the gut mucosa.[1-3]

Patients who develop SSIs may require treatment in the intensive care unit and are also likely to require readmission.[2] Furthermore, SSI nearly doubles the mortality rate compared to those with an uneventful postoperative course. Surgical site infection in addition to causing significant morbidity, adds considerable burden to the healthcare cost due to additional investigations, secondary procedures and prolonged hospitalization.[4] Various risk factors have been identified for surgical site infection and many of them are preventable by optimizing patients in the perioperative period with appropriate glycemic control, maintenance of normothermia, perioperative supplemental oxygen, etc. Surgical antimicrobial prophylaxis is one among several accepted and proven methods to effectively reduce SSI.

PROPHYLACTIC ANTIBIOTIC RECOMMENDATIONS: GENERAL PRINCIPLES

Surgery on the gastrointestinal tract carries higher risk of wound infection due to the high bacterial load in the gut.[5] Majority of the operative procedures in the gastrointestinal (GI) tract falls into the clean-contaminated or contaminated wound class [as per the surgical wound classification of Centers for Disease Control and Prevention (CDC)] and hence the rate of SSI is higher and requires antimicrobial prophylaxis. In addition to the gram-positive skin flora (*Streptococcal species, Staphylococcus aureus,* coagulase negative *staphylococci*), gram-negative rods and Enterococci are frequently isolated from the SSI after GI tract surgery indicating the need for prophylactic cover against these organisms by appropriate antibiotics.

The goal of antimicrobial prophylaxis is to prevent SSI by reducing the burden of microorganisms at the surgical site during the operative procedure.

Efficacy of antibiotic prophylaxis for reducing SSI has been clearly established by multiple randomized trials and meta-analyses.[6,7] The guidelines for selecting appropriate antibiotic have been framed by World Health Organization (WHO), CDC, National Institute of Care and Excellence (NICE), etc. for easy access and reference. Though wound classification gives an estimation of expected rate of SSI, alone it is a poor predictor of overall risk of SSI. Other factors, such as operative technique, length of surgery and pre-existing comorbidity of the patients also influences development of SSI.

The practice of antimicrobial prophylaxis implies the following considerations.

- *Appropriate antibiotic selection:* The aim is to provide serum and tissue concentrations exceeding minimum inhibitory concentration (MIC) for probable organisms at the time of incision and for the duration of procedure. Pharmacokinetics and dynamics of the selected antibiotic as well as patient factors such as allergy, renal/ liver failure etc. need to be kept in mind while selecting the antimicrobial agent.

  Cefazoline is the preferred agent for antimicrobial prophylaxis in majority of GI procedures due to its moderate serum half-life of 2 hours with good anti-staphylococcal activity and activity against gram-negative organisms.[6-8] It's established safety profile and low cost makes it the most commonly used antimicrobial agent for surgical prophylaxis. However, it requires frequent redosing if surgery is prolonged more than 2-3 hours.

  Ceftriaxone is used in many centers in the place of cefazoline due to its longer half-life (8 hours). The plasma concentration of ceftriaxone remains higher than the MIC even after 24 hours for most pathogens. Due to its high protein binding, no redosing is needed even after massive bleeding or reopening within 24 hours. The main limitation for using ceftriaxone is the higher cost. It's also less effective than cefazoline against *S. aureus.*

- *Second line prophylaxis:* Patients with known allergy to beta-lactam antibiotics with the history of developing urticarial rash or anaphylaxis within 72 hours of administration of beta lactam antibiotics or previous documented drug fever or serious drug reactions such as toxic epidermal necrolysis are considered for second line antimicrobial prophylaxis.[9] Patients who are colonized with methicillin-resistant *S. aureus (MRSA)* or with methicillin-resistant coagulase-negative *staphylococci* are also candidates for second line antimicrobial prophylaxis. These patients may be given vancomycin (15-20 mg/kg) or clindamycin (40-60 mg/kg/day or 600-900 mg eight hourly). Gentamicin and ciprofloxacin are also considered depending on the local antimicrobial resistance pattern of the hospital.

- *Adequate dosing and redosing:* Standard dose in adults are easier to follow; however, weight based higher dosing may be required in obese patients.[10] For example, the standard dose of cefazoline is 1g; however, if the body weight is >80 kg, it is recommended to give 2 g dose, and if weight >120 kg, 3 g dose is recommended. Special consideration is also required for obese patients as lipophilic drugs such as vancomycin might fail in low dose, whereas aminoglycosides (hydrophilic) might result in excess concentration. Redosing is generally recommended if the operative procedure is longer than 2 hours or exceeds two half-lives of the antimicrobial agent given. Redosing is also to be considered in case of excessive bleeding (>1,500 mL).[6-10] Redosing may be deferred in cases where elimination of drug may be delayed as in renal insufficiency.

- *Route of administration:* Intravenous administration is recommended for rapid, reliable, and predictable serum concentration with maximum bioavailability. Oral route may be considered for colonic surgery for *Clostridium difficile* infection or pseudomembranous colitis.
- *Optimum timing for antibiotic administration:* Many studies have evaluated the optimum timing of the initial dose of prophylactic antibiotics. Classen et al. studied the occurrence of SSIs in 2,847 patients who underwent clean or clean-contaminated surgical wound and found that the rate of SSI was lowest when the prophylactic antibiotic was given 0–2 hours before the incision compared to earlier preoperative or intraoperative or postoperative dosing.[11] Excepting the drugs requiring infusion such as vancomycin and ciprofloxacin, CDC recommends prophylactic antibiotic to be given within 60 minutes prior to the skin incision so as to achieve the MIC in the blood at the time of incision.

    Studies comparing less than 30 minutes versus 30–60 minutes before skin incision for prophylactic antibiotic administration failed to prove any further reduction in the rate of SSIs.[12-14] Additional prophylaxis with antimicrobial agents should be administered before surgery even in patients who are getting therapeutic antibiotics (e.g., diagnosed acute appendicitis or diverticulitis) in order to achieve the MIC during the skin incision.
- *Duration of antimicrobial prophylaxis:* It is recommended to not repeat the antibiotic dose after skin closure, as it does not provide additional protection against SSI. McDonald et al. in their meta-analysis showed that multiple doses after surgery do not provide any benefit compared to the single dose of antimicrobial dose before surgery.[15] Bernatz et al. have shown that unwarranted antibiotic administration is one of the major risk factors for *C. difficile* infection among surgical patients.[16]

ANTIBIOTICS FOR BILIARY PROCEDURES

Elective Laparoscopic Cholecystectomy

Laparoscopic cholecystectomy is considered as the gold standard for symptomatic gall stone disease and is the most commonly performed minimally invasive procedure in the elective setting. It is reported to have lesser rates of SSI.[17,18] Traditionally, one dose of prophylactic antibiotic was given in the past to all the patients undergoing laparoscopic cholecystectomy. This practice was questioned by many studies as antibiotic prophylaxis was not shown to offer any benefit in low risk elective laparoscopic cholecystectomy and was shown to increase the cost of the treatment.[19-21] The rate of SSI with prophylactic antibiotic was shown to be 0–4% whereas it was 0–7% without prophylaxis with no statistical significance in SSI rates between the two groups.[19-21]

Prophylaxis is generally recommended only for high-risk patients, which include age more than 70 years, ASA classification of 3 or greater, pregnancy, diabetes mellitus, obesity, nonfunctioning gallbladder, and immunosuppression. Common organisms isolated from SSI following laparoscopic cholecystectomy include gram-negative bacilli *Escherichia coli*, *Klebsiella species* and *Enterococci*. The recommended prophylaxis for high-risk laparoscopic cholecystectomy is shown in **Table 1**.

The role of prophylactic antibiotic for low risk laparoscopic cholecystectomy has regained interest in recent years as some studies have shown benefit in terms of reduced rate of SSIs.[22,23] Liang et al. in their meta-analysis of 21 randomized controlled trials (RCTs), concluded that prophylactic antibiotic administration significantly reduces the SSI.[24] Meta-analysis by Kim et al. also supports administering prophylactic antibiotic in elective low risk cholecystectomy.[25] A more practical approach for giving antimicrobial prophylaxis for elective laparoscopic cholecystectomy would be to identify subset of patients who are likely to benefit with prophylactic antibiotics.

In addition to the high-risk group mentioned earlier, those with increased risk of infectious complications should be considered for prophylaxis. High risk for infectious complications includes patients who had biliary colic within 30 days before surgery, patients with jaundice or common bile duct stones and expected risk of conversion to open cholecystectomy, intraoperative rupture of gall bladder and spillage of bile or gallstones, reintervention for noninfectious complication within a month and acute cholecystitis.

TABLE 1: Antimicrobial prophylaxis for laparoscopic cholecystectomy.

	Antibiotic	Dose	Half-life* (Hours)	Redosing interval (Hours)
First line	Cefazoline	2 g IV 3 g for >120 kg BW	1.2–2.2	4
Second line (For patients with beta-lactam allergy)	Clindamycin or vancomycin + Gentamicin Metronidazole + Gentamicin	Clindamycin 900 mg Vancomycin 15 mg/kg Gentamicin 5 mg/kg Metronidazole 500 mg	2–4 4–8 2–3 6–8	6 NA NA NA

*In adults with normal renal and liver function

As it is difficult to predict many of these high-risk factors preoperatively, proponents of routine antibiotic prophylaxis consider one dose of preoperative antibiotic in all elective laparoscopic cholecystectomy a rational choice.

Other Biliary Procedures

Antimicrobial prophylaxis is not recommended in patients subjected to endoscopic retrograde cholangio-pancreatography, both diagnostic and therapeutic for retrieval of stone even in the presence of stone or a stricture.[26] However, if the patient has features of cholangitis or obstructive jaundice due to bile duct obstruction, they may be considered for antibiotic prophylaxis.[26,27] The rate of SSIs reported in other biliary surgeries including open cholecystectomy, bile duct exploration and bilio-enteric anastomoses ranges from 1 to 19%.[27,28] In addition to wound infection, significant proportion of septic complications is also reported following biliary surgery. Cainzos et al. studied 280 patients who underwent various biliary procedures and demonstrated a rate of 7.5% of septic complications with a significantly prolonged length of hospitalization including an incidence of 1.8% of intra-abdominal abscess.[29]

Common organisms encountered in postoperative infection following open biliary surgery include enteric gram-negative bacilli *E. coli*, *Klebsiella* species, and *Enterococci*.[28-30] Bacteriological studies have also revealed *Clostridium* species isolated by anaerobic culture from postoperative wound infections after open cholecystectomy and bile duct surgery. Less commonly, skin isolates streptococci and staphylococci are attributed as the cause of postoperative SSI following biliary tract surgery.

Though bile culture obtained intraoperatively has demonstrated similar microbial flora, positive culture did not significantly correlate with postoperative wound infection.[31,32] Wound infection and septic complications have been shown to be significantly high in patients not receiving prophylactic antibiotics compared to the antimicrobial prophylaxis group in most biliary tract procedures except the low risk laparoscopic cholecystectomy. Current guidelines advocate that any open biliary surgical procedures require prophylactic antibiotic administration to reduce the wound complication. The recommended antimicrobial prophylaxis is given in **Table 2**.

Antibiotics for Acute Cholecystitis

Acute cholecystitis is associated with the presence of biliary infection with significant physiological derangement. Considering the presence of acute infection and the probability of progression to severe septic complications in untreated patients, biliary tract infections are treated as per guidelines for complicated intra-abdominal infections.[33] Though the magnitude of infection is lesser compared to the severe biliary infections such as cholangitis, patients with cholecystitis experience considerable morbidity.

TABLE 2: Antimicrobial prophylaxis for biliary tract procedures.

	Antibiotic	Dose	Half-life* (Hours)	Redosing interval (Hours)
First line	Cefazoline	2 g for < 120 kg 3 g for > 120 kg	1.2–2.2	4
	Ampicillin-sulbactam	3 g (ampicillin 2 g/ sulbactam 1 g)	0.8–1.3	2
Second line (For patients with beta-lactam allergy)	Clindamycin or vancomycin + Gentamicin	Clindamycin 900 mg Vancomycin 15 mg/kg Gentamicin 5 mg/kg	2–4 4–8 2–3	6 NA NA
	Metronidazole + Gentamicin	Metronidazole 500 mg	6–8	NA

*In adults with normal renal and liver function

Tokyo guidelines 2018 (TG 18) provide severity classification to categorize cholecystitis patients according to the disease severity.[34] This classification is widely used to assess morbidity and mortality among cholecystitis patients and also to identify the subset of population who will benefit by prophylactic antibiotics.[34,35] Grade I patients are otherwise healthy patients without any evidence of organ dysfunction and only mild gallbladder inflammation. Laparoscopic cholecystectomy remains the choice for mild acute cholecystitis patients presenting within 72 hours and who are low risk patients (ASA 1 or II).[36,37] One dose of prophylactic antibiotic is recommended for mild cholecystitis before surgery. Studies have shown no benefit of administering further dose of antibiotics postoperatively after emergency cholecystectomy for mild cholecystitis in terms of postoperative wound complications.[38,39] Grade II patients in TG18 include those with signs of systemic inflammation evident from elevated total count and local complications such as gangrenous or emphysematous cholecystitis, peri-cholecystic or hepatic abscess and biliary peritonitis. Mortality among these patients is reported to be as high as 4.7%; all moderately severe cholecystitis patients should receive empirical antibiotic course and followed by culture-based antibiotic till the gallbladder is removed or the inflammation/infection subsides.[35,40] Grade III patients with severe cholecystitis show evidence of one or more organ failure and carry 8.4% mortality due to severe sepsis.[41] Emergency cholecystectomy for acute cholecystitis carries a higher rate of postoperative wound complications due to presence of systemic inflammation and infection.[42]

The organisms isolated from the biliary tract infections include predominantly enteric gram-negative organisms. *E. coli* (62%) and *Klebsiella spp.* (28%) are the frequent isolate from the bile culture; less commonly, *Pseudomonas* (14%). *Enterobacter* (7%) and *Acinetobacter* (3%) are also isolated from biliary tract infections.[43] Third generation cephalosporins ceftriaxone or

TABLE 3: Antimicrobial prophylaxis for acute cholecystitis.				
	Antibiotic	Dose	Half-life* (Hours)	Re-dosing interval (Hours)
Mild acute cholecystitis (TG18 Grade I)	Ceftriaxone or Cefotaxime	2 g 1 g	5.4–10.9 0.9–1.7	NA 3
Moderately severe (TG18 Grade II and III)	Piperacillin- Tazobactam or Cefoperazone-Sulbactam	4.5 g 3 g	0.7–1.2 1.6-3	NA NA

*In adults with normal renal and liver function

cefotaxime are considered reasonable choice for the prophylaxis for patients undergoing emergency cholecystectomy for mild acute cholecystitis.[35,44] Ceftriaxone antimicrobial prophylaxis should also be given for suspected acute biliary tract infections that may not have been diagnosed prior to elective laparoscopic cholecystectomy.[45] Moderately severe and severe cholecystitis patients in addition to antibiotics, require more intense treatment including fluid resuscitation, source control by drainage or surgery and management for organ dysfunction. Antibiotics with broad spectrum of coverage (Piperacillin and tazobactam) for extended duration are generally advocated for these patients.[33] Intravenous administration of Imipenem 500 mg, 6 hourly orMeropenem 1 g, 8 hourly also are considered in patients in severe sepsis with organ failure.[46] Recommendations for antimicrobial prophylaxis for patients undergoing emergency laparoscopic cholecystectomy for mild acute cholecystitis (TG18 Grade I) and therapeutic antibiotic recommendations for moderately severe and severe acute cholecystitis (TG 18 Grade II and III) are shown in **Table 3**.

ANTIBIOTICS FOR ACUTE APPENDICITIS

Acute appendicitis is the most common emergency operation performed and appendectomy still remains the mainstay of treatment for both simple and complex appendicitis.[47] The presentation ranges from uncomplicated simple appendicitis in up to 80%, presenting with migrating abdominal pain to complex appendicitis presenting with gangrene, perforation, intra-abdominal or pelvic abscess formation and less commonly with signs of peritonitis.[48] Presence of fecolith increases the likelihood of perforation and gangrene due to luminal obstruction.

Common organisms isolated from appendectomy wound infections include anaerobic and aerobic gram-negative enteric organisms. Among the anaerobes *Bacteroides fragilis* is the most frequently cultured from the wound. *E. coli* is the most commonly isolated aerobe. Less frequently isolated organisms include aerobic and anaerobic *Streptococci, Staphylococcus spp.*, and *Enterococcus*.[49] Many controlled trials have evaluated the role of prophylactic antibiotics in appendectomy and have shown clear benefit of administering antimicrobial prophylaxis to reduce postoperative wound complications.[50,51] The rate of SSI after appendectomy without antimicrobial prophylaxis has been reported to be as high as 30%. National Healthcare Safety Network (NHSN) in 2009 reported a mean SSI rate of 1.2% for risk categories 0 and 1 and 3.5% for risk categories 2 and 3 following appendectomy.[2] Complex appendicitis increases the chance of postoperative SSIs and other complications fourfold compared to the simple appendicitis.

Laparoscopic appendectomy has been shown to have low postoperative wound complications in terms of superficial and deep SSI compared to open appendectomy; however, there are also reports of higher organ space infection after laparoscopic appendectomy.[17,52,53] The current recommendation is to give prophylactic antibiotics in both simple and complex appendectomy.[45,54] There is no evidence to show any benefit of continuing antibiotics in the postoperative period for simple appendicitis; however, it has been shown in many studies that continuing antibiotic after surgery for complex appendicitis considerably reduces postoperative complications including SSI.[55] Complicated appendicitis is treated as complicated intra-abdominal infection with the therapeutic course of antibiotics for a longer duration.[33]

Considering the mixed aerobic and anaerobic spectrum of bacteria implicated in appendectomy wound infection, monotherapy using second-generation cephalosporin with anaerobic activity or a first-generation cephalosporin in combination with metronidazole is considered a reasonable choice. Third generation cephalosporins with partial anaerobic activity have also been shown to reduce the rate of SSIs to <5%. Morris et al., in their randomized placebo-controlled trial, randomly allocated 271 patients with appendicitis to receive either cefazoline or metronidazole monotherapy or in combination. They found that the combination of cefazoline and metronidazole significantly reduces wound complications compared to the other three arms.[56] The recommended antimicrobial prophylaxis is given in **Table 4**.

ACUTE PANCREATITIS

Acute pancreatitis is a common abdominal emergency associated with high morbidity and mortality primarily due to septic complications. While majority of patients have mild self-limiting acute pancreatitis, a small proportion develop severe acute pancreatitis.[57] Early phase (first 2 weeks) of severe pancreatitis is characterized by early systemic inflammatory response syndrome with or without multiple organ dysfunction syndrome. Approximately one-fifth of patients develop secondary bacterial infection and septic complications that usually occurs 2-3 weeks after the onset of pancreatitis.[58] As infection is a major cause of mortality, the role of antibiotics has been extensively studied. To determine the timing and type of antibiotics it is important to understand the pathogenesis of infection in acute pancreatitis.

TABLE 4: Antimicrobial prophylaxis for acute appendicitis.

	Antibiotic	Dose	Half-life* (Hours)	Re-dosing interval (Hours)
First line	Cefazoline Or Metronidazole	2 g for < 120 kg 3 g for > 120 kg Metronidazole 500 mg	1.2–2.2 6–8	4 NA
Second line (For patients with beta-lactam allergy)	Clindamycin + Gentamicin Metronidazole + Gentamicin	Clindamycin 900 mg Gentamicin 5 mg/kg Metronidazole 500 mg	2–4 2–3 6–8	6 NA NA

*In adults with normal renal and liver function

Pathogenesis of Infection in Acute Pancreatitis

The routes of infection in acute pancreatitis are:[59]
- Bacterial translocation from the gut to the portal system and systemic circulation due to impaired gut mucosal defense mechanism.
- From the biliary system especially in patients with biliary pancreatitis secondary to stones in the biliary tract
- Ascending infection from the duodenum through the ampulla and pancreatic duct
- Infection from the colon due to bacterial translocation through lymphatics

Implication of gut organisms as the primary source of infection is supported by the fact that commonly isolated microbes in infected pancreatic necrosis are Gram-negative bacteria (*E. coli, Klebsiella*) normally seen in the intestinal lumen. Gram positive bacteria (*Enterococcus, S. aureus*), anaerobes and fungi (anaerobes) have also been implicated as the source of infection in approximately 20–30% of patients with acute pancreatitis.[60]

Role of Prophylactic Antibiotics in Acute Pancreatitis

The use of antibiotics to prevent infection is still controversial; many authors have advocated their routine use while others decry it. The proponents of prophylactic antibiotics suggest that close to 50% of patients with severe acute pancreatitis develop infection and it contributes to mortality in three-fourths of patients with necrotizing pancreatitis.[61]

Golub et al. published the first meta-analysis of eight RCTs on the role of prophylactic antibiotics in acute severe pancreatitis and concluded that they reduce mortality by reducing the pancreatic and extra pancreatic infections.[62] Two more meta-analysis of RCTs published in 2001 and 2006 by Sharma et al. and Villatoro et al. also supported the beneficial role of prophylactic antibiotics.[63,64] A Cochrane review by Bassi et al. published in 2003 concluded that parenteral antibiotic prophylaxis for 10–14 days reduced the risk of superinfection of pancreatic tissue and its associated mortality.[65] An updated meta-analysis of eleven RCTs published by Jiang et al. in the year 2012, however, concluded that routine use of prophylactic antibiotics in patients with severe acute pancreatitis is not to be recommended.[66] Interestingly in the funnel plot analysis the authors found asymmetric distribution of RCTs published before 2000, suggesting a possibility of publication bias,[66] viz., publication of trials with positive results as they were accepted easily for publication compared to trials with negative results that were less easily published. The pooled analysis of four RCTs published before 2000 found a significant reduction in mortality in the antibiotics arm (5.26%) compared to the placebo/no antibiotics group (18.18%).[66] However, there was no significant difference in the mortality between two groups (15.0% vs. 15.7%) in the pooled analysis of seven well designed RCTs published after 2000.[10] In clinical practice as evidenced by multiple surveys of international scientific associations, prophylactic antibiotics are still used by 40–70% of physicians in different regions of the globe.[67] The emergence of multiresistant gram-positive and fungal infections is a major problem with the nonindicated use of prophylactic antibiotics. Hence, the 2019 World Society for Emergency Surgery (WSES) guidelines for the management of severe acute pancreatitis gave a Level IA recommendation that routine prophylactic antibiotics should not be administered for severe acute pancreatitis as it is not associated with significant reduction in morbidity and mortality.[68]

Therapeutic Antibiotics for Infected Pancreatic Necrosis

Unlike sterile pancreatic necrosis there is no controversy in the role of antibiotics for infected acute pancreatitis. However, definite diagnosis of infected pancreatic necrosis remains a challenge as systemic inflammatory response seen in patients with severe pancreatitis often mimics infection. The investigation of choice to document infection is CT-guided fine needle aspiration cytology (FNAC) from the area of pancreatic necrosis as it will also guide management by selecting appropriate antibiotics.[69] However, it is an invasive procedure and is associated with high false negative results. Presence of gas within the necrotic areas on cross sectional imaging also signifies infection. However, this finding is seen only in a small proportion of patients with infected pancreatic necrosis.[69] Hence, serum markers are commonly used to determine infection. Although inflammatory biomarkers namely the CRP and WBC are highly sensitive, they are nonspecific to determine infection. Serum procalcitonin, an inactive 116 amino acid propeptide of the biologically active hormone calcitonin has been found to be a reliable serum marker to determine infected pancreatic necrosis.[70]

In patients with infected pancreatic necrosis antibiotics known to penetrate pancreatic necrosis should be used.[71] Aminoglycosides have poor penetration; acyl ureidopenicillins and third generation cephalosporins have an intermediate penetration whereas Quinolones and carbapenems have shown good pancreatic tissue penetration. In view of widespread resistance to quinolones, carbapenems remain the antibiotic of choice for critically ill patients with infected pancreatic necrosis.[71] In addition to their activity against commonly implicated gram-negative organisms they are also effective against anaerobes. Of the antibiotics with intermediate penetration, piperacillin/tazobactam is effective against gram-positive bacteria and anaerobes in addition to its efficacy against gram negative bacteria and may be the initial empiric antibiotic in patients with acute pancreatitis. Probiotics are no longer recommended in acute pancreatitis as they do not reduce infective complications. Selective gut decontamination with oral antibiotics is of uncertain benefit.[72] Like antibiotics, there is no role for prophylactic antifungal treatment in acute pancreatitis. However, infection with candida species is common in patients receiving antibiotics and treatment with azoles/echinocandins (caspofungin/anidulafungin) for a minimum duration of 2 weeks is recommended.[73]

ABDOMINAL SEPSIS

As per the third International Consensus Definitions for Sepsis and Septic Shock (Sepsis-3) published in February 2016, sepsis is defined as "life-threatening organ dysfunction caused by a dysregulated host response to infection".[74] Sequential Organ Failure Assessment (SOFA) score is used to objectively determine organ dysfunction. An increase in the sepsis related SOFA score by ≥2 points is considered life threatening.[75] As per the current recommendations abdominal sepsis is defined as an "increase of the SOFA score of ≥2 points due to intra-abdominal infection".[74] In patients with abdominal sepsis, if there is requirement of vasopressors to maintain a mean arterial pressure of ≥65 mm Hg and the serum lactate is ≥ 2 mmol/L, it is defined as septic shock.[76] It is recommended to avoid the term severe sepsis suggested by previous guidelines. In clinical practice secondary peritonitis due to loss of integrity of the gastrointestinal tract (as in hollow viscus perforations) is the common source of abdominal sepsis.[77] Primary peritonitis or spontaneous bacterial peritonitis typically seen in children and cirrhotic patients with ascites is characterized by abdominal sepsis without intestinal perforation. Tertiary peritonitis refers to recurrent intra-abdominal sepsis that occurs 48 hours after successful source control of secondary peritonitis.[77] It usually occurs in critically ill patients and associated with multidrug resistant pathogens acquired in the hospital setting.

The principles of management of patients with abdominal sepsis are:
- Early diagnosis
- Source control in the form of debridement
- Removal of infected devices, drainage of purulent cavities, and decompression of the abdominal cavity

- Antibiotic therapy: In this section the focus will be on antibiotic therapy for abdominal sepsis due to secondary peritonitis. The Surviving Sepsis Campaign (SSC) guidelines for antimicrobial therapy in patients with abdominal sepsis are:[78]
  - Early administration of parenteral antibiotics within 1 hour after admission
  - Choice of initial empirical antimicrobial therapy before the availability of culture and antibiotic susceptibility results should be based on potential causative organisms, local trend of antibiotic resistance, patient risk factors, severity and source of infection
  - Once the culture and antibiotic susceptibility results are available the antibiotic spectrum should be narrowed
  - De-escalation or withdrawal of antimicrobial therapy should be considered as soon as possible based on multidisciplinary, daily reevaluation of the critically ill patient.

  The aim of these guidelines and antibiotic stewardship program is to prevent the emergence of multidrug resistant bacteria and superinfection with fungal pathogens.

Guidelines for Empirical Antibiotics Therapy in Abdominal Sepsis

Community acquired intra-abdominal sepsis (secondary peritonitis) is usually due to polymicrobial infection of gut origin that includes aerobic gram-negative bacteria, anaerobes and gram-positive aerobes.[79,80] Frequently isolated aerobic gram-negative bacteria include *E. coli, Klebsiella, Enterobacter* and *Proteus. Bacteroides species* accounts for majority of anaerobic infection. Aerobic gram-positive bacteria include *Streptococcus* and *Enterococcus*. Ideally the empiric therapy should cover these common organisms. Extended-spectrum beta-lactamases (ESBL) producing *Enterobacteriaceae*, a common source of antibiotic resistance is frequently isolated in patients with community acquired intra-abdominal sepsis especially in those exposed to beta-lactams or fluoroquinolones within 3 months of intra-abdominal sepsis.[81] Recent publications have shown that commonly isolated organisms in patients with abdominal sepsis are resistant to ampicillin/sulbactam.[82]

The proposed empiric antibiotic therapy based on the current prevalence of resistance pattern is summarized in **Table 5**. Use of fluroquinolones as empiric therapy should be restricted to low risk patients with allergy to beta-lactam antibiotics as their prolonged use promotes growth of ESBL producing *Enterobacteriaceae* with prolonged use.[83] Inappropriate use of carbapenems should be avoided to prevent widespread emergence of carbapenem resistant *Enterobacteriaceae*. Ceftolozane/tazobactam and ceftazidime/avibactam in combination with metronidazole has been promoted as carbapenem sparing regimens.[84] In patients with tertiary peritonitis, infection with vancomycin

TABLE 5: Antimicrobial therapy for abdominal sepsis.

Diagnosis	Antibiotic regimen – Low risk	Antibiotic regimen – High risk
Secondary peritonitis	Piperacillin + Tazobactam Cefoperazone + Sulbactam Ceftolozane + tazobactam + metronidazole Ceftazidime + avibactam + metronidazole Moxifloxacin Levofloxacin/ciprofloxacin + metronidazole	Imipenem + Cilastatin Meropenem
Primary peritonitis	Cefotaxime	Piperacillin + Tazobactam Cefoperazone + Sulbactam Imipenem + Cilastatin Meropenem
Tertiary peritonitis	Imipenem + Cilastatin (+linezolid) Meropenem (+linezolid) Ceftolozane + tazobactam + metronidazole (+linezolid) Ceftazidime + avibactam + metronidazole (+linezolid) Tigecycline	

resistant enterococci is common.[85] Linezolid (mono-microbial infection) or tigecycline (polymicrobial infection) is recommended in these patients. Antifungal therapy is not routinely indicated as empiric therapy except in secondary peritonitis patients with septic shock and patients with tertiary peritonitis.[86] As *Candida glabrata* is resistant to azoles, echinocandins (caspofungin/anidulafungin) are recommended as empiric antifungal therapy in these patients. For treating infection with *C. parapsilosis* Fluconazole can be used.[86]

Duration of Antimicrobial Therapy

In patients with abdominal sepsis, traditionally antibiotics are given for a minimum period of one week. However, studies have shown that in patients with abdominal sepsis who are not severely ill and in whom adequate source control has been achieved a shorter course of antibiotics (3–5 days) is as effective as a long course.[87] Use of antibiotics for short duration minimizes drug-related adverse events, avoids selection of antibiotic resistance, and significantly reduces health care costs. However, in patients with staphylococcus septicemia (positive blood culture) antibiotics should be given for two (uncomplicated infection) to four (complicated infection) weeks.[88] In the presence of on-going abdominal sepsis, the duration of antibiotics should be based on the clinical assessment. Serum markers of sepsis such as procalcitonin can guide in the determination of duration of antimicrobial therapy. For systemic candidiasis antifungals should be administered for a minimum duration of 2 weeks after negative blood culture.[88] Antimicrobial prophylaxis recommendations for abdominal sepsis are shown in **Table 5**.

High-risk patients include critically ill patients or patients prone for infection with multidrug resistant pathogens.

COLORECTAL SURGERY

Surgical site infection is the most common cause of postoperative morbidity in patients undergoing surgery for colorectal diseases.[89] While the advent of minimally invasive surgery has reduced the morbidity related to SSI, SSIs still remain a common postoperative complication in approximately 25% of patients.[89] The evolution of antibiotics usage and its current recommendations in patients undergoing surgery for elective and emergency colorectal disorders will be covered in this section.

Evolution of Antibiotic Therapy in Colorectal Surgery

Postoperative infectious complication in patients undergoing colorectal surgery has been attributed to fecal flora and hence the initial efforts to mitigate infectious complications were focused on reducing fecal load. In the preantibiotic era, diverting stoma to divert feces away from the anastomosis was employed in almost all patients. By the mid-20th century, mechanical bowel preparation (MBP) became the commonly used strategy to reduce fecal load. With the discovery of antibiotics, the focus shifted on microbiological preparation. With the landmark publication of Nichols et al., the combination of oral antibiotics and MBP became the standard preoperative bowel preparation in the late twentieth century.[90] In the Nichols regimen, the combination of oral neomycin (1 g) and erythromycin (1 g) is given 19, 18 and 9 hours before surgery along with mechanical bowel preparation using bisacodyl and magnesium sulfate started 3 days before surgery.[90] In the landmark RCT, neomycin–erythromycin combination was selected as it is effective against both aerobes and anaerobes. Compared to MBP, Nichols regimen significantly reduced fecal bacterial load and postoperative infectious complications. The impressive results were confirmed in a subsequent study and it was suggested that further RCTs on preoperative bowel preparation should not have a placebo arm or an arm without antibiotics.[91,92]

Toward the end of the twentieth century, the advent of parenteral antibiotics with better bioavailability and convenient dosing regimen tempted researchers to shift to parenteral antibiotics instead of oral antibiotics. Song et al. in a meta-analysis of 147 trials on antimicrobial prophylaxis reported that a single dose of parenteral antibiotics is effective in reducing postoperative infectious complications.[93] At the same time, poor tolerability of MBP and recognition of its harmful effects such as fluid and electrolyte imbalance combined with studies documenting the safety of primary colonic repair in trauma setting without MBP, have raised questions on the role of preoperative MBP.[94,95]

Multiple RCTs and guidelines on ERAS in colorectal surgery, mainly from Europe, supported the hypothesis that MBP does not reduce postoperative infectious complications.[96-98] Oral antibiotics are always administered along with MBP as it was thought that reduced fecal load was a prerequisite for the effectiveness of oral antibiotics. Hence, in the majority of the RCTs published in early 21st century, oral antibiotics were not part of preoperative preparation and the trial arms are generally parenteral antibiotics with or without MBP.[96-98] The lack of beneficial effect of MBP could be explained by the fact that administration of MBP alone without oral antibiotics reduces only intraluminal bacteria without significant effect on mucosa-associated bacteria found within epithelium adherent to the colonic mucus lining.[99] This hypothesis was supported by two recently published large observational studies and one RCT that MBP has no significant effect on colonic bacterial count.[100-102]

Current evidence supports the combination of mechanical and microbiological preparation using parenteral antibiotics, oral antibiotics and MBP for patients undergoing elective colorectal surgery, especially for left colon and rectal surgery.[103] The antibiotic prophylaxis in colorectal surgery has moved a complete circle and we are moving toward the regimen proposed in the 1970s.

It is important to understand that current evidence is primarily influenced by the studies originating from the American College of Surgeons National Surgical Quality Improvement Program (ACS NSQIP) database. As it is derived from a database, the dose, type, and duration of oral antibiotics and the type of parenteral antibiotics used were different. Also, current evidence is not clear whether oral antibiotics alone are effective without MBP. Only a large-scale multicenter study with three arms, namely parenteral + oral antibiotics + MBP; parenteral + oral antibiotics; parenteral antibiotics alone can give a definite answer about ideal preoperative antibiotic prophylaxis in colorectal surgery. The recommendations given here are based on current evidence which could change in future.

Antibiotic Prophylaxis for Elective Colorectal Surgery

There is level 1 evidence for intravenous antibiotic prophylaxis administered within 60 min before incision.[104] The currently recommended regimen is second or third generation cephalosporin combined with metronidazole to cover both gram-negative aerobes and anaerobes. Additional intraoperative or postoperative doses are not recommended when the antibiotics are given for prophylaxis in the elective setting as it increases the risk of *C. difficile* colitis. Oral antibiotics are recommended in patients receiving MBP, although the evidence is not as robust as with parenteral antibiotics.[105] Usage of oral antibiotics in patients not receiving MBP is under evaluation and no definite recommendations could be given with the available evidence. Also, there is no consensus on the appropriate oral antibiotic regimen as regards its dosage and duration. While the neomycin-erythromycin combination was used in Nichol's regimen, recent trials have used a combination of kanamycin/tobramycin (oral non-absorbable aminoglycosides) with metronidazole 1-3 days before surgery.

Song et al. have shown that if the regimen covers gram-negative, gram-positive and anaerobic bacteria, individual drug differences in different regimens do not influence postoperative infection rate.[93] Hence, the chosen antibiotic regimen should be based on the availability of antibiotics in the institute, institutional antimicrobial protocol and the prevalence of local antibiotic resistance.

Antibiotics for Emergency Colorectal Surgery

Emergency surgery is usually performed for obstruction or perforation. In patients presenting with obstruction without signs of systemic sepsis, the parenteral antibiotic regimen is similar to prophylactic antibiotics given for elective surgery.[106] The evidence for oral antibiotics in an emergency setting is limited as MBP is not given in these patients. Patients undergoing surgery for colorectal perforation should receive therapeutic antibiotics covering Gram-negative bacteria (*Enterobacteriaceae*) and anaerobes (*Bacteroides fragilis*). Similar to the recommendations given in the section on abdominal sepsis, initial empiric antibiotic therapy should cover these organisms taking into account the local resistance pattern **(Table 5)**.

INTESTINAL ISCHEMIA

Intestinal ischemia is a life-threatening complication secondary to abrupt interruption of the vascular supply to a segment of bowel. Globally, the incidence of intestinal ischemia is increasing due to the increase in an aging population.[107] Broadly, intestinal ischemia is classified as occlusive or nonocclusive types.[108] Occlusive type of intestinal ischemia could be due to arterial embolism, arterial thrombosis, or venous thrombosis. Irrespective of the etiology the manifestations of intestinal ischemia are dependent on the duration and severity of vascular occlusion. Ischemia could be full thickness resulting in gangrene or partial thickness involving mucosa and submucosa that usually results in stricture. Early diagnosis and prompt intervention can reverse the ischemic process leading to a full recovery of bowel function. As diagnosis is difficult in the early stages, a high index of suspicion is essential, especially in the elderly population to prevent irreversible damage to the bowel.

As three-fourths of mesenteric blood flows to the mucosa and submucosa, intestinal ischemia affects the mucosa in the early stage.[109] Microscopic changes of ischemia can be detected in the intestinal mucosa within minutes of vascular occlusion. Ischemic damage to mucosa affects intestinal barrier resulting in bacterial translocation. Studies have shown that bacteria translocate through the intercellular route between the intestinal epithelial cells or through ulcerations left by denuded epithelial cells in patients with ischemic damage.[110] In contrast to intracellular bacterial translocation seen in patients with an intact intestinal barrier, intercellular route allows bacteria to enter blood bypassing the lymph nodes. Gram-negative, facultative anaerobic *Enterobacteriaceae*, such as *E. coli*, *Klebsiella pneumoniae*, and Proteus mirabilis, translocate at a higher rate compared to obligatory anaerobic bacteria, such as *Bacteroides* and *Fusobacterium* due to their sensitivity to oxygen.[110] As the risk of bacterial sepsis outweighs the risk of antibiotic resistance, broad-spectrum antibiotics as outlined in the **Table 5** for secondary peritonitis should be administered early in the course of treatment.[111]

CONCLUSION

Abdominal surgery forms the bulk of general surgical procedures. In view of the GI tract being resident to a number of species of bacteria, both aerobic and anaerobic, most procedures on the GI tract are classified in the clean contaminated group and may require antibiotic coverage. The practice regarding the choice of the antibiotic and the duration of administration remains controversial with wide disparity between health care institutions. However, there are well-defined clinical guidelines which are periodically updated to cater to this particular situation. This chapter will review all the guidelines available for this purpose and summarize their findings to guide practice in India.

REFERENCES

1. Lewis SS, Moehring RW, Chen LF, Sexton DJ, Anderson DJ. Assessing the relative burden of hospital-acquired infections in a network of community hospitals. Infect Control Hosp Epidemiol. 2013;34:1229-30.
2. Edwards JR, Peterson KD, Mu Y, Banerjee S, Allen-Bridson K, Morrell G, et al. National Healthcare Safety Network (NHSN) report: data summary for 2006 through 2008, issued December 2009. Am J Infect Control. 2009;37:783-805.
3. Leaper D and Ousey K. Evidence update on prevention of surgical site infection. Curr Opin Infect Dis. 2015;28:158-63.
4. Vegas AA, Jodra VM, Garcia ML. Nosocomial infection in surgery wards: a controlled study of increased duration of hospital stays and direct cost of hospitalization, Eur J Epidemiol. 1993;9:504-10.
5. Culver DH, Horan, TC, Gaynes RP, Martone WJ, Jarvis WR, Emori TG, et al. Surgical wound infection rates by wound class, operative procedure, and patient risk index. National Nosocomial Infections Surveillance System. Am J Med. 1991;91;152S-7S.
6. Berríos-Torres SI, Umscheid CA, Bratzler DW, Leas B, Stone EC, Kelz RR, et al. Centers for Disease Control and Prevention Guideline for the Prevention of Surgical Site Infection, 2017. JAMA Surg. 2017;152:784-91.
7. Bratzler DW, Dellinger EP, Olsen KM, Perl TM, Auwaerter PG, Bolon MK, et al. Clinical practice guidelines for antimicrobial prophylaxis in surgery. Surg Infect (Larchmt). 2013;14:73-156.
8. Antimicrobial prophylaxis for surgery. Treat Guide Med Lett. 2012;10:73-8.
9. Blumenthal KG, Ryan EE, Li Y, Lee H, Kuhlen JL, Shenoy ES. The Impact of a Reported Penicillin Allergy on Surgical Site Infection Risk. Clin Infect Dis. 2018;66:329-36.
10. Falagas ME, Karageorgopoulos DE. Adjustment of dosing of antimicrobial agents for bodyweight in adults. Lancet. 2010;375:248-51.
11. Classen DC, Evans RS, Pestotnik SL, Horn SD, Menlove RL, Burke JP. The timing of prophylactic administration of antibiotics and the risk of surgical-wound infection. N Engl J Med. 1992;326:281-6.

12. Weber WP, Mujagic E, Zwahlen M, Bundi M, Hoffmann H, Soysal SD, et al. Timing of surgical antimicrobial prophylaxis: a phase 3 randomised controlled trial. Lancet Infect Dis. 2017;17:605-14.
13. Hawn MT, Richman JS, Vick CC, Deierhoi RJ, Graham LA, Henderson WG, et al. Timing of surgical antibiotic prophylaxis and the risk of surgical site infection. JAMA Surg. 2013;148:649-57.
14. Steinberg JP, Braun BI, Hellinger WC, Kusek L, Bozikis MR, Bush AJ, et al. Timing of antimicrobial prophylaxis and the risk of surgical site infections: results from the Trial to Reduce Antimicrobial Prophylaxis Errors. Ann Surg. 2009;250:10-6.
15. McDonald M, Grabsch E, Marshall C, Forbes A. Single- versus multiple-dose antimicrobial prophylaxis for major surgery: a systematic review. Aust N Z J Surg. 1998;68:388-96.
16. Bernatz JT, Safdar N, Hetzel S, Anderson PA. Antibiotic Overuse is a Major Risk Factor for Clostridium difficile Infection in Surgical Patients. Infect Control Hosp Epidemiol. 2017;38:1254-57.
17. Varela JE, Wilson SE, Nguyen NT. Laparoscopic surgery significantly reduces surgical-site infections compared with open surgery. Surg Endosc. 2010;24:270-6.
18. Siddiqui K, Khan AF. Comparison of frequency of wound infection: open vs laparoscopic cholecystectomy. J Ayub Med Coll Abbottabad. 2006;18:21-4.
19. Chang WT, Lee KT, Chuang SC, Wang SN, Kuo KK, Chen JS, et al. The impact of prophylactic antibiotics on postoperative infection complication in elective laparoscopic cholecystectomy: a prospective randomized study. Am J Surg. 2006; 191:721-5.
20. Koc M, Zulfikaroglu B, Kece C, Ozalp N. A prospective randomized study of prophylactic antibiotics in elective laparoscopic cholecystectomy. Surg Endosc. 2003;17:1716-8.
21. Passos MA, Portari-Filho PE. Antibiotic prophylaxis in laparoscopic cholecystectomy: is it worth doing?. Arq Bras Cir Dig. 2016;29(3):170-2.
22. Matsui Y, Satoi S, Kaibori M, Toyokawa H, Yanagimoto H, Matsui K, et al. Antibiotic Prophylaxis in Laparoscopic Cholecystectomy: A Randomized Controlled Trial. PLoS ONE. 2014;9(9):e106702.
23. Vohra RS, Hodson J, Pasquali S, Griffiths EA. CholeS Study Group and West Midlands Research Collaborative. Effectiveness of antibiotic prophylaxis in non-emergency cholecystectomy using data from a population-based cohort study. World J Surg 2017;41:2231-9.
24. Liang B, Dai M, Zou Z. Safety and efficacy of antibiotic prophylaxis in patients undergoing elective laparoscopic cholecystectomy: a systematic review and meta-analysis. J Gastroenterol Hepatol. 2016;31:921-8.
25. Kim SH, Yu HC, Yang JD, Ahn SW, Hwang HP. Role of prophylactic antibiotics in elective laparoscopic cholecystectomy: a systematic review and meta-analysis. Ann Hepatobiliary Pancreat Surg. 2018;22(3):231-47.
26. Harris A, Chan AC, Torres-Viera C, Hammett R, Carr-Locke D. Meta-analysis of antibiotic prophylaxis in endoscopic retrograde cholangiopancreatography (ERCP). Endoscopy. 1999;31:718-24.
27. Meijer WS, Schmitz PI, Jeekel J. Meta-analysis of randomized, controlled clinical trials of antibiotic prophylaxis in biliary tract surgery. Br J Surg. 1990;77:282-90.
28. Den Hoed PT, Boelhouwer RU, Veen HF, Hop WC, Bruining HA. Infections and bacteriological data after laparoscopic and open gallbladder surgery. J Hosp Infect. 1998;39:27-37.
29. Cainzos M, Sayek I, Wacha H, Pulay I, Dominion L, Aeberhard PF, et al. Septic complications after biliary tract stone surgery: a review and report of the European Prospective Study. Hepatogastroenterology. 1997;44:959-67.
30. Lee WJ, Chang KJ, Lee CS, Chen KM. Surgery in cholangitis: bacteriology and choice of antibiotic. Hepatogastroenterology 1992;39:347-9.
31. Kanter MA, Geelhoed GW. Biliary antibiotics: clinical utility in biliary surgery. South Med J. 1987;80:1007-15.

32. Lewis RT, Goodall RG, Marien B, Park M, Lloyd-Smith W, Wiegand FM. Biliary bacteria, antibiotic use, and wound infection in surgery of the gallbladder and common bile duct. Arch Surg. 1987;122:44.
33. Solomkin JS, Mazuski JE, Bradley JS, Rodvold KA, Goldstein EJ, Baron EJ, et al. Diagnosis and management of complicated intra- abdominal infection in adults and children: guidelines by the Surgical Infection Society and the Infectious Diseases Society of America. Surg Infect. 2010;11:79-109.
34. Yokoe M, Hata J, Takada T, Strasberg SM, Asbun HJ, Wakabayashi G, et al. Tokyo guidelines 2018: diagnostic criteria and severity grading of acute cholecystitis (with videos). J Hepatobiliary Pancreat Sci. 2018;25 (1):41-54.
35. Gomi H, Solomkin JS, Schlossberg D, Okamoto K, Takada T, Strasberg SM, et al. Tokyo guidelines 2018: antimicrobial therapy for acute cholangitis and cholecystitis. J Hepatobiliary Pancreat Sci. 2018;25:3-16.
36. Wu XD, Tian X, Liu MM, Zhao S, Chen L. Meta-analysis comparing early versus delayed laparoscopic cholecystectomy for acute cholecystitis. Br J Surg. 2015;102:1302-13.
37. Blohm M, Österberg J, Sandblom G, Lundell L, Hedberg M, Enochsson L. The Sooner, the Better? The Importance of Optimal Timing of Cholecystectomy in Acute Cholecystitis: data from the National Swedish Registry for Gallstone Surgery, GallRiks. J Gastrointest Surg. 2017;21:33-40.
38. Regimbeau JM, Fuks D, Pautrat K, Mauvais F, Haccart V, Msika S, et al. Effect of postoperative antibiotic administration on postoperative infection following cholecystectomy for acute calculouscholecystitis: a randomized clinical trial. JAMA. 2014;312:145-54.
39. de Santibañes M, Glinka J, Pelegrini P, Alvarez FA, Elizondo C, Giunta D, et al. Extended antibiotic therapy versus placebo after laparoscopic cholecystectomy for mild and moderate acute calculouscholecystitis: a randomized double-blind clinical trial. Surgery. 2018;164(1): 24-30.
40. Strasberg SM. Clinical practice. Acutecalculouscholecystitis. N Engl J Med. 2008;358:2804–11.
41. Yokoe M, Takada T, Strasberg SM, Solomkin JS, Mayumi T, Gomi H, et al. New diagnostic criteria and severity assessment of acute cholecystitis in revised Tokyo guidelines. J HepatobiliaryPancreat Sci. 2012;19:578-85.
42. Cao AM, Eslick GD, Cox MR. Early cholecystectomy is superior to delayed cholecystectomy for acute cholecystitis: a meta-analysis. J Gastrointest Surg. 2015;19:848-57.
43. Lee CC, Chang IJ, Lai YC, Chen SY, Chen SC. Epidemiology and prognostic determinants of patients with bacteremiccholecystitis or cholangitis. Am J Gastroenterol. 2007;102:563-9.
44. Coccolini F, Sartelli M, Catena F, Montori G, Di Saverio S, Sugrue M, et al. Antibiotic resistance pattern and clinical out- comes in acute cholecystitis: 567 consecutive worldwide patients in a prospective cohort study. Int J Surg. 2015;21:32-7.
45. Bratzler DW, Dellinger EP, Olsen KM, Perl TM, Auwaerter PG, Bolon MK, et al. Clinical practice guidelines for antimicrobial prophylaxis in surgery. Am J Health-Syst Pharm. 2013;70:195-283.
46. Fuks D, Regimbeau JM, Cosse C. Antibiotic therapy in acute calculous cholecystitis. J Visc Surg. 2013;150:3-8
47. Stewart B, Khanduri P, McCord C, Ohene-Yeboah M, Uranues S, Vega Rivera F, et al. Global disease burden of conditions requiring emergency surgery. Br J Surg. 2014;101(1):e9-22.
48. Bratzler DW, Hunt DR. The surgical infection prevention and surgical care improvement projects: national initiatives to improve outcomes for patients having surgery. Clin Infect Dis. 2006;43:322-30.
49. Stone HH. Bacterial flora of appendicitis in children. J Pediatr Surg. 1976;11:37-42.
50. Andersen BR, Kallehave FL, Andersen HK. Antibiotics versus placebo for prevention of postoperative infection after appendicectomy. Cochrane Database Syst Rev. 2005;3: CD001439.

51. Bauer T, Vennits B, Holm B, Hahn-Pedersen J, Lysen D, Galatius H, et al. Antibiotic prophylaxis in acute non-perforated appendicitis. The Danish Multicenter Study Group III. Ann Surg. 1989;209(3):307-11.
52. Sauerland S, Lefering R, Neugebauer EA. Laparoscopic versus open surgery for suspected appendicitis. Cochrane Database Syst Rev. 2004:CD001546.
53. Hemmila MR, Birkmeyer NJ, Arbabi S, Osborne NH, Wahl WL, Dimick JB. Introduction to propensity scores: a case study on the comparative effectiveness of laparoscopic vs open appendectomy. Arch Surg. 2010;145:939-45.
54. Antimicrobial prophylaxis for surgery. Treat Guide Med Lett. 2009;7:47-52.
55. Mui LM, Ng CS, Wong SK, Lam YH, Fung TM, Fok KL, et al. Optimum duration of prophylactic antibiotics in acute non-perforated appendicitis. Aust N Z J Surg. 2005;75;425-8.
56. Morris WT, Innes DB, Richardson RA, Rodvold KA, Goldstein EJ, Baron EJ, et al. The prevention of post-appendicectomy sepsis by metro- nidazole and cefazolin: a controlled double-blind trial. Aust N Z J Surg. 1980;50:429-33.
57. Van Santvoort HC, Bakker OJ, Bollen TL, Besselink MG, Ahmed Ali U, Schrijver AM, et al. A conservative and minimally invasive approach to necrotizing pancreatitis improves outcome. Gastroenterology. 2011; 141:1254-63.
58. Werge M, Novovic S, Schmidt PN, Gluud LL. Infection increases mortality in necrotizing pancreatitis: a systematic review and meta-analysis. Pancreatology. 2016;16: 698-707.
59. Schmid SW, Uhl W, Friess H, Malfertheiner P, Büchler MW. The role of infection in acute pancreatitis. Gut. 1999;45:311-6.
60. Dervenis C, Johnson CD, Bassi C, Bradley E, Imrie CW, McMahon MJ, et al. Diagnosis, objective assessment of severity, and management of acute pancreatitis. Santorini consensus conference. Int J Pancreatol. 1999;25:195-210.
61. Mourad MM, Evans R, Kalidindi V, Navaratnam R, Dvorkin L, Bramhall SR. Prophylactic antibiotics in acute pancreatitis: endless debate. Ann R Coll Surg Engl. 2017;99:107-12.
62. Golub R, Siddiqi F, Pohl D. Role of antibiotics in acute pancreatitis: a meta-analysis. J Gastrointest Surg 1998;2:496-503.
63. Sharma VK, Howden CW. Prophylactic antibiotic administration reduces sepsis and mortality in acute necrotizing pancreatitis: a meta-analysis. Pancreas. 2001;22:28-31.
64. Villatoro E, Bassi C, Larvin M. Antibiotic therapy for prophylaxis against infection of pancreatic necrosis in acute pancreatitis. Cochrane Database Syst Rev. 2006;(4):CD002941.
65. Bassi C, Larvin M, Villatoro E. Antibiotic therapy for prophylaxis against infection of pancreatic necrosis in acute pancreatitis. Cochrane Database Syst Rev. 2003;(4):CD002941.
66. Jiang K, Huang W, Yang XN, Xia Q. Present and future of prophylactic antibiotics for severe acute pancreatitis. World J Gastroenterol. 2012;18(3):279-84.
67. Párniczky A, Lantos T, Tóth EM, Szakács Z, Gódi S, Hágendorn R, et al. Hungarian Pancreatic Study Group. Antibiotic therapy in acute pancreatitis: from global overuse to evidence-based recommendations. Pancreatology. 2019;19:488-99.
68. Leppäniemi A, Tolonen M, Tarasconi A, Segovia-Lohse H, Gamberini E, Kirkpatrick AW, et al. 2019 WSES guidelines for the management of severe acute pancreatitis. World J Emerg Surg. 2019;14:27.
69. Stigliano S, Sternby H, de Madaria E, Capurso G, Petrov MS. Early management of acute pancreatitis: a review of the best evidence. Dig Liver Dis. 2017;49:585-94.
70. Mofidi R, Suttie SA, Patil PV, Ogston S, Parks RW. The value of procalcitonin at predicting the severity of acute pancreatitis and development of infected pancreatic necrosis: systematic review. Surgery. 2009;146:72-81.
71. Otto W, Komorzycki K, Krawczyk M. Efficacy of antibiotic penetration into pancreatic necrosis. HPB (Oxford). 2006;8:43-8.

72. Besselink MG, van Santvoort HC, Buskens E, Boermeester MA, van Goor H, Timmerman HM, et al. Dutch Acute Pancreatitis Study Group. Probiotic prophylaxis in predicted severe acute pancreatitis: a randomised, double-blind, placebo-controlled trial. Lancet. 2008;371:651-9.
73. Reuken PA, Albig H, Rödel J, Hocke M, Will U, Stallmach A, et al. Fungal infections in patients with infected pancreatic necrosis and pseudocysts: risk factors and outcome. Pancreas. 2018;47:92-8.
74. Cecconi M, Evans L, Levy M, Rhodes A. Sepsis and septic shock. Lancet. 2018;392:75-87.
75. Vincent JL, Moreno R, Takala J, Willatts S, De Mendonça A, Bruining H, et al. The SOFA (Sepsis-related Organ Failure Assessment) score to describe organ dysfunction/failure. On behalf of the Working Group on Sepsis-Related Problems of the European Society of Intensive Care Medicine. Intensive Care Med. 1996;22:707-10.
76. Singer M, Deutschman CS, Seymour CW, Shankar-Hari M, Annane D, Bauer M, et al. The Third International Consensus Definitions for Sepsis and Septic Shock (Sepsis-3). JAMA. 2016;315:801-10.
77. Menichetti F, Sganga G. Definition and classification of intra-abdominal infections. J Chemother. 2009;21(Suppl 1):3-4.
78. Rhodes A, Evans LE, Alhazzani W, Levy MM, Antonelli M, Ferrer R, et al. Surviving Sepsis Campaign: international guidelines for management of sepsis and septic shock: 2016. Intensive Care Med. 2017;43:304-77.
79. Jeon HG, Ju HU, Kim GY, Jeong J, Kim MH, Jun JB. Bacteriology and changes in antibiotic susceptibility in adults with community-acquired perforated appendicitis. PLoS One. 2014;9:e111144.
80. Van Ruler O, Kiewiet JJ, Van Ketel RJ, Boermeester MA. Dutch Peritonitis Study Group. Initial microbial spectrum in severe secondary peritonitis and relevance for treatment. Eur J Clin Microbiol Infect Dis. 2012;31:671-82.
81. Al-Hasan MN, Eckel-Passow JE, Baddour LM. Impact of healthcare-associated acquisition on community-onset Gram-negative bloodstream infection: a population-based study. Eur J Clin Microbiol Infect Dis. 2012;31:1163-71.
82. Hackel MA, Badal RE, Bouchillon SK, Biedenbach DJ, Hoban DJ. Resistance rates of intra-abdominal isolates from intensive care units and non-intensive care units in the United States: the study for monitoring antimicrobial resistance trends 2010-2012. Surg Infect. 2015;16:298-304.
83. Ortega M, Marco F, Soriano A, Almela M, Martínez JA, Muñoz A, et al. Analysis of 4758 Escherichia coli bacteraemia episodes: predictive factors for isolation of an antibiotic-resistant strain and their impact on the outcome. J Antimicrob Chemother. 2009;63:568-74.
84. Solomkin J, Hershberger E, Miller B, Popejoy M, Friedland I, Steenbergen J, et al. Ceftolozane/tazobactam plus metronidazole for complicated intra-abdominal infections in an era of multidrug resistance: results from a randomized, double-blind, phase 3 trial (ASPECT-cIAI). Clin Infect Dis. 2015;60:1462-71.
85. Dupont H, Friggeri A, Touzeau J, Airapetian N, Tinturier F, Lobjoie E, et al. Enterococci increase the morbidity and mortality associated with severe intra-abdominal infections in elderly patients hospitalized in the intensive care unit. J Antimicrob Chemother. 2011;66:2379-85.
86. Pappas PG, Kauffman CA, Andes DR, Clancy CJ, Marr KA, Ostrosky-Zeichner L, et al. Executive summary: clinical practice guideline for the management of Candidiasis: 2016 update by the Infectious Diseases Society of America. Clin Infect Dis. 2016;62:409-17.
87. Sawyer RG, Claridge JA, Nathens AB, Rotstein OD, Duane TM, Evans HL, et al. Trial of short-course antimicrobial therapy for intra-abdominal infection. N Engl J Med. 2015;372:1996-2005.
88. Hecker A, Reichert M, Reuß CJ, Schmoch T, Riedel JG, Schneck E, et al. Intra-abdominal sepsis: new definitions and current clinical standards. Langenbecks Arch Surg. 2019;404:257-71.

89. Bellows CF, Mills KT, Kelly TN, Gagliardi G. Combination of oral non-absorbable and intravenous antibiotics versus intravenous antibiotics alone in the prevention of surgical site infections after colorectal surgery: a meta-analysis of randomized controlled trials. Tech Coloproctol. 2011;15:385-95.
90. Nichols RL, Broido P, Condon RE, Gorbach SL, Nyhus LM. Effect of preoperative neomycin-erythromycin intestinal preparation on the incidence of infectious complications following colon surgery. Ann Surg. 1973;178:453-62.
91. Goldring J, McNaught W, Scott A, Gillespie G. Prophylactic oral antimicrobial agents in elective colonic surgery. A controlled trial. Lancet. 1975;2:997-1000.
92. Proud G, Chamberlain J. Antimicrobial prophylaxis in elective colonic surgery. Lancet. 1979;2:1017-8.
93. Song F, Glenny AM. Antimicrobial prophylaxis in colorectal surgery: a systematic review of randomized controlled trials. Br J Surg. 1998;85:1232-41.
94. Sasaki LS, Allaben RD, Golwala R, Mittal VK. Primary repair of colon injuries: a prospective randomized study. J Trauma. 1995;39:895-901.
95. Nelson R, Singer M. Primary repair for penetrating colon injuries. Cochrane Database Syst Rev. 2003;(3):CD002247.
96. Slim K, Vicaut E, Launay-Savary MV, Contant C, Chipponi J. Updated systematic review and meta-analysis of randomized clinical trials on the role of mechanical bowel preparation before colorectal surgery. Ann Surg. 2009;249:203-9.
97. Gustafsson UO, Scott MJ, Schwenk W, Demartines N, Roulin D, Francis N, et al. Guidelines for perioperative care in elective colonic surgery: Enhanced Recovery after Surgery (ERAS®) Society recommendations. Clin Nutr. 2012;31:783-800.
98. Nygren J, Thacker J, Carli F, Fearon KC, Norderval S, Lobo DN, et al. Guidelines for perioperative care in elective rectal/pelvic surgery: Enhanced Recovery after Surgery (ERAS®) Society recommendations. Clin Nutr. 2012;31:801-16.
99. Smith MB, Baliga P, Sartor WM, Goradia VK, Holmes JW, Nichols RL. Intraoperative colonic lavage: failure to decrease mucosal microflora. South Med J. 1991;84:38-42.
100. Klinger AL, Green H, Monlezun DJ, Beck D, Kann B, Vargas HD, et al. The Role of Bowel Preparation in Colorectal Surgery: Results of the 2012-2015 ACS-NSQIP Data. Ann Surg. 2019;269:671-7.
101. Koller SE, Bauer KW, Egleston BL, Smith R, Philp MM, Ross HM, et al. Comparative Effectiveness and Risks of Bowel Preparation before Elective Colorectal Surgery. Ann Surg. 2018;267:734-42.
102. Sadahiro S, Suzuki T, Tanaka A, Okada K, Kamata H, Ozaki T, et al. Comparison between oral antibiotics and probiotics as bowel preparation for elective colon cancer surgery to prevent infection: prospective randomized trial. Surgery. 2014;155:493-503.
103. Rollins KE, Javanmard-Emamghissi H, Acheson AG, Lobo DN. The role of oral antibiotic preparation in elective colorectal surgery: a meta-analysis. Ann Surg. 2019;270:43-58.
104. Nelson RL, Gladman E, Barbateskovic M. Antimicrobial prophylaxis for colorectal surgery. Cochrane Database Syst Rev. 2014;(5):CD001181.
105. Gustafsson UO, Scott MJ, Hubner M, Nygren J, Demartines N, Francis N, et al. Guidelines for Perioperative Care in Elective Colorectal Surgery: Enhanced Recovery After Surgery (ERAS®) Society Recommendations: 2018. World J Surg. 2019;43:659-95.
106. Pisano M, Zorcolo L, Merli C, Cimbanassi S, Poiasina E, Ceresoli M, et al. 2017 WSES guidelines on colon and rectal cancer emergencies: obstruction and perforation. World J Emerg Surg. 2018;13:36.
107. Tilsed JV, Casamassima A, Kurihara H, Mariani D, Martinez I, Pereira J, et al. ESTES guidelines: acute mesenteric ischaemia. Eur J Trauma Emerg Surg. 2016;42:253-70.
108. Sise MJ. Mesenteric ischemia: the whole spectrum. Scand J Surg. 2010;99:106-10.
109. Robinson JW, Mirkovitch V, Winistörfer B, Saegesser F. Response of the intestinal mucosa to ischaemia. Gut. 1981;22:512-27.
110. Berg RD. Bacterial translocation from the gastrointestinal tract. Adv Exp Med Biol. 1999;473:11-30.
111. Bala M, Kashuk J, Moore EE, luger Y, Biffl W, Gomes CA, et al. Acute mesenteric ischemia: guidelines of the World Society of Emergency Surgery. World J Emerg Surg. 2017;12:38.

CHAPTER 9

Malignant Melanoma

SVS Deo, Manoj Gowda

INTRODUCTION

Melanoma is the most serious form of skin cancer. According to GLOBOCAN-2018, worldwide the incidence and mortality of melanoma accounts for 3.8 and 0.8 per 100,000 population, respectively. Compared to worldwide figures the incidence and mortality rates are 0.23 and 0.15 per 100,000 population, respectively in India. Worldwide Australia has highest incidence with 57.6 per 100,000 population and mortality of 6.5 per 100,000 population.[1] The overall survival and disease free survival for people with melanoma is determined by the stage at diagnosis. Stage 0 and I patients can be cured by surgery and have prolonged disease free survival. Whereas those with stage II to IV are more likely to develop early relapse.[2]

CLINICAL PROGRESSION OF MELANOMA

Melanomas arise as superficial tumors that are confined to epidermis. It may have two types of spread **(Fig. 1)**:

1. *Horizontal or radial spread:* During early stages the melanoma is confined to epidermis and usually has radial spread. It will not extend in to dermis. During this phase the melanomas are curable by surgical excision.

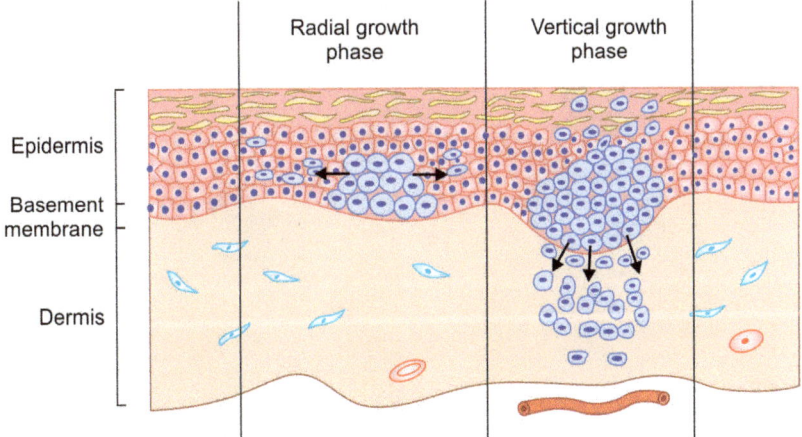

Fig. 1: Types of progression of melanoma.

2. *Vertical spread:* Once the melanoma extends to the dermis, they are considered invasive and have vertical growth pattern. These tumors have metastatic potential. Nodular melanomas will have vertical growth phase from its inception. This lead to worse prognosis of nodular melanoma. Breslow's thickness is the marker of this vertical spread which in turn determines the probability of metastasis.

SUBTYPES OF MELANOMA

There are four major subtypes of cutaneous melanoma **(Figs. 2A to D)**:
1. *Superficial spreading melanoma:* It is the most common subtype, accounting for approximately 70% of all melanomas. They have variable presentation in the form of pigmented macule or thin plaque with irregular border. These melanomas can occur anywhere in the body, but has high predilection for back. These tumors have more of radial spread and less vertical spread. Because of less vertical spread they have good cure rates.
2. *Nodular melanoma:* It is the second most common type of melanoma accounting for 15–30% of all melanomas. They present as darkly pigmented pedunculated or polypoidal papules or nodules with relatively small

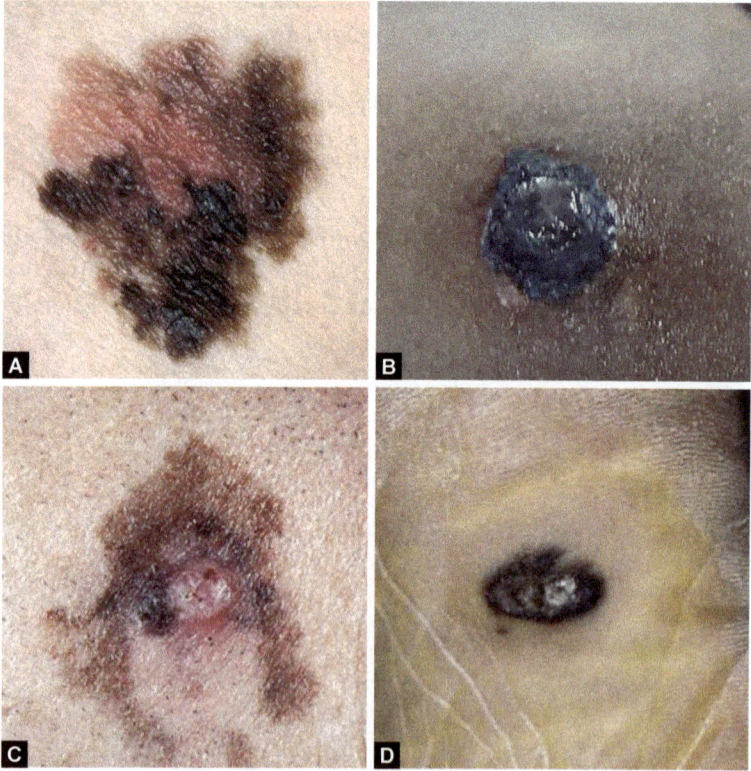

Figs. 2A to D: (A) Superficial spreading melanoma; (B) Nodular melanoma; (C) Lentigo maligna melanoma; (D) Acral lentiginous melanoma.

diameter. Since it has vertical spread from the time of inception, the Breslow's thickness will be greater than 2 mm at the time of diagnosis.
3. *Lentigo maligna melanoma:* It accounts for 10-15% of all melanomas. It develops from "lentigo maligna—a slow growing form of in situ melanoma" and hence the name lentigo maligna melanoma. The lesion enlarges over the years and may develop asymmetric, darker pigmentation and color variegation.
4. *Acral lentiginous melanoma:* It accounts for <5% of all melanomas. It is more common in dark skinned individuals. The most common locations are on palms, plantar and subungual surfaces.
5. *Other rare subtypes:*
    a. *Amelanotic melanoma:* It accounts for 2-10% of all melanomas. As the name suggests, it presents as amelanotic or hypomelanotic lesions. Clinically it presents as pink or red macules, plaques or nodules.
    b. *Spitzoid melanoma:* These tumors have morphological resemblance to Spitz tumors both clinically and histologically. Although spitzoid melanomas have more severe atypia than spitz tumors, the histologic differentiation is challenging and may require additional molecular tests to differentiate them.
    c. *Desmoplastic melanoma:* As the name suggests, it presents as a scar, nonmelanoma skin cancer or other benign process. Clinically it looks like a scar like growth in a sun exposed areas of older patients.
    d. *Pigment synthesizing (animal-type) melanoma:* It is also called melanocytoma. It has indolent growth pattern with low incidence of metastasis and low mortality rate despite high frequency of positive sentinel lymph nodes. They presented as pigmented slow growing nodule, which on histology is seen as a heavily pigmented dermal epithelioid and spindled melanocytes.

CLINICAL DIAGNOSIS

Clinical diagnosis of melanoma is very challenging. Clinical suspicion and high risk history should alert the physician to order for biopsy.
1. *History and risk factors:* The key questions which should be asked to the patient while taking history are:
    a. When the lesion was first noticed?
    b. Is there any change in the size or color of the lesion?
    c. Does the patient has any personal or family history of melanoma?
    d. Does patient's occupation expose him to excess sun exposure or does the patient has history of sun bathing?
    e. Any history of genetic syndrome or familial cancer syndrome: Xeroderma pigmentosum or familial atypical mole-melanoma syndrome
    f. History of any transplant/use of immunosuppressants/HIV
    g. Psoralen plus ultraviolet A (PUVA) therapy

2. *General examination features:* These features should raise the suspicion for melanoma
   a. Fair complexion
   b. Red or blond hair
   c. Light eye color
   d. Presence of large number of melanocytic nevi (>50)
   e. Presence of atypical melanocytic nevi (benign nevi that clinically share some of the clinical features of melanoma, such as large diameter, irregular borders, and multiple colors)
3. *Visual examination:* Visual examination is the most important step in identifying the high risk lesion which requires biopsy or serial examinations. Various clinical prediction checklists have been developed to help the clinician in identifying high risk lesions.
   a. *ABCDE Rule* **(Fig. 3)**: This rule was developed by the dermatologists from New York City. ABCDE is an acronym which stands for:
      I. *Asymmetry:* Bisect the lesion in to two equal halves. If one half of the lesion is not identical to the other half, it is considered as asymmetric.
      II. *Border irregularity:* The borders of the nevus are irregular
      III. *Color variegation:* Presence of multiple shades of color in the same lesion
      IV. *Diameter:* Any lesion with diameter ≥6 mm
      V. *Evolution:* Recent change in size, shape or color. Appearance of new lesion.

      Many studies have been conducted to find out the sensitivity and specificity of ABCDE clinical tool in identifying melanoma. Using the principle of "biopsy the lesion: even if one criteria is positive" is sensitive

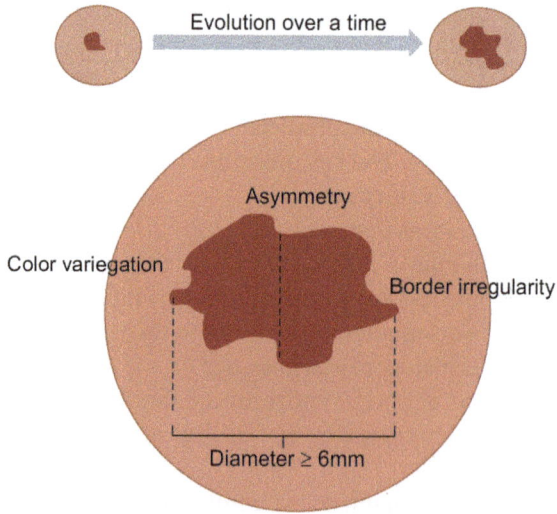

Fig. 3: ABCDE of melanoma.

but not specific, i.e., many benign lesions would be biopsied. On the other hand if we biopsy lesions when it meets ≥2 criteria increases specificity but may increase the chance of missing some high risk lesions with atypical presentation.

In a study reported by Thomas et al. which includes 1,140 lesions, including 460 melanomas the sensitivity and specificity of identifying a melanoma were 97% and 36%, respectively when single criterion was used. By contrast the sensitivity and specificity were 43% and 100% when all five criteria were used.[3]

In a primary care setting, any patient with evolution of the lesion with any one of the ABCD criteria should be referred to the oncologist for examination and biopsy.

b. *Glasgow revised seven point checklist:* It was developed by clinicians in United Kingdom to help the general practitioners in referring the melanoma patients to the specialists.[4] It includes seven points checklist which should by checked by the physician whenever he/she come across a suspicious lesion.

   I. Major:
      - Change in size/new lesion
      - Change in shape
      - Change in color
   II. Minor:
      - Diameter ≥7 mm
      - Inflammation
      - Crusting or bleeding
      - Sensory change

   The presence of one major or three minor criteria is an indication for referral to the specialist. The sensitivity and specificity of this tool is 92% and 33% respectively when one major or three minor rule is applied.[5]

c. *The "ugly duckling" sign:* It is the central component of intrapatient comparative analysis. In a patient with multiple nevi, they tend to exhibit common morphologic features. This specific profile is called the signature nevi. Any lesion that does not match the signature nevi should be biopsied even if they do not fulfill ABCDE criterion.[5]

d. *Difficult melanomas:* Any of the melanomas which vary from the usual clinical presentation are difficult to diagnose clinically. Clinician should be aware of such scenarios, so that he/she will not miss the diagnosis.

   I. *Melanomas in children:* ABCDE criterion is not applicable in children. Since onset of new nevi/evolution of the old nevi is common in growing children the evolution of lesion also cannot be used as a criteria. To diagnose melanomas in children an alternative criteria is proposed: ABCD and CUP.[6]
      - Amelanotic
      - Bleeding, Bump

- Color uniformity
- De novo, any diameter
- Color pink/red, changing
- Ulceration, upward thickening
- Pyogenic granuloma like lesions, pop-up of new lesions

II. *Nodular melanomas:* Due to its vertical growth pattern, early nodular melanomas do not follow ABCDE rule. To help in diagnosing these melanomas EFG criteria is used.[7]
- Elevation
- Firm on palpation
- Continuous growth for 1 month

III. *Subungual melanomas:* These melanomas are buried below the nail. So it does not follow the ABCDE rule. An alternative ABCDEF criteria is proposed to diagnose this condition.[8]
- Age >50 years, African-Americans, Asians and native Americans
- Brown to black band
- Change in nail bed
- *Digit most commonly involved:* Great toe or thumb
- Extension of pigment on to proximal and/or lateral nail fold
- Family or personal history of melanoma

Biopsy of the lesion should be considered if any of the above criteria are present in a patient.

4. *Other noninvasive diagnostic aids:* Imaging technologies, including dermoscopy, confocal microscopy, and multispectral imaging, may improve the early recognition of melanoma. Among them, dermoscopy is the most widely used and studied diagnostic tool.

Histopathological Diagnosis

- *Biopsy:* Biopsy can be a full thickness excision biopsy or partial incisional biopsy. Full thickness excision biopsy includes complete excision of the suspicious lesion with 1–3 mm margin and part of subcutaneous fat. Partial incisional biopsy is recommended for large lesions or for lesions in cosmetic areas, e.g., face or in lesions with low suspicion for melanoma. Various types of biopsy which can be used in malignant melanoma are described in **Table 1**.
- *Histopathology:* The definitive diagnosis of melanoma is always done by histopathological examination. The presence of atypical melanocytes and architectural distortion are required for diagnosis.

PROGNOSTIC FACTORS AND STAGING

The eighth edition of the American Joint Committee on Cancer (AJCC) tumor, node, metastasis (TNM) staging system is based upon an evaluation of the primary tumor, the regional lymph nodes and lymphatic drainage, and the

TABLE 1: Various types of biopsies in a case of suspicious lesion.

Types of biopsy	Description	Indications
Excisional biopsy	It can be an elliptical excision or punch biopsy or saucerization. Whole lesion is excised with a margin of 2 mm	Preferred method for biopsy of any suspicious lesion
Incisional biopsy	A full thickness biopsy is taken from the thickest portion of the lesion	Method of choice when biopsy is being done from cosmetic areas and functionally critical areas, e.g., face, ear, digits, large lesions where excisional biopsy is difficult
Punch biopsy	A full thickness biopsy is taken as a punch	Same as incisional biopsy
Shave biopsy	Includes removal of superficial layers of skin using a blade	Not an ideal method if melanoma is suspected. Depth analysis is not possible. Indicated when suspicion of melanoma is low

presence or absence of distant metastases. The information from TNM staging is then combined to classify patients into AJCC prognostic stage groups.[9] The 8th edition of AJCC staging for melanoma is described in **Table 2**.

Other Prognostic Factors

- *Age:* Old age is associated with worse prognosis. In spite of aggressive tumor features, young patients do better than old age patients.
- *Gender:* Females do better than males for similar stage.
- *Anatomic location*: Melanomas arising on head and neck area, trunk and lower extremity have worse prognosis compared to melanomas arising from upper extremity.
- *Pathologic factors not included in AJCC staging:*
    a. *Tumor burden within a sentinel lymph node:* Larger tumor burden is associated with worse disease free survival and melanoma specific survival.[10]
    b. *Growth pattern:* Tumors with predominant vertical growth pattern have worse prognosis.
    c. *Lymphatic invasion:* Lymphatic invasion of tumor is an important negative prognostic factor.
    d. *Nevus associated melanoma:* Nevus associated melanoma are associated with a better prognosis than melanomas arising de novo.[11]
    e. *Desmoplastic melanoma:* They are locally aggressive but still the prognosis is better when compared to other forms of melanoma.

Staging Workup

Clinical stage I and II: Melanoma can metastasize to any organ in the body. Common sites include skin, subcutaneous tissues, lymph nodes, lungs, liver,

TABLE 2: American Joint Committee on Cancer (AJCC) 8th edition tumor-node-metastasis (TNM) staging of melanoma.

T Category	Thickness	Ulceration status
TX: Primary tumor thickness cannot be assessed (e.g., diagnosis by curettage)	Not applicable	Not applicable
T0: No evidence of primary tumor (e.g., unknown primary or completely regressed melanoma)	Not applicable	Not applicable
Tis (melanoma in situ)	Not applicable	Not applicable
T1	≤ 1 mm	Unknown or unspecified
T1a	<0.8 mm	Without ulceration
T1b	<0.8 mm	With ulceration
	0.8–1.0 mm	With or without ulceration
T2	>1.0–2.0 mm	Unknown or unspecified
T2a	>1.0–2.0 mm	Without ulceration
T2b	>1.0–2.0 mm	With ulceration
T3	>2.0–4.0 mm	Unknown or unspecified
T3a	>2.0–4.0 mm	Without ulceration
T3b	>2.0–4.0 mm	With ulceration
T4	>4.0 mm	Unknown or unspecified
T4a	>4.0 mm	Without ulceration
T4b	>4.0 mm	With ulceration

	Extent of regional lymph node and/or lymphatic metastasis	
N Category	Number of tumor-involved regional lymph node	Presence of in-transit, satellite and/or microsatellite metastases
NX	Regional nodes not assessed (eg. SLN biopsy not performed, regional nodes previously removed for another reason) *Exception:* When there are no clinically detected regional metastases in a pT1 cM0 melanoma, assign cN0 instead of pNX	No
N0	No regional metastases detected	No
N1	One tumor-involved node or in-transit, satellite, and/or microsatellite metastases with no tumor-involved nodes	
N1a	One clinically occult (i.e., detected by SLN biopsy)	No
N1b	One clinically detected	No
N1c	No regional lymph node disease	Yes
N2	Two or three tumor-involved nodes or in-transit, satellite, and/or microsatellite metastases with one tumor-involved node	
N2a	Two or three clinically occult (i.e., detected by SLN biopsy)	No

Contd...

Contd...

N Category	Extent of regional lymph node and/or lymphatic metastasis	
	Number of tumor-involved regional lymph node	Presence of in-transit, satellite and/or microsatellite metastases
N2b	Two or three, at least one of which was clinically detected	No
N2c	One clinically occult or clinically detected	Yes
N3	Four or more tumor-involved nodes or in-transit, satellite, and/or microsatellite metastases with two or more tumor-involved nodes, or any number of matted nodes without or with in-transit, satellite, and/or microsatellite metastases	
N3a	Four or more clinically occult (i.e., detected by SLN biopsy)	No
N3b	Four or more, at least one of which was clinically detected, or presence of any number of matted nodes	No
N3c	Two or more clinically occult or clinically detected and/or presence of any number of matted nodes	Yes

M Category	Anatomic site	LDH level
M0	No evidence of distant metastasis	Not applicable
M1	Evidence of distant metastasis	See below
M1a	Distant metastasis to skin, soft tissue including muscle, and/or nonregional lymph node	Not recorded or unspecified
M1a(0)		Not elevated
M1a(1)		Elevated
M1b	Distant metastasis to lung with or without M1a sites of disease	Not recorded or unspecified
M1b(0)		Not elevated
M1b(1)		Elevated
M1c	Distant metastasis to non-CNS visceral sites with or without M1a or M1b sites of disease	Not recorded or unspecified
M1c(0)		Not elevated
M1c(1)		Elevated
M1d	Distant metastasis to CNS with or without M1a, M1b, or M1c sites of disease	Not recorded or unspecified
M1d(0)		Not elevated
M1d(1)		Elevated

- Serum lactate dehydrogenase (LDH)
- Suffixes for M category. (0) LDH not elevated. (1) LDH elevated.
- No suffix is used if LDH is not recorded or is unspecified.

	Clinical staging (cTNM)*		
	T	N	M
Stage 0	Tis	N0	M0
Stage IA	T1a	N0	M0
Stage IB	T1b	N0	M0
	T2a	N0	M0

Contd...

Contd...

	Clinical staging (cTNM)*		
	T	N	M
Stage IIA	T2b	N0	M0
	T3a	N0	M0
Stage IIB	T3b	N0	M0
	T4a	N0	M0
Stage IIC	T4b	N0	M0
Stage III	Any T, Tis	≥N1	M0
Stage IV	Any T	Any N	M1

*Clinical staging includes microstaging of the primary melanoma and clinical/radiologic/biopsy evaluation for metastases. By convention, clinical staging should be used after biopsy of the primary melanoma, with clinical assessment for regional and distant metastases. Note that pathological assessment of the primary melanoma is used for both clinical and pathological classification. Diagnostic biopsies to evaluate possible regional and/or distant metastasis also are included. Note there is only one stage group for clinical Stage III melanoma.

	Pathological staging (pTNM)**		
	T	N	M
Stage 0†	Tis	N0	M0
Stage IA	T1a	N0	M0
	T1b	N0	M0
Stage IB	T2a	N0	M0
Stage IIA	T2b	N0	M0
	T3a	N0	M0
Stage IIB	T3b	N0	M0
	T4a	N0	M0
Stage IIC	T4b	N0	M0
Stage IIIA	T1a/b.T2a	N1a, N2a	M0
Stage IIIB	T0	N1b. N1c	M0
	T1a/b, T2a	N1b/c. N2b	M0
	T2b, T3a	N1a/b/c. N2a/b	M0
Stage IIIC	T0	N2b/c. N3b/c	M0
	T1a/b, T2a/b, T3a	N2c, N3a/b/c	M0
	T3b. T4a	Any N ≥ N1	M0
	T4b	N1a/b/c. N2a/b/c	M0
Stage IIID	T4b	N3a/b/c	M0
Stage IV	Any T, Tis	Any N	M1

**Pathological staging includes microstaging of the primary melanoma, including any additional staging information from the wide-excision (surgical) specimen that constitutes primary tumor surgical treatment and pathological information about the regional lymph nodes after SLN biopsy or therapeutic lymph node dissection for clinically evident regional lymph node disease.
†Pathological Stage 0 and pathological T1 without clinically detected regional or distant metastases (pTis/pT1 cN0 cM0) do not require pathological evaluation of lymph nodes to complete pathological staging: use cN0 to assign pathological stage.

bone, and brain. Since stage I and II are clinically node negative and there is very less chance of distant metastasis there is no role of routine imaging studies. Sentinel lymph node biopsy (SLNB) is indicated in intermediate thickness and thick melanoma. PET scan is not a useful modality in stage I and II melanoma. This is due to low sensitivity and rarity of distant metastasis in stage I and II melanoma. In addition they have high false positive rates. In a retrospective series published by Arrangoiz R et al. they found that only 7% of patients with T4 primary and clinically node negative disease had distant metastasis.[12]

Stage III disease: Stage III disease is defined by the presence of regional disease in the form of lymph node metastasis, in transit nodules and satellite lesions. Patients with clinical stage I and II disease who have positive sentinel node will also be upgraded to stage III disease. Patients with clinically detected stage III disease are at high risk for distant relapse. These patients need to be thoroughly evaluated with complete blood count, serum lactate dehydrogenase (LDH) and chest radiography. Imaging studies in the form of computed tomography (CT) scan or positron emission tomography-CT (PET-CT) is routinely done in symptomatic patients to rule out distant metastasis **(Figs. 4A and B)**. Routine use of CT/PET-CT in asymptomatic patients and SLNB positive patients is still controversial. Many centers still recommend these imaging modalities in asymptomatic patients to have a base line imaging for follow up. Since the introduction of PET-CT as a single modality of imaging, it has replaced PET alone and CT scan as the imaging modality of choice.

Stage IV: Any patient with known systemic disease should be evaluated thoroughly to identify other sites of metastasis. Whole body PET-CT and MRI brain are the investigations of choice to identify additional sites of metastasis. CT scan of chest, abdomen, and pelvis is used as an alternative to PET-CT if it is not available. Serum LDH is obtained in all patients, which will be used as a prognostic marker and as the marker of response to therapy. Rest of the investigations are based on the symptoms of the patient, e.g., MRI spine for back pain.

SURGICAL MANAGEMENT

The goal of surgical management is to excise the primary tumor with negative margins and assessment of regional nodal basin either by SLNB or therapeutic lymph node dissection **(Figs. 5A to C)**. Historically melanoma was treated by wide excision with 3–5 cm margin and routine regional lymph node dissection. This was based on the principle that any patient who underwent resection with narrow margins and in whom regional nodal basin was not addressed developed locoregional recurrence which was difficult to treat. In the past few decades lot of advances has taken place in the management of melanoma. The treatment has become more conservative and more scientific.[13]

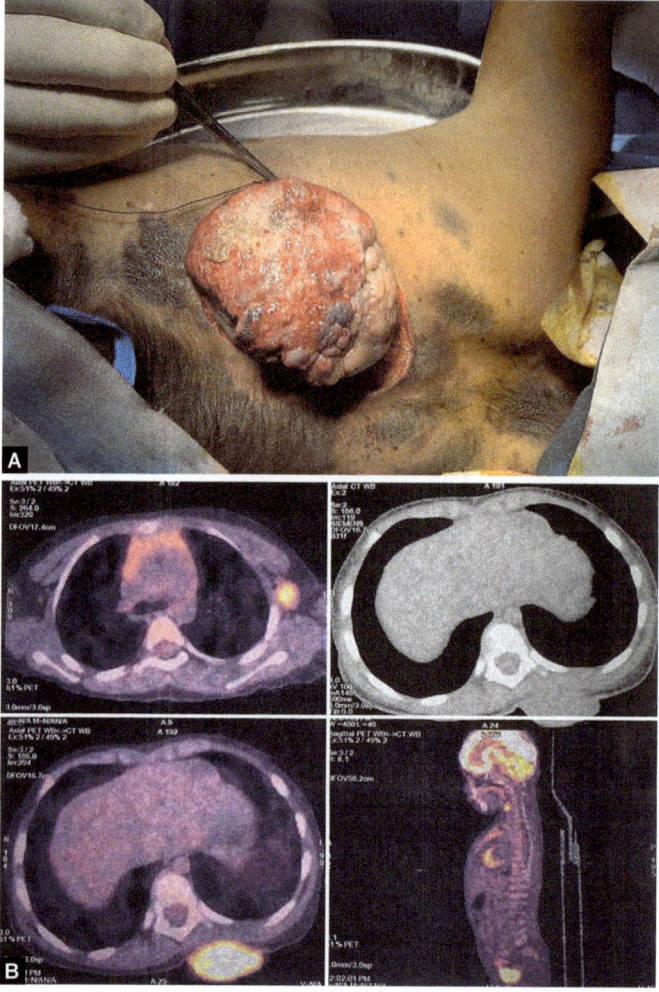

Figs. 4A and B: (A) A 6-year-old kid with multiple dysplastic nevi over back with nodular melanoma; (B) Positron emission tomography-computed tomography (PET-CT) showing hypermetabolic lesion over back and left axillary lymph node metastasis.

1. Surgical excision:
    a. *Primary goal:* Margin free resection
    b. Secondary goals:
        i. preserve function and cosmesis
        ii. Minimum surgical morbidity
        iii. Minimal hospital stay
    c. Margins:
        i. *Old concept (Oslen's theory):* Oslen published her experience of 500 patients in the year 1967. She proposed that atypical melanocytes will be present up to 5 cm from the primary tumor. If these melanocytes are left behind, it will lead to local recurrence.

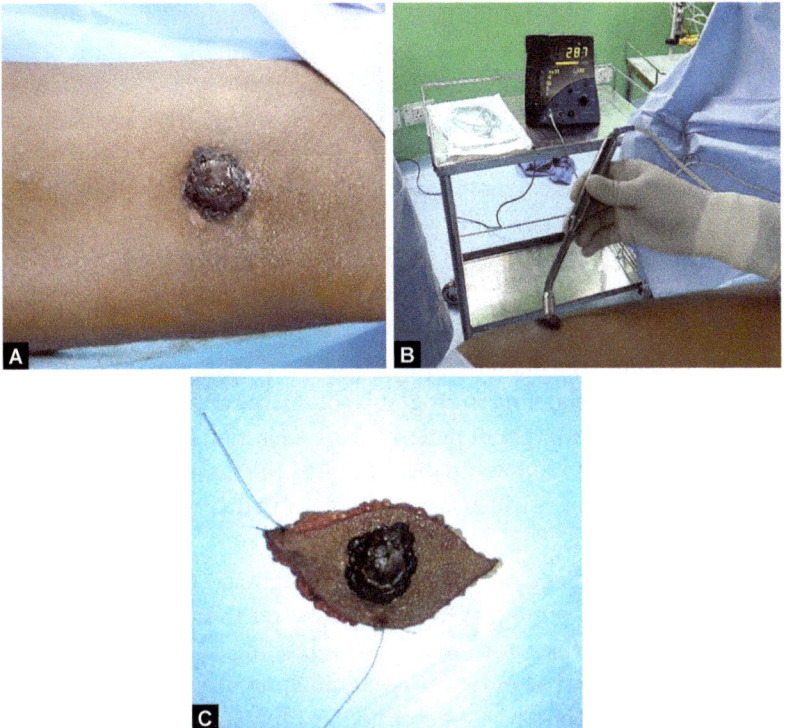

Figs. 5A to C: (A) Nodular melanoma over right thigh; (B) Intraoperative sentinel node identification using gamma probe; (C) Wide excision specimen of melanoma.

Hence wider margin resections were emphasized to decrease local recurrence.[14] Based on her findings wider resections with margins up to 5 cm became the standard of care.

ii. *New concept:* With many studies proving that, the depth of the tumor is most important prognostic indicator in melanoma and not the width. The traditional concept of wide excision was challenged. Later many randomized controlled trials (RCTs) were conducted to find out adequate margins in a case of melanoma.

One of the first studies conducted was the World Health Organization Melanoma Program trial. They included 612 patients with primary melanoma less than 2 mm thickness. They randomized patients into two groups: (1) 305 patients underwent excision with 1 cm margin and (2) 307 underwent excision with 3 cm margin. At a median follow-up of 90 months there was no difference in disease free survival or overall survival between the two groups.[15] However, they found that the local recurrence was higher (3.3%) in patients with tumor thickness between 1.1 and 2.0 mm. Thus, it was concluded that melanomas with thickness less than or equal to 1 mm could be adequately treated with a margin of 1 cm.

Later a multi-institutional randomized study was done in United States to compare a new 2 cm margin with the standard of care 4 cm margin in patients with intermediate thickness melanoma (1–4 mm). At a median follow-up of 6 years there was no difference in local recurrence (0.8% for 2-cm margins and 1.7% for 4-cm margins), rate of in-transit metastases [2.1% and 2.5%, respectively (p = NS)] and overall survival [5-year survival rate was 79.5% for the 2-cm margin patients and 83.7% for the 4-cm margin patients (p = NS)]. The need for skin grafting was reduced from 46% with 4-cm surgical margins to 11% with 2-cm surgical margins (p <0.001).[16]

To reduce the margins further, British association of plastic surgeons and UK melanoma study group conducted an RCT comparing 1 cm with 3 cm margin in patients with melanoma thicker than 2 mm. At a median follow-up of 60 months the group with 1 cm margin had a higher risk of local recurrence. But there was no difference in overall survival.[17]

Above studies clearly show that a margin of 1 cm is recommended for thin melanomas (<1 mm). However there is no clear data to define margins for intermediate thickness (1–4 mm) and thick melanomas (>4 mm). Current guidelines across various countries and organizations are described in **Table 3**.

2. *Management of lymph nodes:* Initial evaluation of lymph node is done by physical examination. Physical examination is often inaccurate, since 20% of cN0 patients still harbor microscopic disease and 20% of patients with cN+ will be pathologically negative. To obtain more definite information fine needle aspiration cytology (FNAC) and SLNB are used.

   a. *SLNB:* Lymphatic mapping using SLNB is the standard method for evaluation of regional lymph nodes in cN0 patients with significant risk of regional lymph node metastasis **(Table 4)**. Tc-99 can be used for both preoperative mapping and for sentinel node identification in the operating room using a hand-held gamma probe (*see* **Figs. 5A to C**). The Multicenter Selective Lymphadenectomy Trial (MSLT-I) was a prospective, randomized trial which began accrual in 1994 with the goal

TABLE 3: Recommended margin for various thicknesses of melanoma.

Breslow's thickness (mm)	T stage	Recommended margin of excision (cm)
Melanoma in situ	Tis	0.5–1
<1.0	T1	1
1.01–2.0	T2	1–2
2.01–4.0	T3	2
>4.0	T4	2

TABLE 4: Sentinel lymph node biopsy (SLNB) recommendations: The National Comprehensive Cancer Network (NCCN) guidelines.

Melanoma thickness (mm)	NCCN recommendations regarding SLNB
Melanoma in situ	Not recommended
<0.76	Not recommended
0.76–1.0 (no ulceration and mitotic rate <1/mm^2)	Considered
0.76–1.0 (ulcerated or mitotic rate ≥1/mm^2)	Discussed and offered
≥1.0–4.0	Discussed and offered

of determining whether SLNB provided a survival benefit to patients with primary melanoma. The patients were assigned to either undergo wide local excision alone with observation of nodal basin or wide local excision with SLNB and immediate therapeutic lymph node dissection if SLNB was positive. In patients with intermediate thickness melanoma 10 year disease free survival was significantly improved in SLNB group compared to the observation group (71.3 ± 1.8% vs. 64.7 ± 2.3%; hazard ratio for recurrence or metastasis, 0.76; P = 0.01). Similar results was also observed in thick melanomas (50.7 ± 4.0% vs. 40.5 ± 4.7%; hazard ratio, 0.70; P = 0.03).[18]

The current standard of care is to do completion lymph node dissection in all patients found to have SLNB positive on pathological evaluation. In patients who underwent completion lymph node dissection only 15–18% had metastatic disease in the nonsentinel nodes. To study if observation after SLNB is an effective modality, MSLT-II study was designed. Patients who were found to be positive on SLNB were randomly assigned to two groups: (1) group 1 underwent completion lymph node dissection; (2) group 2 was kept under observation with ultrasonography (USG). At the end of 3 years, disease free survival rate was higher in dissection group compared to observation group (68±1.7% and 63±1.7%, respectively; P = 0.05 by the log-rank test). The disease control at the regional nodal basin was also higher in the dissection group (92±1.0% vs. 77±1.5%; P <0.001 by the log-rank test). It should be noted that only 11.5% patients had nonsentinel lymph node metastasis. Lymphedema rates were higher in dissection group (24.1% vs 6.3%).[19]

b. *Macroscopic disease:* Any clinically or radiologically identified lymph node should be confirmed pathologically by FNAC. Individuals with positive FNAC should be advised a staging evaluation to rule out distant metastasis before advising for lymph node dissection. In the absence of distant metastasis and a FNAC proven lymph node metastasis, therapeutic lymph node dissection is the standard of care.

LOCOREGIONAL THERAPIES IN MELANOMA

Hyperthermic isolated limb perfusion (HILP) and isolated limb infusion (ILI) are indicated in locoregionally unresectable recurrence and in patients with in-transit metastasis. Some unresectable recurrences may become resectable following a response to HILP or ILI therapy. Although no RCTs have been conducted, theoretically regional chemotherapy will prevent further in-transit recurrences.

Hyperthermic Isolated Limb Perfusion

As the name suggests a high dose of chemotherapy drug is circulated in the extremity in a hyperthermic setting. The vessels supplying the extremity are dissected and cannulated at the root of the limb. The limb vasculature is isolated from the systemic circulation using a tourniquet. Femoral vessels are used in case of lower limb melanoma and axillary vessels are used in upper limb disease. The temperature of the limb is raised up to 39–41°C using a HILP pump and warm blankets. Once the ideal temperature is reached the chemotherapy drug is circulated for a period of 60 minutes. Flow rates are typically maintained between 400 and 600 mL/min and a pump oxygenator is used to oxygenate the perfusate. During the procedure, systemic leakage of the chemotherapy is monitored with a precordial probe used to detect radiolabeled red blood cells in the circuit that may leak into the systemic circulation. The overall response rates to HILP is reported between 80 and 90% and complete response rates (CR) are as high as 55–65%.[20]

Melphalan is the most common drug used in HILP. Many centers in Europe are using Melphalan and tumor necrosis factor-alpha (TNF-α) as combination. But a large multicenter trial American College of Surgeons Oncology Group (ACOSOG) Z0020 trial conducted in United States compared Melphalan alone with Melphalan + TNF-α in HILP. The addition of TNF-α did not improve the complete response rate (25% vs. 26%) and increased the regional toxicity.[21]

Lymphedema has been reported in 12–36% of patients after HILP.[22] Acute skin reactions are classified under Wieberdink grading system **(Table 5)**.[23]

Grade IV and V toxicities are reported in 3–5% of patients after HILP.[21,22] Apart from the regional toxicities, melphalan and TNF-α can lead to systemic

TABLE 5: Wieberdink toxicity grading system for severity of complications following regional therapies.

Grade I	No reaction
Grade II	Slight erythema or edema
Grade III	Considerable edema or erythema with some blistering
Grade IV	Toxicities may result in functional impairment or even compartment syndrome requiring fasciotomy
Grade V	Severe tissue necrosis or vascular catastrophe that often results in amputation

TABLE 6: Comparison between hyperthermic isolated limb perfusion (HILP) and isolated limb infusion (ILI).

HILP	ILI
High flow rates: 400–600 mL/min	Low flow rate: 80–120 mL/min
Hyperthermia >38°C	Normothermia to mild hyperthermia 37-40°C
Open, surgical cannulation of vessels	Minimally invasive, percutaneous cannulation of vessels
Difficult to repeat the procedure	Easy to repeat the procedure
Aerobic, oxygenated, mildly acidotic perfusate	Ischemic, anaerobic and acidotic perfusate
Melphalan ± TNF-α	Melphalan and actinomycin D
Overall response rates 80–90%	Overall response rates 80%

toxicity such as GI disturbance, myelosuppression, hypotension and liver dysfunction when it leaks in to systemic circulation.

Isolated Limb Infusion

Isolated limb infusion is the less invasive counterpart of HILP. ILI is a low flow perfusion conducted in a hyperthermic, acidotic and hypoxic environment. The comparison between HILP and ILI is shown in **Table 6**.

Beasley et al. reported a complete response rate of 30% and a partial response rate of 14% with ILI. ILI was associated with less morbidity compared to HILP.[24]

Intralesional Therapies

Intralesional therapy is indicated in patients with unresectable, multiple and locally advanced stage IIIb and IIIc melanoma. First reports of use of intralesional therapy dates back to 1960s, when BCG was used in melanomas to treat dermal and subcutaneous melanoma. Due to significant toxicities associated with this treatment, it did not gain much of popularity.

Other intralesional agents that have been studied include the cytokines IL-2, interferon gamma, and interferon alpha. Generally, these agents are associated with high response rates locally at the site of injection but no systemic response.

Three compounds that are of increased interest currently are talimogene laherparepvec (T-VEC), HLA-B7 gene therapy (allovectin 7), and PV-10 because of the perception that they may generate a specific antitumor immune response and be associated with a higher systemic response rate than is seen with other compounds injected into tumors.

Talimogene laherparepvec—an attenuated oncolytic herpes simplex virus that contains granulocyte macrophage colony stimulating factor (GM-CSF) gene is injected directly in to the tumor to induce induction of systemic immune response and local lytic replication in the tumor.

A phase III trial was conducted comparing T-VEC versus GM-CSF in patients with melanoma which were not amenable for surgical resection. The T-VEC was given as intralesional injections once every 2 weeks, while the GM-CSF was given subcutaneously daily for 14 days in each 28 day cycle. The primary end point was to assess the durable response rate which was defined as an objective response lasting continuously for ≥6 months. Secondary endpoints were overall survival and overall response rate. The durable response rate was 16.3% in T-VEC group compared to 2.1% in GM-CSF group. Overall response rate also favored T-VEC (26.4% vs. 5.7%).[25]

Further studies are now being conducted to study combination of other immunotherapy drugs with T-VEC.

MANAGEMENT OF ADVANCED CUTANEOUS MELANOMA

Treatment options available for the management of advanced melanoma are: surgical metastasectomy, immunotherapy, targeted therapy and radiation therapy to the symptomatic sites of metastasis **(Flowchart 1)**. Cytotoxic chemotherapy has no established role in management of metastatic melanoma.

- *Surgical metastasectomy:* Metastasectomy can be used as an upfront treatment strategy in patients with limited metastasis and to eradicate the residual disease after good response to systemic therapy. Adjuvant systemic therapy should be considered in all patients undergoing upfront metastasectomy.
- *Immunotherapy:* Checkpoint inhibition with an antiprogrammed cell death 1(PD-1) antibody in combination with anti-cytotoxic T-lymphocyte

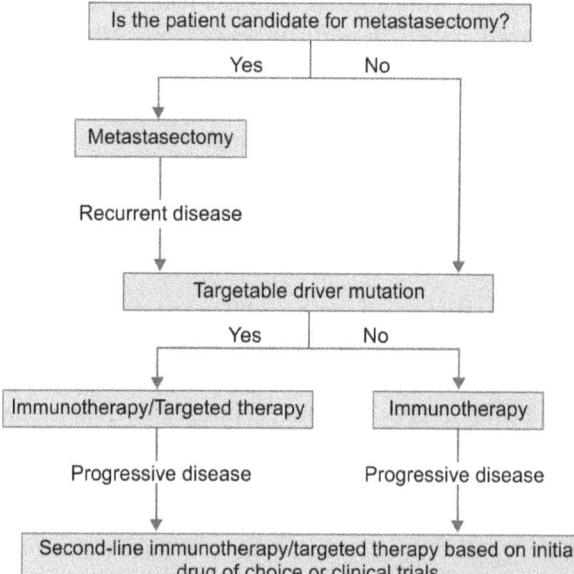

Flowchart 1: Management of stage IV melanoma.

associated protein 4 (CTLA-4) antibody has a proven efficacy in improving the progression free survival in patients with metastatic melanoma. In an RCT conducted in UK, they found that the combination of nivolumab plus ipilimumab significantly increased the response rate and extent of tumor shrinkage compared with either nivolumab alone or ipilimumab alone.[26]

- *Targeted therapy:* Nearly 50% of patients of cutaneous melanoma have a V600 mutation in *BRAF gene* and 15% have mutation in NRAS. BRAF inhibition induces rapid tumor regression. Addition of MEK inhibitors which is a downstream signal in the MAPK pathway reduced the toxicity of BRAF inhibitors and also reduces the resistance to MEK inhibitors.[27] Simultaneous inhibition of BRAF and MEK improves response rates and survival compared with BRAF inhibition alone. The rapid tumor regression is especially important for patients with extensive tumor burden and disease-related symptoms. As a result, combined BRAF plus MEK inhibitor therapy has replaced the use of single-agent BRAF inhibitors. Options include dabrafenib plus trametinib, vemurafenib plus cobimetinib, and encorafenib plus binimetinib. Treatment is generally well tolerated.
- *Radiation therapy:* Radiation therapy may have a palliative role for symptomatic localized areas of disease. Radiation therapy, especially stereotactic radiosurgery, may be particularly important for patients with brain metastases.
- *Cytotoxic chemotherapy*: Cytotoxic chemotherapy (single agent or combination) has not been shown to improve overall survival in patients with advanced melanoma. Response rates are typically less than 20%, and median response durations are 4-6 months. Its role is limited to patients who have progressed after optimal treatment with other systemic therapy options.

MANAGEMENT OF LOCAL RECURRENCE

Local recurrence is defined as a tumor regrowth within 2 cm of the surgical scar following definitive excision of a primary melanoma with appropriate surgical margins. Recurrences that are more than 2 cm from the primary lesion but are not beyond the regional nodal basin are termed in-transit metastases **(Fig. 6)**.

Surgery is the treatment of choice for most melanoma local recurrences. There is no evidence to employ extensive margins in case of recurrent setting. Most melanoma surgeons recommend the use of resection margins for recurrences that are sufficient to ensure a grossly and microscopically clear margin, although there are no data that definitively address this issue.

Strong consideration should be given to performing lymphatic mapping and a sentinel lymph node (SLN) biopsy in appropriate patients with isolated local recurrence or in-transit disease, because of its prognostic significance and the potential for additional therapeutic options if the SLN biopsy is positive. Factors influencing this decision should be similar to those for patients with an aggressive primary melanoma.

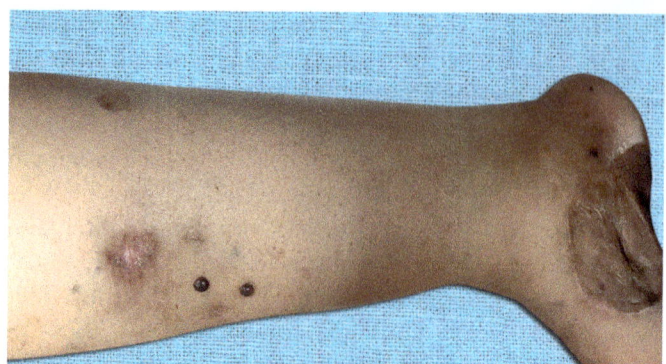

Fig. 6: In-transit nodules over leg away from the primary site (foot).

Patients with melanoma local recurrences are at high risk for the development of disseminated disease. Randomized clinical trials are not available to address the value of adjuvant immunotherapy in patients who are rendered disease free following resection of a local recurrence. However, patients who have undergone resection of a local recurrence and have no other evidence of disease should be considered for adjuvant therapy after discussion with the patient.

For patients with a local recurrence and no evidence of systemic disease, but the local recurrence is felt to be unresectable, options include neoadjuvant systemic therapy to downstage the recurrence, isolated limb infusion, isolated limb perfusion, and/or intralesional therapy with talimogene laherparepvec.

For patients with a local recurrence and evidence of systemic disease elsewhere, systemic therapy using targeted agents or immunotherapy as a first line of therapy is suggested. Use of intralesional therapy with talimogene laherparepvec may be considered in patients who are felt not to be candidates for systemic therapy. Surgery is occasionally utilized in a palliative fashion for control of locoregional recurrences in the presence of distant disease.

SURVEILLANCE AFTER TREATMENT

The main objective of follow-up is to detect locoregional recurrences, distant recurrences, and second primary melanomas in a potentially curable stage. Since there is no clear cut evidence to decide the frequency and duration of follow-up, it should be determined based on the available resources and patient preferences in conjunction with the preferences of the treating doctor. Nearly half of patients treated for melanoma will have recurrence in their life time. Among these, 20% are local recurrences, 50% are in regional lymph nodes and rest 30% are distant relapses.[28] The incidence of second melanomas range from 2 to 5% over a period of 5–20 years after the initial diagnosis.[29]

Early detection of the recurrence has its own clinical implications. An isolated local recurrence can be treated with repeat excision without affecting the overall survival. Prognosis in patients with regional relapse depends on the tumor burden at the time of detection. By the time the tumor is detected by physical examination or when the patient becomes symptomatic, the tumor burden will be high.[30]

Melanoma can metastasize to any organ in the body. Lungs are the most common site of metastasis. For patients with lung metastasis, the 5 year overall survival is 4%.[31] One-fourth of these patients who are suitable for surgical metastasectomy had an improved 5 year survival up to 30%.[31-33]

Most of local recurrences in melanoma can be effectively diagnosed by clinical examination. Up to 95% of local recurrences can be picked up by either self-detection or clinical examination.[32,33]

Regional lymph node relapses can be effectively evaluated using USG. Ultrasonography has highest sensitivity (60%; 95% CI, 33-83%), specificity (97%; 95% CI, 88-99%), and diagnostic odds ratio (42; 95% CI, 8.08-249.8) for the surveillance of regional lymph nodes[34] and is therefore superior to physical examination in detecting regional nodal recurrences.[35]

For the surveillance of distant metastasis, PET/CT had the highest sensitivity (80%; 95% CI, 53-93), specificity (87%; 95% CI, 54-97%), and diagnostic odds ratio (1675; 95% CI, 226.5-15,920).[34]

Follow-up schedules are tailored by risk of recurrence. NCCN recommends the following follow-up schedule based on stage of melanoma at diagnosis.[36]

1. Stage Ia-IIa:
   a. History and physical examination every 6-12 months for 5 years and annually thereafter.
   b. No need of imaging to detect asymptomatic recurrences.
   c. Imaging as indicated to investigate specific signs and symptoms.
2. Stage IIb-IV:
   a. History and physical examination every 3-6 months for 2 years, then every 3-12 months for 3 years and annually thereafter.
   b. Imaging as indicated to investigate specific signs or symptoms.
   c. Consider imaging every 3-12 months to screen for recurrence or metastatic disease(Category 2B recommendation)
   d. Routine imaging to screen for asymptomatic recurrence or metastatic disease is not recommended after 3-5 years.

CONCLUSION

Malignant Melanoma is the most aggressive type of skin cancer with distinct clinical features. Early detection is of paramount importance in determining the overall outcome of melanoma. Clinical suspicion and high risk history should alert the physician to refer the patient to an expert for examination and biopsy. Greater efforts should be made in improving awareness among both public and health care providers to facilitate early detection. Surgery plays an important role in the management of melanoma. Recent studies are showing promising outcomes with immunotherapy. Multidisciplinary approach is crucial for optimal diagnosis, staging and management of melanoma patients.

REFERENCES

1. Bray F, Ferlay J, Soerjomataram I, Siegel RL, Torre LA, Jemal A. Global cancer statistics 2018: GLOBOCAN estimates of incidence and mortality worldwide for 36 cancers in 185 countries. CA Cancer J Clin. 2018;68(6):394-424.
2. Balch CM, Soong SJ, Gershenwald JE, Thompson JF, Reintgen DS, Cascinelli N, et al. Prognostic factors analysis of 17,600 melanoma patients: validation of the American Joint Committee on Cancer melanoma staging system. J Clin Oncol Off J Am Soc Clin Oncol. 2001;19(16):3622-34.
3. Thomas L, Tranchand P, Berard F, Secchi T, Colin C, Moulin G. Semiological value of ABCDE criteria in the diagnosis of cutaneous pigmented tumors. Dermatol Basel Switz. 1998;197(1):11-7.
4. National Collaborating Centre for Cancer (UK). Melanoma: Assessment and Management (National Institute for Health and Care Excellence: Clinical Guidelines). London: National Institute for Health and Care Excellence (UK); 2015.
5. Gaudy-Marqueste C, Wazaefi Y, Bruneu Y, Triller R, Thomas L, Pellacani G, et al. Ugly Duckling Sign as a Major Factor of Efficiency in Melanoma Detection. JAMA Dermatol. 2017;153(4):279-84.
6. Cordoro KM, Gupta D, Frieden IJ, McCalmont T, Kashani-Sabet M. Pediatric melanoma: results of a large cohort study and proposal for modified ABCD detection criteria for children. J Am Acad Dermatol. 2013;68(6):913-25.
7. Chamberlain AJ, Fritschi L, Kelly JW. Nodular melanoma: patients' perceptions of presenting features and implications for earlier detection. J Am Acad Dermatol. 2003;48(5):694-701.
8. Levit EK, Kagen MH, Scher RK, Grossman M, Altman E. The ABC rule for clinical detection of subungual melanoma. J Am Acad Dermatol. 2000 Feb;42(2 Pt 1):269-74.
9. Gershenwald JE, Scolyer RA, Hess KR, Sondak VK, Long GV, Ross MI, et al. Melanoma staging: evidence-based changes in the American Joint Committee on Cancer eighth edition cancer staging manual. CA Cancer J Clin. 2017;67(6):472-92.
10. van der Ploeg AP, van Akkooi AC, Haydu LE, Scolyer RA, Murali R, Verhoef C, et al. The prognostic significance of sentinel node tumour burden in melanoma patients: an international, multicenter study of 1539 sentinel node-positive. Eur J Cancer. 2014;50(1):111-20.
11. Cymerman RM, Shao Y, Wang K, Zhang Y, Murzaku EC, Penn LA, et al. De Novo vs Nevus-Associated Melanomas: Differences in Associations With Prognostic Indicators and Survival. J Natl Cancer Inst. 2016;108(10).
12. Arrangoiz R, Papavasiliou P, Stransky CA, Yu JQ, Tianyu L, Sigurdson ER, et al. Preoperative FDG-PET/CT Is an Important Tool in the Management of Patients with Thick (T4) Melanoma. Dermatol Res Pract. 2012;2012:614349.
13. Thompson JF, Scolyer RA, Uren RF. Surgical management of primary cutaneous melanoma: excision margins and the role of sentinel lymph node examination. Surg Oncol Clin N Am. 2006;15(2):301-18.
14. Olsen G. The malignant melanoma of the skin. New theories based on a study of 500 cases. Dan Med Bull. 1967;14(9):229-38.
15. Veronesi U, Cascinelli N. Narrow excision (1-cm margin). A safe procedure for thin cutaneous melanoma. Arch Surg Chic Ill 1960. 1991;126(4):438-41.
16. Balch CM, Urist MM, Karakousis CP, Smith TJ, Temple WJ, Drzewiecki K, et al. Efficacy of 2-cm surgical margins for intermediate-thickness melanomas (1 to 4 mm). Results of a multi-institutional randomized surgical trial. Ann Surg. 1993;218(3):262-9.
17. Thomas JM, Newton-Bishop J, A'Hern R, Coombes G, Timmons M, Evans J, et al. Excision margins in high-risk malignant melanoma. N Engl J Med. 2004;350(8):757-66.
18. Morton DL, Thompson JF, Cochran AJ, Mozzillo N, Nieweg OE, Roses DF, et al. Final trial report of sentinel-node biopsy versus nodal observation in melanoma. N Engl J Med. 2014;370(7):599-609.

19. Faries MB, Thompson JF, Cochran AJ, Andtbacka RH, Mozzillo N, Zager JS, et al. Completion Dissection or Observation for Sentinel-Node Metastasis in Melanoma. N Engl J Med. 2017;376(23):2211-22.
20. Fraker DL. Management of in-transit melanoma of the extremity with isolated limb perfusion. Curr Treat Options Oncol. 2004;5(3):173-84.
21. Cornett WR, McCall LM, Petersen RP, Ross MI, Briele HA, Noyes RD, et al. Randomized multicenter trial of hyperthermic isolated limb perfusion with melphalan alone compared with melphalan plus tumor necrosis factor: American College of Surgeons Oncology Group Trial Z0020. J Clin Oncol Off J Am Soc Clin Oncol. 2006 1;24(25): 4196-201.
22. Möller MG, Lewis JM, Dessureault S, Zager JS. Toxicities associated with hyperthermic isolated limb perfusion and isolated limb infusion in the treatment of melanoma and sarcoma. Int J Hyperth Off J Eur Soc Hyperthermic Oncol North Am Hyperth Group. 2008;24(3):275-89.
23. Wieberdink J, Benckhuysen C, Braat RP, van Slooten EA, Olthuis GA. Dosimetry in isolation perfusion of the limbs by assessment of perfused tissue volume and grading of toxic tissue reactions. Eur J Cancer Clin Oncol. 1982;18(10):905-10.
24. Beasley GM, Petersen RP, Yoo J, McMahon N, Aloia T, Petros W, et al. Isolated limb infusion for in-transit malignant melanoma of the extremity: a well-tolerated but less effective alternative to hyperthermic isolated limb perfusion. Ann Surg Oncol. 2008;15(8):2195-205.
25. Andtbacka RH, Kaufman HL, Collichio F, Amatruda T, Senzer N, Chesney J, et al. Talimogene Laherparepvec Improves Durable Response Rate in Patients With Advanced Melanoma. J Clin Oncol Off J Am Soc Clin Oncol. 2015;33(25):2780-8.
26. Larkin J, Chiarion-Sileni V, Gonzalez R, Grob JJ, Cowey CL, Lao CD, et al. Combined Nivolumab and Ipilimumab or Monotherapy in Untreated Melanoma. N Engl J Med. 2015;373(1):23-34.
27. Eroglu Z, Ribas A. Combination therapy with BRAF and MEK inhibitors for melanoma: latest evidence and place in therapy. Ther Adv Med Oncol. 2016;8(1):48-56.
28. Leiter U, Meier F, Schittek B, Garbe C. The natural course of cutaneous melanoma. J Surg Oncol. 2004;86(4):172-8.
29. Goggins WB, Tsao H. A population-based analysis of risk factors for a second primary cutaneous melanoma among melanoma survivors. Cancer. 2003;97(3):639-43.
30. Garbe C, Paul A, Kohler-Späth H, Ellwanger U, Stroebel W, Schwarz M, et al. Prospective evaluation of a follow-up schedule in cutaneous melanoma patients: recommendations for an effective follow-up strategy. J Clin Oncol Off J Am Soc Clin Oncol. 2003;21(3):520-9.
31. Harpole DH, Johnson CM, Wolfe WG, George SL, Seigler HF. Analysis of 945 cases of pulmonary metastatic melanoma. J Thorac Cardiovasc Surg. 1992;103(4):743-50.
32. Moore Dalal K, Zhou Q, Panageas KS, Brady MS, Jaques DP, Coit DG. Methods of detection of first recurrence in patients with stage I/II primary cutaneous melanoma after sentinel lymph node biopsy. Ann Surg Oncol. 2008;15(8):2206-14.
33. Meyers MO, Yeh JJ, Frank J, Long P, Deal AM, Amos KD, et al. Method of detection of initial recurrence of stage II/III cutaneous melanoma: analysis of the utility of follow-up staging. Ann Surg Oncol. 2009;16(4):941-7.
34. Xing Y, Bronstein Y, Ross MI, Askew RL, Lee JE, Gershenwald JE, et al. Contemporary diagnostic imaging modalities for the staging and surveillance of melanoma patients: a meta-analysis. J Natl Cancer Inst. 2011;103(2):129-42.
35. Bafounta ML, Beauchet A, Chagnon S, Saiag P. Ultrasonography or palpation for detection of melanoma nodal invasion: a meta-analysis. Lancet Oncol. 2004;5(11): 673-80.
36. National Comprehensive Cancer Network. Cutaneous melanoma. Available from: https://www.nccn.org/professionals/physician_gls/pdf/cutaneous_melanoma.pdf. [Last Accessed January, 2021].

CHAPTER 10
Surgical Safety Checklist

Arunima Verma, Sharad Kumar, Vinita Singh, Sunil Kumar

INTRODUCTION

Every surgeon has a story to narrate to another, often about the shock of the unexpected and at times about the regret over missed possibilities. As surgeons we talk about our great saves but discuss less about our failures. There are two reasons described for the failures. One is ignorance and the other is ineptitude. Ignorance can be overcome by gaining knowledge. In the past, most of the lives lost were due to ignorance. We had little knowledge about the causative factors of illnesses. Causes of fever were unknown. Infections were difficult to treat. Over the years, we have acquired stupendous knowledge. In the present era, where more than 13,000 diseases and 10,000 remedies (drugs and intervention processes) have been described, the knowledge is no more a deterrent to saving lives. Now, ineptitude is more common a cause for failures in medicine. If we have the knowledge and still fail to execute correctly in need, it is bound to invite trouble both for the patient and the treating physician. In the era of quality assurance, strategy development to overcome avoidable human errors has become imperative. Increasing complexities of the procedure has led to evolution of what is called *checklists*. Checklists are meant to reduce failure by compensating for potential limits of human memory and attention.[1] Surgical Safety Checklist (SSC) aids in standardization of protocols as well as minimizes medical errors.

NEED FOR A SURGICAL CHECKLIST

The report on the safety of American health care system released in 1999 by the Institute of Medicine titled "To Err is Human: Building a Safer Health System," revealed that annually 44,000–98,000 patients die in United States due to preventable medical errors.[2] This report also highlighted that the high intensity settings, such as the intensive care units (ICU), emergency departments and surgical operating rooms were highly prone to these errors. Approximately 234 million surgeries are performed worldwide annually. Studies show that half to two-thirds of the adverse events in hospitals are related to surgery and drug administration. About one-half of them are preventable.[3-8] Looking at the huge number of surgeries being performed, and the potential impact of these unwanted errors on health care system, both in terms of quality of services and financial burden is immense. Counteracting the processes leading to errors seems the most vital step in improving the health care system. As a part of the "Safe Surgery Saves Life" campaign, the World Health Organization (WHO), in 2009, launched the Surgical Safety Checklist (SSC) adapted from the field of aviation.[9]

HISTORY OF SURGICAL SAFETY CHECKLIST

History of safety checklists dates back to 1935. It was first introduced by the aviation department of US army. In aviation, checklist was introduced as a response to an air crash that killed an experienced pilot who was operating a new model. This new version was more sophisticated with additional features and required additional gears to fly. The pilot forgot to pull one of the gears during takeoff and landed in a crash. This embarked the development of checklist as the people understood that experience is not the sole criteria to fly safe.[9] The same theory applies in other fields as well including medicine and surgery.

The first checklist was introduced in the John Hopkins Hospital in ICU by Pronovost. It started with central line care checklist and then followed to include all aspects of ICU care. Slowly other hospitals started adapting similar steps to reduce ICU morbidity and mortality. In 2002, WHO Patient Safety Group was formed and was meant to address global safety challenges in surgery. Later under the supervision of Professor Atul Gawande, WHO launched its guidelines on safe surgery. The SSC propagates a safety culture, team work, better communication between team members in order to effect reduction in complications, morbidity and mortality. This translates into cost cutting in terms of handling preventable complications. Gradually, this safety measure was accepted by a number of hospitals across the globe. By 2014, the WHO SSC was being followed in nearly 2,000 institutions worldwide.

CONTENTS OF THE SURGICAL SAFETY CHECKLIST

The WHO SSC has been developed, tested and revised multiple times over the past decade (**Fig. 1**). It is used as a reference for hospitals to customize and make the checklist catering to their needs. The points enumerated in SSC aims at preventing uncommon but serious errors. When the patient reaches the theater, the team should follow the checklist every time confirming patient's identity, surgical site, important comorbid conditions and any anticipated complications. The checklist has three components: *sign in, time out* and *sign out*. Going through the checklist at these three stages during surgery of a patient is important:
1. An attempt to confirm the right patient, the right surgery with the right surgical site during *sign in*
2. Whole team being aware of the comorbid conditions of that particular patient and prepared for handling any complications preemptively during *time out*, and

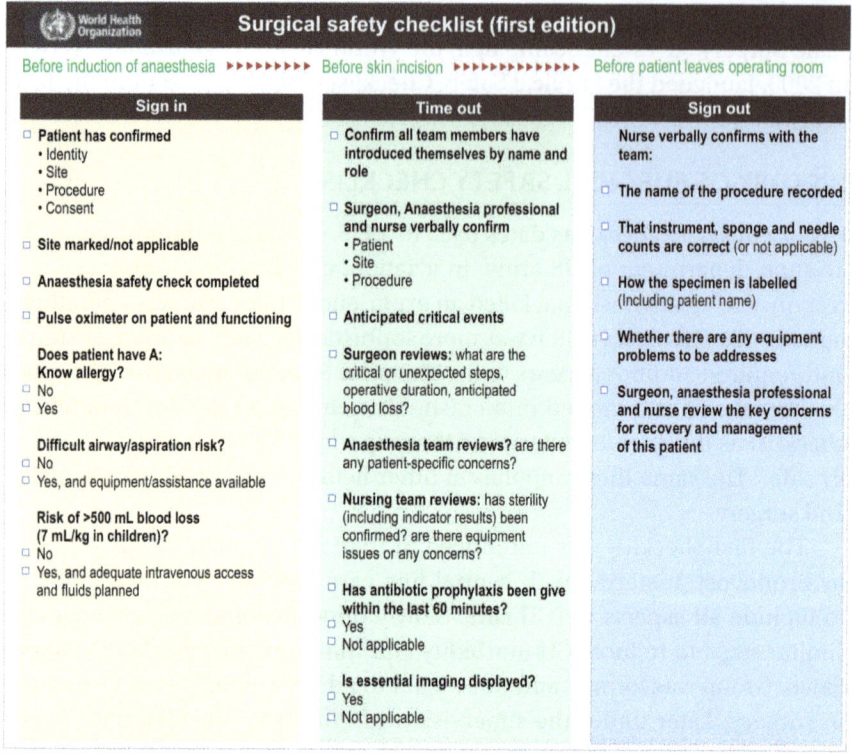

Fig. 1: World Health Organization (WHO) surgical safety checklist (first edition).

3. Confirming the surgery done, counts of instruments and sponges, specimen retrieved and plan for the postoperative period is made during the *sign out*.[10]

Besides the WHO SSC, other checklists are also in practice. The use of checklist for time-out is one of The Joint Commission's 2016 National Patient Safety Goals and is defined under UP.01.03.01. The Universal Protocol applies to all surgical and nonsurgical invasive procedures. It is based on the principles of prevention of wrong-person, wrong-site and wrong-procedure in surgery using multiple complementary strategies to achieve the goal. Involvement and empowerment of each team member and to an extent the patient and family as and when needed, is important for its success. Use of standardized protocols and its consistent implementation is most effective means to achieve safety. **Figure 2** shows an example of the UP checklist. It can be customized by hospitals and institutes according to their facility requirements. The amount and type of documentation can be determined by the institute, but ensuring clinical and operational accuracy at par with the standards set by The Joint Commission.[11]

Another checklist in use is the SURgical PAtient Safety System (SURPASS). It was created to reduce the in-hospital mortality and surgical complications

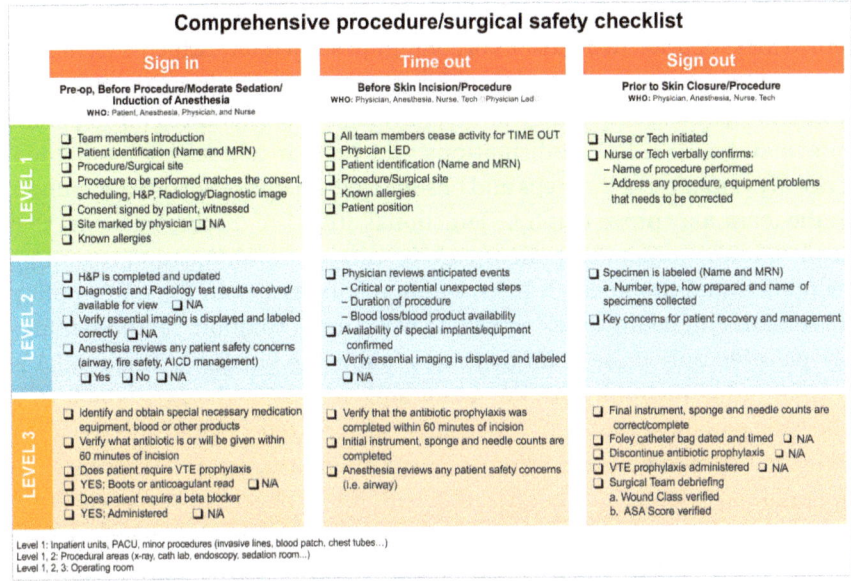

Fig. 2: Comprehensive procedure/surgical safety checklist.

by standardizing the operative process of all procedures along with designated responsibilities and specific checks. This checklist accompanies patient during each step of the surgical pathway and is split into different stages—*outpatient, preoperative ward, holding area, operating room, recovery or intensive care unit, postoperative-ward, home.* The SURPASS has been validated in various studies for the entire surgical pathway.[12] It is widely accepted in hospitals in Netherlands. It can be downloaded from the website: https://www.surpass-checklist.nl/en/checklist.html. Recently a study was conducted in 11 Dutch health care centers accredited by various Dutch agencies for safety standards. The SURPASS strategy was followed in all the hospitals and a drop in overall morbidity from 27.3 to 16.7 per 100 patients was recorded.[13] It also showed significant decrease in mortality, multiple complications, temporary disability and need for multiple surgeries.[14]

SURGICAL SAFETY CHECKLIST AND COMMUNICATION

Patient care is negatively impacted by dysfunctional communication among the members of the surgical team. Research has shown that surgeons, anesthesiologists and nurses have rather varied concepts of teamwork and communication in the operating room (OR). Communication failures occur almost every 7–8 minutes and affect about 30% of the interactions in the OR.[15,16] Hence, during the development of the WHO SSC, major attention has been paid to avoid communication lapse as it is a huge contributor to surgical errors. Unfortunately, these lapses are only observed when they result in an adverse event or complication. This "invisibility" can be addressed through proactive discussions among the team members. Lingard et al.[16] did a pair of studies in which they reported two versions of communication utility, which is facilitated by the checklists: informational and functional utility. "Informational" utility implies improvement in the team's knowledge and awareness through new information, detailed confirmations and regular educational activities. Critical evaluation of the steps and observing the activities of other members in the team may prove helpful. "Functional utility" of discussing a checklist implies improvement in patient care by direct communication regarding patient related problems. It helps in identifying issues in time, prompting discussion and taking quick actions to bring out a solution. All these things are possible only if the team members follow the checklist. This model is helpful in highlighting both the latent and the visible dangers which may affect the patient's outcome.[16-18] Lingard et al. reported a significant ($p < 0.001$) reduction in miscommunication events from an average of 3.95 events per operation to 1.31 events per operation with use of checklist. Use of checklist also resulted in 64% reduction in miscommunication that led to at least one visible consequence and 34% improvement in functional utility.[17] Various studies have reported better recognition of team members leading to better communication in the OR with an improved likelihood of staff speaking up when a problem is noticed.[19-21]

TEAMWORK ENHANCEMENT

Preventable adverse events in surgery are common. Majority can be avoided by good communication. The association between interaction among team members in the OR and patient outcome is well recognized. Collaborative approach in the OR is a challenge due to multiple factors: a hierarchical environment, team members not acquainted to each other, and different communication pattern each time. The surgical staff has stoicism due to the hierarchy, which to an extent is influenced by the level of education and experience of individuals in the operating team. Traditionally, the surgeon leads the operation and the anesthesiologist, OR nurses, radiologists and other personnel assist in the progression of the operation.[14] This kind of environment is detrimental for a team approach due to compromises in open communication. With use of SSC, communication among the members is facilitated. It renders the OT environment discussion friendly as the completion of the checklist requires the inputs from all team members. The whole team should introduce themselves by speaking aloud at the beginning of the operative day, and any new member who joins the team later should begin with an introduction to reinforce team communication. Every member of the team is involved in execution of the checklist, but a single person should be responsible for leading the discussion of all components of the SSC. This could be any health care professional participating in the operation, usually the circulating nurse. Evidence shows that once an individual has spoken aloud, they are more likely to speak up if they find any ambiguity during the operation, especially the junior members of the team.[22] Numerous studies have shown the positive impact of checklists on temperament of the OR team members. According to a report on the use of SSC in OR,[17] it was found that 73% surgical, anesthesia and nursing staff agreed on the fact that checklists help in strengthening of the team. Its regular use improves the team quality which in turn enhances patient safety. It also reduces staff turnover, especially nursing staff, as they feel themselves to be a part of a group. This makes every member equally important and at the same time imparts a sense of responsibility among the members to produce their best. This translates into other long-term benefits such as increase in team efficiency which would lead to performing more number of safer operations during the same hours.[23]

Decrease in Surgical Adverse Events

Majority of errors that emerge during the preoperative period of patient care are the surgical adverse events. A pilot study was conducted by WHO between October 2007 and September 2008 in eight hospitals, in eight different cities, representing a wide variety of health care settings, diverse patient population and differing economic circumstances. Use of WHO SSC was reported to reduce the deaths and surgical complications by more than one-third across all the eight centers. A drop in rate of major patient complications from 11% to 7% and the inpatient death rate following major operations from 1.5% to 0.8% was recorded.[24] Besides this landmark study, many smaller studies also confirmed the reduction in complications and death by the use of WHO SSC. In a cluster randomized control trial from Norway on the use of SSC, complication rates decreased from 19.9% to 11.5%, mean length of stay decreased by 0.8 days and in-hospital mortality decreased from 1.6% to 1.0%.[25] Yuan et al. in their study in two Liberian hospitals found that use of SSC resulted in significantly fewer surgical site infections [adjusted OR (AOR) 0.28; 95% CI 0.15–0.54] and surgical complications (AOR 0.45; 95% CI 0.26–0.78).[26] Askarian et al., in their study on use of SSC in a hospital in Iran also reported a decrease in surgical complications from 22.9% to 10%.[27] The use of a comprehensive surgical checklist by the Netherland's Surgical Patient Safety System also found a significant reduction in in-hospital mortality (1.5% to 0.5%) and overall complication(27.3% to 16.7% per 100).[28] A study on an orthopedic group of patients reported a similar effect of SSC with a significant reduction in postoperative fever after implementation of the same. This was attributed to the improved usage of preoperative prophylactic antibiotic due to the checklist.[13] On the other hand, a study published from Canada concluded that the implementation of SSC was not associated with significant reduction in mortality or complications.[29] However, the study did emphasize on the fact that simply asking people to follow SSC does not work. It needs a lot of effort, motivation and time to show effects.

DISADVANTAGES OF THE CHECKLIST

While SSC has been found to be useful for decreasing surgical adverse events, few studies have raised concerns regarding its harmful effects as well. Sewell et al. reported an increase in the rate of lower respiratory tract infection from 2.1 to 2.5%,[21] though it was not significant. Kearns et al. found that 30% staff felt that following the checklist during an emergency was inconvenient and painful.[20] It increases the reaction time due to duplication of routine safety measures and few unnecessary steps which can prove detrimental in exigencies. Calling the patient's name several times in the OR before the patient is anesthetized for the purpose of checklist increases the patient's anxiety.[30,31] Though direct harms have not been reported by the use of SSC, the users have expressed concerns about the potential harms.

IMPLEMENTATION AND COMPLIANCE OF THE SURGICAL SAFETY CHECKLIST

Surgical safety checklist has been adapted in a wide variety of settings and has shown improvement in the patient safety culture and perioperative care. However, the challenge is the implementation of the culture to follow checklists. The barriers to implementation include:

- *Lack of resources at small centers:* Marker pens, drugs including antibiotics, ample staff in the theaters
- *Lack of support and dismissive attitude of the teams members:* Members not ready to accept that they can ever miss routine tasks, hierarchy in the OR discouraging open communication, lack of engagement and support from the leaders
- *Practical issues:* Duplication with existing checklist leading to confusion among the members and checklist fatigue, absence of leaders or key members, time consuming, undue delay during emergencies.

World Health Organization describes various ways to effective implementation and compliance of the SSC. One of them is identification of local champions. The chief surgeon, anesthetist or the nursing staff plays an instrumental role. They should act as leaders and should encourage an honest and transparent culture. They should be approachable to all the members. The support staff should feel free to communicate at every level in their presence. People from the administration should also be engaged to ensure regular supply of resources such as paper for checklists, pens, boards, antibiotics and necessary instruments. In addition, the checklists should be implemented in a phasic manner to increase compliance. Teaching sessions should be organized to educate the members about the need and importance of following checklist. Examples from previous mistakes and miss-outs should be used to reinforce the ideology. In addition to training sessions, posters, newsletters and pamphlets can be helpful in raising awareness. Local antibiotic protocols should be standardized to avoid confusion among members of the team.

The whole OR team should be encouraged to remain attentive at the time of checks. They should refrain from distracting activities. Regular feedbacks from the members of the team are important to analyze and correct the mistakes. The role of fully engaged staff who brings in local modifications relevant to the checklist, along with commitment of the senior hospital leaders to implement the checklist, cannot be over emphasized. Besides these, there are ready presentations and step by step guide on the WHO website for the implementation of SSC on the WHO website which may be a useful adjunct to initiate the implementation. Starting the use of SSC with an enthusiastic and receptive clinician followed by collecting data on its compliance and effects on outcome of surgery, may be a very powerful motivating tool for other clinicians at that center to adopt the checklist. All these different factors were studied in various studies. Vats et al. reported that the anesthetist and nurses were "largely supportive" while some surgeons were "not very enthusiastic".[30] Coney et al. emphasized on the role of local champions and their role in persuasion and education in using the SSC.[32] Styer et al. and Bohmer et al. suggested the role of senior leaders of institution as local champions and incorporating real-time feedback in the checklist protocol to be useful.[19,33]

VALIDITY OF SURGICAL SAFETY CHECKLIST

Various studies and meta-analysis have been done to check for the effectiveness of the use of SSC in terms of communication, reduction of morbidity and mortality. The results indicate that surgical safety checklists improve teamwork and communication, reduce morbidity and mortality, and improve compliance with safety measures.[34] A Latin American report on the effectiveness of the WHO SSC showed a decrease in postoperative death rates and decrease in length of stay after implementation of the SSC in surgical patients.[35] A systematic review on the effectiveness of WHO SSC on postoperative complications reported a reduction in postoperative complications and mortality following implementation of WHO SSC but due to absence of higher-quality studies cannot be regarded as definitive.[36] Compliance to the SSC varies significantly and depends on the staff perceptions, training, implementation strategies, and effective senior leadership.

CONCLUSION

Modern surgical era includes complex procedures. Communication errors during long procedures are common, especially at the end of long shifts, when even simple tasks are easily missed. Checklists intend to serve two purposes: (1) ensure consistency in patient safety; and (2) maintain a culture that helps to achieve this goal. Successful implementation of the same is not possible without sincere commitment by the team leaders and the team members. Attention should be paid toward regular training, feedbacks, availability of resources and encourage customization to fit the local needs. With the burgeoning evidence on the role of SSC in increasing communication, teamwork enhancement, reduction in surgical adverse events and validity of SSC, we can conclude that SSC is a strong and simple tool to make health care safer, especially in the developing countries.

REFERENCES

1. Wikipedia. Checklist. Available from https://en.wikipedia.org/wiki/Checklist. [Last Accessed November, 2020].
2. Kohn LT, Corrigan JM, Donaldson MS. To err is human: building a safer health system. Washington (DC): National Academies Press (US); 2000.
3. Weiser TG, Regenbogen SE, Thompson KD, Haynes AB, Lipsitz SR, Berry WR, et al. An estimation of the global volume of surgery: a modeling strategy based on available data. Lancet. 2008;372:139-44.
4. Gawande AA, Thomas EJ, Zinner MJ, Brennan TA. The incidence and nature of surgical adverse events in Colorado and Utah in 1992. Surgery. 1999;126:66-75.
5. Leape LL, Brennan TA, Laird N, Lawthers AG, Localio AR, Barnes BA, et al. The nature of adverse events in hospitalized patients. Results of the Harvard Medical Practice Study II. N Engl J Med. 1991;324:377-84.
6. Thomas EJ, Studdert DM, Burstin HR, Orav EJ, Zeena T, Williams EJ, et al. Incidence and types of adverse events and negligent care in Utah and Colorado. Med Care. 2000;38:261-71.
7. Wilson RM, Runciman WB, Gibberd RW, Harrison BT, Newby L, Hamilton JD. The Quality in Australian Health Care Study. Med J Aust. 1995;163:458-71.
8. Thomas EJ, Studdert DM, Newhouse JP, Zbar BI, Howard KM, Williams EJ, et al. Costs of medical injuries in Utah and Colorado. Inquiry. 1999;36:255-64.
9. Pugel AE, Simianu VV, Flum DR, Patchen Dellinger E. Use of the surgical safety checklist to improve communication and reduce complications. J Infect Public Health. 2015;8(3):219-25.
10. World Health Organization. (2012). Surgical safety web map. Available from: http://maps.cga.harvard.edu/surgical_safety/. [Last Accessed November, 2020].
11. Hess CT. Review of 2016 National Patient Safety Goal "Time-out". Adv Skin Wound Care. 2016;29(11):528.
12. de Vries EN, Hollmann MW, Smorenburg SM, Gouma DJ, Boermeester MA. Development and validation of the SURgical PAtient Safety System (SURPASS) checklist. Qual Saf Health Care. 2009;18(2):121-6.
13. de Vries EN, Prins HA, Crolla RM, den Outer AJ, van Andel G, van Helden SH, et al. Effect of a comprehensive surgical safety system on patient outcomes. N Engl J Med. 2010;363:1928-37.
14. McConnell DJ, Fargen KM, Mocco J. Surgical checklists: a detailed review of their emergence, development, and relevance to neurosurgical practice. Surg Neurol Int. 2012;3:2.
15. Hu YY, Arriaga AF, Peyre SE, Corso KA, Roth EM, Greenberg CC. Deconstructing intra-operative communication failures. J Surg Res. 2012;177(1):37-42.
16. Lingard L, Espin S, Whyte S, Regehr G, Baker GR, Reznick R, et al. Communication failures in the operating room: an observational classification of recurrent types and effects. Qual Saf Health Care. 2004;13(5):330-4.
17. Lingard L, Regehr G, Orser B, Reznick R, Baker GR, Doran D, et al. Evaluation of a preoperative checklist and team briefing among surgeons, nurses, and anesthesiologists to reduce failures in communication. Arch Surg. 2008;143:12-8.
18. Lingard L, Whyte S, Espin S, Baker GR, Orser B, Doran D. Towards safer interprofessional communication: Constructing a model of "utility" from preoperative team briefings. J Interprof Care. 2006;20:471-83.

19. Bohmer AB, Wappler F, Tinschmann T, Kindermann P, Rixen D, Bellendir M, et al. The implementation of a perioperative checklist increases patients' perioperative safety and staff satisfaction. Acta Anaesthesiol Scand. 2012;56:332-8.
20. Kearns RJ, Uppal V, Bonner J, Robertson J, Daniel M, McGrady EM. The introduction of a surgical safety checklist in a tertiary referral obstetric centre. BMJ Qual Saf. 2011;20:818-22.
21. Sewell M, Adebibe M, Jayakumar P, Jowett C, Kong K, Vemulapalli K, et al. Use of the WHO surgical safety checklist in trauma and orthopaedic patients. Int Ortho (SICOT). 2010;35:897-901.
22. World Health Organization. Safe Surgery Saves Lives Frequently Asked Questions. Available from: https://www.who.int/patientsafety/safesurgery/faq_introduction/en/. [Last Accessed November, 2020].
23. Nundy S, Mukherjee A, Sexton JB, Pronovost PJ, Knight A, Rowen LC, et al. Impact of preoperative briefings on operating room delays: A preliminary report. Arch Surg. 2008;143:1068-72.
24. Haynes AB, Weiser TG, Berry WR, Lipsitz SR, Breizat AH, Dellinger EP, et al. A Surgical Safety Checklist to Reduce Morbidity and Mortality in a Global Population. N Engl J Med. 2009;360:491-9.
25. Haugen AS, Søfteland E, Almeland SK, Sevdalis N, Vonen B, Eide GE, et al. Effect of the World Health Organization Checklist on Patient Outcomes: A Stepped Wedge Cluster Randomized Controlled Trial. Ann Surg. Ann Surg. 2015;261(5):821-8.
26. Yuan CT, Walsh D, Tomarken JL, Alpern R, Shakpeh J, Bradley EH. Incorporating the World Health Organization Surgical Safety Checklist into practice at two hospitals in Liberia. Jt Comm J Qual Patient Saf. 2012;38:254-60.
27. Askarian M, Kouchak F, Palenik CJ. Effect of surgical safety checklists on postoperative morbidity and mortality rates, Shiraz, Faghihy Hospital, a 1-year study. Qual Manag Health Care. 2011;20:293-7.
28. Boaz M, Bermant A, Ezri T, Bermant A, Ezri T, Lakstein D, et al. Effect of Surgical Safety checklist implementation on the occurrence of postoperative complications in orthopedic patients. Isr Med Assoc J. 2014;16(1):20-5.
29. Urbach DR, Govindarajan A, Saskin R, Wilton AS, Baxter NN. Introduction of Surgical Safety Checklists in Ontario, Canada. N Engl J Med. 2014;370(11):1029-38.
30. Vats A, Vincent CA, Nagpal K, Davies RW, Darzi A, Moorthy K. Practical challenges of introducing WHO surgical checklist: UK pilot experience. BMJ. 2010;340:133-5.
31. Fourcade A, Blache JL, Grenier C, Bourgain JL, Minvielle E. Barriers to staff adoption of a surgical safety checklist. BMJ Qual Saf. 2012;21:191-7.
32. Conley DM, Singer SJ, Edmondson L, Berry WR, Gawande AA. Effective surgical safety checklist implementation. J Am Coll Surg. 2011;212:873-9.
33. Styer KA, Ashley SW, Schmidt I, Zive EM, Eappen S. Implementing the World Health Organization surgical safety checklist: a model for future perioperative initiatives. AORN J 2011;94:590-8.
34. Lyons VE, Popejoy LL. Meta-analysis of surgical safety checklist effects on teamwork, communication, morbidity, mortality, and safety. West J Nurs Res. 2014;36(2):245-61.
35. Lacassie HJ, Ferdinand C, Guzmán S, Camus L, Echevarria GC. World Health Organization (WHO) surgical safety checklist implementation and its impact on perioperative morbidity and mortality in an academic medical center in Chile. Medicine (Baltimore). 2016;95(23):e3844.
36. Bergs J, Hellings J, Cleemput I, Zurel Ö, De Troyer V, Van Hiel M, et al. Systematic review and meta-analysis of the effect of the World Health Organization surgical safety checklist on postoperative complications. Br J Surg. 2014;101(3):150-8.

CHAPTER 11

Management of Penile Carcinoma

Sameer Trivedi, Sabby Dias

INTRODUCTION

Penile cancer, although considered to be a rare malignancy in developed countries with an annual incidence of less than 1% of all male malignancies, is much more common in India and certain other countries in Asia, South America and Africa with reported incidence of up to 10% of all cancers in men. More than 95% of penile cancers are squamous cell carcinomas (SCC) and the peak age of incidence is in 5th to 7th decades of life.[1] The shame and embarrassment coupled with ignorance and lack of accessible health care has been reported to produce a delay in seeking treatment by an average of 1 year while nearly one-fourth patients present with advanced disease.

In the last two decades, several important advancements have ensued in the management of penile cancer due to a better understanding of etiopathological processes, improved diagnostic modalities, refinements in surgical procedures, innovative minimally invasive lymph node dissection techniques and introduction of new classes of drugs such as targeted therapies and immune checkpoint inhibitors for systemic therapy of advanced penile cancer. Moreover, the increasing role of multidisciplinary approach in management of penile cancer has greatly improved the oncological outcomes and quality of life while reducing the overall morbidity and mortality.

EPIDEMIOLOGY

Penile cancer has a widely variable incidence with very low rates in developed countries, with annual incidence below 1 case per 100,000 men, i.e., less than 1% of all male malignancies, while in many Asian, African, and South American countries, the reported incidence is up to 10% of all male cancers.[2] India has one of the highest incidence of penile cancer in the world, with rates of 1.8–3.32 per 100,000 men in different regions. The age-standardized incidence rates in different countries have ranged from 0.3 to 1.8/100,000 (United States), 2.8/100,000 (Uganda) and 1.5–3.7/100,000 (Brazil). The lowest incidence worldwide has been reported in Israeli Jews (0.1/100,000).[2]

Historically, the peak incidence of penile cancer is seen in 5th to 7th decades of life;[3] however, recent studies have reported that approximately 7% patients are below 30 years and 19% patients are less than 40 years old.[3] A socioeconomic correlation has been reported in the incidence of penile carcinoma with a 43% greater risk in countries with greater proportion of populations below the poverty line.

RISK FACTORS

Phimosis

The role of phimosis in etiopathology of penile cancer has been extensively studied and documented. The extreme rarity of the disease in populations which practice neonatal circumcision, like in Israeli-born Jewish population and other Asian and African communities which practice religious circumcision provides strong corroborative evidence toward the role of intact preputial skin in etiology of penile cancer. The incidence of phimosis in patients with penile cancer has been reported in the range of 25-60%.[3] A study comparing 110 cases of penile cancer with 355 controls described a 3.5-fold higher risk associated with phimosis.[4]

Circumcision

While circumcision has been widely reported to have a preventive effect in etiopathology of penile cancer, the timing of circumcision is believed to play a key role in the magnitude of the protection offered. Overall reduction in risk of penile cancer in the circumcised populace is reported to be approximately 70%, particularly in the neonatal circumcision groups. In one study, uncircumcised men had a 3.2 times higher risk of developing penile cancer as compared to neonatally circumcised men, while the risk in men who underwent circumcision later in life was 3 times higher.[4] Interestingly, uncircumcised men have been shown to have a higher incidence of glanular location of cancer vis-à-vis men who were circumcised at birth.

Cigarette Smoking

Tobacco consumption, either in form of smoking or as oral tobacco chewing, has been directly linked to increased risk of developing penile cancer. The relationship with smoking has been shown to be linear and dose dependent. In a study of over 500 patients and 500 controls, risk of penile cancer was higher in smokers as compared to nonsmokers (OR 1.44), higher in those who smoked more than 10 cigarettes per day (OR 2.14), higher in those with duration of smoking longer than 5 years (OR 1.43), and in those with a cumulative exposure of more than 30 pack years (OR 1.86). Likewise, oral tobacco chewing was an independent significant risk factor for penile cancer in the exposed group (OR 3.11). In isolation, both smoking and oral tobacco chewing conferred a higher risk of penile cancer (OR 2.29), however, the concomitant use of both practices posed a much higher risk (OR 3.39).[5] Likewise, other studies have reported a similar association between smoking and the risk of developing penile cancer—2.4-fold higher risk in smokers, higher risk in heavy smokers with more than 20 cigarettes per day (OR 5.9) as compared to men who smoked less than 20 cigarettes/day (OR 1.2).[6]

Chronic Balanitis and Penile Trauma

Many studies have reported role of penile injuries and infections as a causative factor for both invasive penile cancer and carcinoma in situ. The likelihood of history of penile injury occurring more than 2 years before the diagnosis of penile cancer was much higher for carcinoma in situ (OR 23) as compared to invasive penile cancer (OR 4.6).[6] Another study reported a similar significant association between microabrasions of penis and penile cancer (RR 3.9).[4] Balanitis has also been shown to increase the risk of developing penile cancer (OR 3.07).[7]

Genital Warts

The association between genital warts and penile cancer has been demonstrated by many studies; however, the exact relationship has not been elucidated clearly. In one study, men with genital warts have been demonstrated to harbor a 5.9 times higher risk of penile cancer.[4] Likewise, another study reported a history of genital warts in 27% patients as compared to 4.8% in normal controls (OR 7.6).[8] Moreover, genital or perianal warts that occurred ≥2 years before the reference date increased the rate of both carcinoma in situ (OR 1.7) and invasive penile carcinoma (OR 3.7).[6]

Human Papillomavirus Infection

Role of human papillomavirus (HPV) infection in the etiopathology of penile cancer is well-established although the association is weaker than with cervical cancer. The most commonly implicated subtypes in penile carcinoma include HPV types 16 and 18. The reported overall prevalence of HPV-DNA in patients with penile cancer has been widely variable (22-72%).[9] In various case control studies, incidence of high-risk HPV in penile cancer cases has been reported as 24-65% as opposed to 12% in controls.[7] On subtype analysis, the most commonly associated subtype in penile cancer is HPV-16 (25-94%) followed by HPV-18 (10.5-55.4%).[4,9] Incidentally, the probability of getting infected by HPV is higher in sexually promiscuous individuals while HPV infections are less common in circumcised men.[7]

PREMALIGNANT LESIONS

A variety of lesions have been implicated in the pathogenesis of squamous cell carcinoma of the penis. Only some of these lesions progress to invasive carcinoma, their natural history is unpredictable, and their malignant potential has been under evaluated in the published literature. While some of these lesions have a weak association in the development of squamous cell

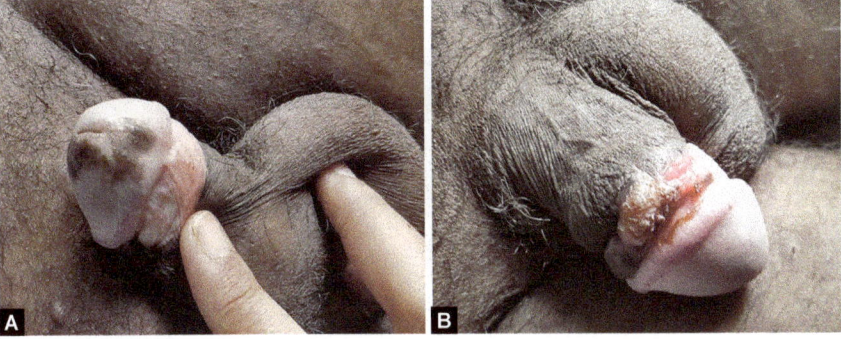

Figs. 1A and B: Patient with Lichen sclerosus associated with penile cancer.

carcinoma, there are certain conditions which have a strong predisposition for malignant transformation.

Conditions which have a weak and infrequent association with penile squamous cell carcinoma and are usually related to chronic inflammation include:
- Lichen sclerosus et atrophicus (earlier called as balanitis xerotica obliterans) **(Figs. 1A and B)**
- Leukoplakia
- Cutaneous horn of the penis
- Pseudoepitheliomatous, keratotic, and micaceous balanitis

Lesions which carry a definite risk of progression to penile carcinoma are related to HPV and include:
1. Erythroplasia of Queyrat ⎫
2. Bowen's disease ⎬ Variants of Carcinoma-in-situ
3. Paget's disease of the penis
4. Bowenoid papulosis of the penis
5. Giant condylomata acuminata (Buschke-Löwenstein tumor)
6. Penile intraepithelial neoplasia (High grade)

Natural History

The patients with penile cancer typically defer getting medical consultation for a variable period ranging from months to years. It has been estimated that at least 25–50% of patients with penile cancer harbor penile lesions for more than one year prior to getting diagnosed.[10] Location wise, the most common sites of penile lesion include glans (48%), prepuce (21%), both the glans and prepuce (9%), coronal sulcus (6%), and penile shaft (less than 2%) **(Fig. 2)**.

Spectrum of clinical appearance in penile cancer extends from an area of imperceptible induration to a small growth, papule, flat ulcerative lesion, exophytic lesion or a fungating ulceroproliferative growth replacing whole of penis **(Figs. 3A to D)**. Patients may also present with inguinal swelling, ulceration or proliferative lesions which may be associated with superimposed infection and seropurulent discharge. The primary lesions are usually painless

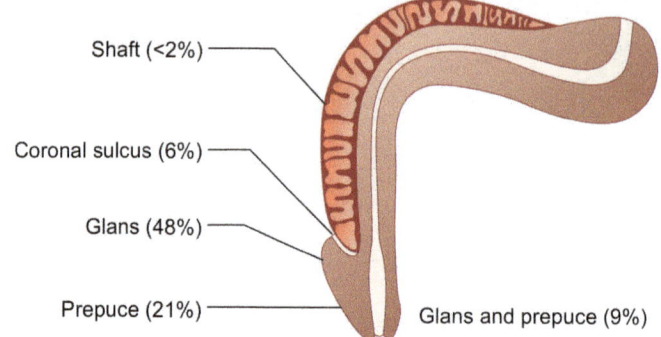

Fig. 2: Penile cancer distribution by anatomical site.

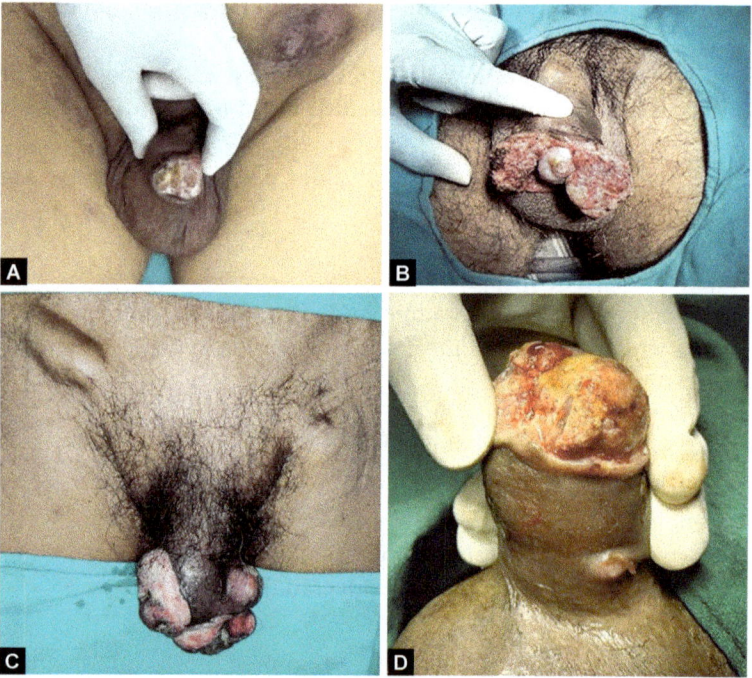

Figs. 3A to D: Spectrum of clinical appearance in penile cancer. (A) Ulcerative growth with left inguinal mass; (B) and (C) Fungating growth with bilateral inguinal nodes; (D) Induration of whole shaft with skin ulceration.

and the most common presenting symptoms are the growth itself, a foul smelling discharge with or without bleeding, itching or burning and rarely urinary symptoms in the unusual scenario of urethral or meatus involvement.[11]

The natural history of the disease involves an onset usually from the glans and then relentless and gradual progression to embroil the entire glans and thence shaft of the penis **(Fig. 4)**. Coexistent phimosis can initially conceal a lesion and allow progression of the disease covertly. In due course, the lesion erodes through the preputial barrier and becomes noticeable. Deeper

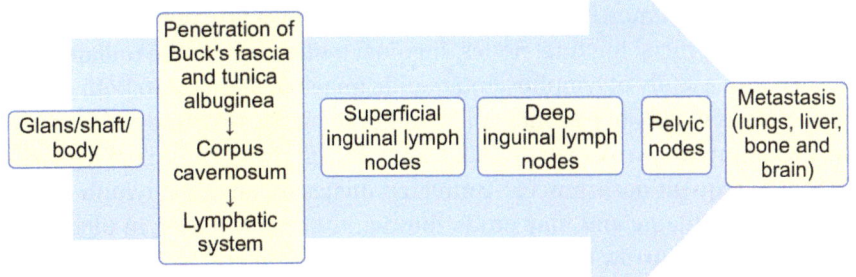

Fig. 4: Natural history of penile cancer.

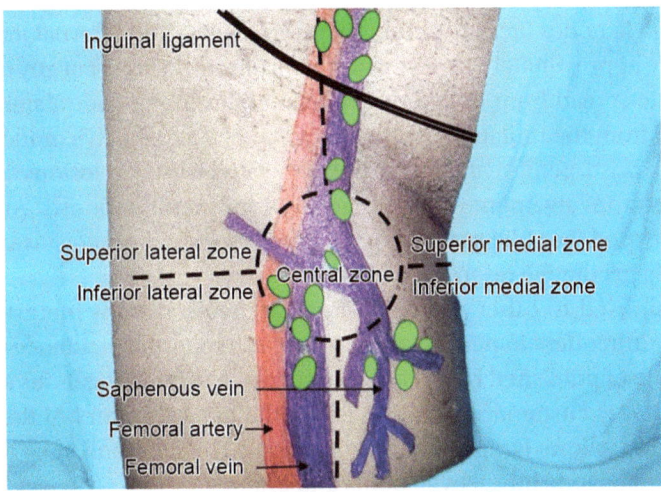

Fig. 5: Lymphatic drainage in penile cancer.

invasion of the lesion into the corporal bodies is prevented till late stages by Buck's fascia which plays the role of a natural barrier to disease progression. Eventual breach in the Buck's fascia and tunica albuginea enables involvement of corpora cavernosa and penetration of the lymphatic channels. In untreated cases, relentless progression of the disease may uncommonly result in penile autoamputation.

The spread of penile cancer occurs almost exclusively in a stepwise manner and lymphatic metastases usually precede hematogenous spread. The lymphatic drainage of penis is in the form of an anastomotic network of channels which freely crosses the midline at the base of penis and along the shaft. These lymphatic channels drain sequentially into superficial inguinal, deep inguinal and then pelvic lymph nodes **(Fig. 5)**. This systematic pattern of lymphatic drainage without any skip drainage has been validated reliably by lymphangiography studies.[12] Approximately 20-25 superficial nodes lie between Scarpa's fascia and the fascia lata whereas around 5-6 deep nodes are found below the fascia lata medial to the femoral vein.

The most common initial landing site of metastasis is in the superomedial group of superficial inguinal nodes. Inguinal metastases can be unilateral or bilateral. In a study of lymphoscintigraphic imaging, drainage to both groins was evident in 80% of patients, unilateral drainage in 18%, and no drainage in 2%.[13] Moreover, crossover drainage from the left to right groin or vice versa is also a frequent occurrence.[14] Untreated metastatic inguinal lymph nodes continue to enlarge and may erode through the skin resulting in ulcerative growth or may burrow into the femoral vessels leading to fatal hemorrhage. Penile cancer follows an unrelenting course and untreated patients typically succumb to disease within 2-3 years.[11]

The second landing sites of lymphatic metastases are the pelvic lymph nodes (LNs) which are invariably involved from the ipsilateral inguinal nodes. These pelvic nodes include obturator, external iliac, and internal iliac nodes which are approximately 12-20 in number. There is no report of any crossover metastatic spread from unilateral inguinal nodes to the contralateral pelvic nodes or from the unilateral pelvic LNs to contralateral pelvic nodes or vice versa. Likewise, penile cancers are not associated with skip lesions, i.e., there is no direct involvement of pelvic nodes from penile lesions.[14] Any nodal spread beyond the pelvic nodes is considered as systemic metastases and not amenable to curative resections.

As opposed to other urological malignancies, distant metastases are relatively infrequent in penile carcinoma, with a reported incidence of 1-10% in majority of published reports. The occurrence of hematogenous spread to distant sites is customarily a late event in the natural history of the disease and usually follows lymph node involvement. The common sites of distant metastases include lungs, liver, bone, and brain.

Pathology

A vast majority of penile cancers are squamous cell carcinomas or their variants (>95% of cases). These include the usual squamous cell carcinoma (48-65%) and the various mixed forms of squamous cell carcinoma, viz., the warty-basaloid variant, hybrid of usual and verrucous forms, usual with warty type, usual with basaloid variant, papillary, sarcomatoid and other infrequent combinations **(Table 1)**. Other rarer primary malignant lesions involving the penis include melanomas, lymphomas, leukemias and mesenchymal tumors such as sarcomas. Secondaries to penis can result from other primary cancers such as prostatic or colorectal malignancies.

Diagnosis and Local Tumor Staging

Physical examination plays a key role in the diagnosis of penile cancer. A thorough clinical examination includes number of lesions, size, location

TABLE 1: Histological subtypes of penile carcinomas in order of frequency.	
Subtype	Frequency (% of cases)
Common squamous cell carcinoma (SCC)	48–65
Papillary carcinoma	5–15
Warty-basaloid carcinoma	9–14
Mixed carcinoma	9–10
Warty carcinoma	7–10
Basaloid carcinoma	4–10
Verrucous carcinoma	3–8
Sarcomatoid carcinoma	1–3
Clear cell variant of penile carcinoma	1–2
Miscellaneous: Pseudohyperplastic, pseudoglandular, adenosquamous, mucoepidermoid, carcinoma cuniculatum	<1

and extent (foreskin, glans, shaft), color, appearance (flat, papillary, nodular, ulcerating, fungating), margins, involvement of adjacent structures (corpus spongiosum, corpora cavernosa, urethra), and edges. However, mismatch between clinical and pathological staging can be present in up to 26% patients.[15] Ultrasonography (USG) has been used for diagnosis and staging of local lesions with varying results. While it may not be accurate for staging of small glanular lesions, it can provide useful information in larger tumors in assessing the involvement of deeper structures.[16] It has been suggested that USG is more useful for lesions over shaft of penis while physical examination is more useful for lesions limited to glans. Likewise, USG can be helpful if physical examination is inconclusive about corporal infiltration.[17]

Contrast enhanced penile MRI has been evaluated for improving the accuracy of local staging. An artificial erection, obtained by intracavernosal injection of vasoactive drugs, improves the accuracy of MRI in this setting. The penile cancer usually appears hypointense as compared to corpora on T1 and T2-weighted images and enhancement after gadolinium administration is lesser than the normal corpora. However, certain factors can influence the results of MRI. These include a flaccid penis, prior radiotherapy, movement artifacts, and concurrent infection.[18] As per the recommendations of National Comprehensive Cancer Network (NCCN) and European Association of Urology (EAU) guidelines, MRI with artificial erection or ultrasound with Doppler is advised in cases with intended organ-sparing surgery.[19,20]

Inguinal Nodes—Clinical Staging

Inguinal lymph node involvement is the single most important determinant of prognosis in penile cancer patients. The incidence of palpable inguinal nodes in penile cancer patients ranges from 28 to 64%. Of these, approximately

47–85% patients will be harboring malignancy. In patients with palpable inguinal nodes, around 75% will have bilateral and 25% will have unilateral palpable nodes.[16]

A thorough physical examination is essential in the diagnosis and clinical staging of inguinal nodes. The groin examination for palpable nodes should include the number, size, uni-/bilaterality, mobility, matting or fixation, adjacent structures such as skin or Cooper's ligaments, tenderness, and swelling over external genitalia or lower limbs. However, physical examination by itself can be misleading with a false-negative rate ranging from 11 to 62%. Various imaging modalities such as USG, computed tomography (CT) and magnetic resonance imaging (MRI) have been used to improve the diagnostic accuracy of nodal staging but the results have not been encouraging. Use of invasive techniques such as fine needle aspiration cytology (FNAC) and dynamic sentinel node biopsy (DSNB) has been shown to improve the pickup rate in many studies.[15] Since 10–20% patients of penile cancer harbor inguinal micrometastases without being clinically palpable, surgical staging of inguinal nodes using prophylactic inguinal lymph node dissection (LND) becomes important. For assessment of the pelvic lymph nodes in patients with palpable inguinal nodes, a CT scan can be used although sub-centimetric nodes are difficult to pick up on cross-sectional imaging. The diagnostic accuracy of 18FDG-PET/CT has been shown to be much superior with a sensitivity of 88–100% and a specificity of 98–100% in this setting.[21]

Assessment for Distant Metastases

All patients with positive inguinal nodes should be assessed for distant metastases. The recommended tests include a chest radiograph, liver function tests and CT abdomen and pelvis. In selected cases with high suspicion of pulmonary metastases, chest CT is preferred over a conventional chest X-ray. Likewise, in patients with palpable inguinal lymph nodes, a positron emission tomography (PET)/CT scan offers a better opportunity of detecting pelvic lymph node involvement and distant metastases.[22] Although penile cancer does not have a recognized tumor marker, studies have evaluated the role of SCC antigen as a tumor marker. The levels of SCC antigen are found to be elevated in approximately 25% patients.[23]

Table 2 summarizes the recommended tests for locoregional and distant staging of penile cancer according to the EAU and NCCN guidelines.

Biopsy and Histopathologic Examination

Histopathological analysis should be performed in all penile lesions. The tissue for biopsy can be obtained using any of the following techniques—excisional biopsy, incisional biopsy, brush biopsy, tissue core biopsy or FNAC. Out of these, a generous wedge biopsy from the edge of the tumor, incorporating a part of normal tissue, provides maximal information regarding prognostic

TABLE 2: Recommended tests for diagnosis and staging in penile cancer.

	Primary tumor		Lymph nodes			Distant metastases	
			cN0	cN+	N+ patients		Patients with systemic disease or with relevant symptoms
EAU guidelines 2018	Physical examination	Penile Doppler ultrasound or MRI with artificial erection in cases with intended organ-sparing surgery	Invasive lymph node staging in intermediate and high-risk patients	Stage with a pelvic computed tomography (CT) or positron emission tomography (PET)/CT	Abdominopelvic CT scan and chest X-ray/ thoracic CT for systemic staging. Alternatively, stage with a PET/CT scan.		Bone scan
Grade of EAU recommendation	Strong	Weak	Strong		Strong		
NCCN guidelines 2018			Low grade (Tis, Ta, T1a) DSNB or surveillance	Abdominal/ pelvic CT or MRI and chest imaging (X-ray or CT)	Systemic chemotherapy or radiotherapy or chemotherapy → Abdominal/pelvic CT or MRI and chest imaging (X-ray or CT).		
			Intermediate/ high grade (T1b, T2 or greater) Abdominal/ pelvic CT or MRI and chest imaging (X-ray or CT). Inguinal lymph node dissection (ILND) or DSNB.				

(DSNB: dynamic sentinel node biopsy; EAU: European Association of Urology; NCCN: National Comprehensive Cancer Network) factors like histological type, depth of invasion, LVI, and grade of tumor.[24] For small lesions, an excisional biopsy can be diagnostic as well as therapeutic.

Grading

A variety of grading systems have been proposed for penile cancer. However, these systems have not been compared head to head to find out the superiority of any particular grading system in terms of prognostic value. The most commonly used grading system for penile cancer is based on the extent of cell differentiation as follows:
1. Grade 1—well differentiated (minimal or no anaplasia)
2. Grade 2—moderately differentiated (<50% anaplasia)
3. Grade 3—poorly differentiated (>50% anaplasia)[25]

A more comprehensive grading and scoring system which takes into consideration cell atypia, mitotic activity, extent of keratinization and the degree of inflammatory cell infiltration has been with put forward which includes 4 grades:
1. *Grade 1:* 8-10 points
2. *Grade 2:* 5-7 points
3. *Grade 3:* 3-4 points
4. *Grade 4:* 0-2 points[26]

TNM Staging System

The traditional Jackson staging system used for penile cancer has been replaced by tumor node metastasis (TNM) staging system since 1968. After multiple periodic revisions, the most recent version of TNM staging has been in use since 2016.[27]

T—Primary Tumor

TX: Primary tumor cannot be assessed
T0: No evidence of primary tumor
Tis: Carcinoma in situ
Ta: Noninvasive verrucous carcinoma
T1: Tumor invades subepithelial connective tissue
T1a: Tumor invades subepithelial connective tissue without lymphovascular invasion and is not poorly differentiated (T1G1-2)
T1b: Tumor invades subepithelial connective tissue with lymphovascular invasion or is poorly differentiated (T1G3-4)
T2: Tumor invades corpus spongiosum with or without invasion of the urethra
T3: Tumor invades corpus cavernosum with or without invasion of the urethra
T4: Tumor invades other adjacent structures

N—Regional Lymph Nodes

NX: Regional lymph nodes cannot be assessed
N0: No palpable or visibly enlarged inguinal lymph nodes
N1: Palpable mobile unilateral inguinal lymph node
N2: Palpable mobile multiple or bilateral inguinal lymph nodes
N3: Fixed inguinal nodal mass or pelvic lymphadenopathy, unilateral or bilateral

M—Distant Metastasis

M0: No distant metastasis
M1: Distant metastasis

SURGICAL MANAGEMENT OF THE PRIMARY TUMOR

The aims of surgical treatment in penile cancer are two-fold—complete excision of the cancerous lesion, and, maximal organ preservation with optimal functional, esthetic and psychological results. Choosing the most suitable surgical technique is subject to a variety of factors including stage, grade and location of the primary lesion, penile length, anticipated length of the penile remnant, patient's age, comorbid conditions and sexual history **(Table 3)**.

Role of Circumcision

Irrespective of the surgical technique chosen, prior circumcision should be performed in all patients for a variety of reasons. Circumcision may be curative by itself in selected cases where the disease is localized to prepuce alone. Moreover, circumcision is helpful in carcinoma in situ (CIS) of the glans as it enables proper examination during follow-up, eradicates chronic inflammation and HPV infection thus precluding disease progression, makes application of topical agents simpler, assists in retaining these agents, and avoids edema of the foreskin during laser treatment.

Surgical Treatment of Penile Carcinoma in Situ

Penile CIS with small, superficial mucosal lesions over the glans or shaft is amenable to topical treatment with 5% 5-fluorouracil or 5% imiquimod cream (applied on alternate days for 4 weeks). The topical treatment is an efficacious minimally invasive first-line modality with reported complete response rates ranging from 50 to 60%.[28] In case of failure of topical treatment, laser treatment is preferred over re-application of topical agents. The commonly used LASERs include CO_2 LASER (2-2.5 mm depth of penetration) and neodymium-doped yttrium-aluminum garnet (Nd: YAG) LASER (3-5 mm depth of penetration). In patients who fail to respond to or comply with both topical and LASER therapy, or in patients with widespread lesions, partial or total glans resurfacing is an effective option. Glans resurfacing

TABLE 3: Management options for the primary penile tumor and inguinal nodes.

	Tis	Ta	T1 Low-risk (G1 or G2; T1a)	T1 High-risk (G3 or G4; T1b)	T2	T3 Without invasion of urethra	T3 With invasion of urethra	T4	Local recurrence
Topical imiquimod/ 5-fluorouracil	✓								
CO₂/Nd:YAG Laser	✓	✓							
Radiotherapy		✓ (For lesions <4 cm)	✓	✓ (For lesions <4 cm)	✓ (For lesions <4 cm)	✓ (For lesions <4 cm)		✓ (For palliation)*	
Glans resurfacing	✓	✓	✓						
Mohs surgery		✓	✓						
Circumcision	✓	✓							
Wide local excision		✓	✓						
Partial or total glansectomy			✓	✓					
Partial penectomy				✓	✓	✓	✓		
Total penectomy					✓		✓	✓*	✓*
Inguinal lymphadenectomy (irrespective of lymph node status)				✓	✓	✓	✓	✓	✓*
Neoadjuvant chemotherapy								✓*	

(Nd:YAG: neodymium-doped yttrium aluminum garnet)
*weak strength rating

involves excision of epithelium and subepithelial connective tissue from the involved glanular surface and covering the resultant raw area with a split skin thickness graft.[29]

This organ preserving approach is suitable for sexually active males in terms of improved cosmesis and also has the potential for preserving glanular innervation and sensation in partial glans resurfacing. Moreover, the technique offers the advantages of complete removal of the disease, organ preservation, and precise histopathological findings without producing disfigurement.

Surgical Treatment of Ta/T1 Disease

Majority of Ta/T1 lesions (approximately 75-80%) are located on glans and prepuce and are ideally suited for organ preserving surgical approaches. However, high grade tumors or presence of lymphovascular invasion (LVI) warrants a more aggressive approach with partial penile amputation. When organ sparing resection is considered, frozen section evaluation of surgical margins should be practiced.

If the lesion is limited to the prepuce, then a circumcision by itself may be curative if frozen section reveals negative surgical margins. In case of lesions involving less than 50% of glans, particularly low grade tumors (grades 1 and 2) without LVI (stage T1a), a wide local excision or hemiglansectomy may be considered, although the patients need to be counseled about higher chances of local recurrence and a more intense follow-up. In case of more extensive local disease (involving more than half of glans) or high-grade lesions with LVI (stage T1b), it is advisable to perform a total glansectomy with circumcision, as it offers the best oncological outcomes. The defects produced following glans preserving approaches can be dealt with by either a primary repair or by use of split thickness skin grafts. Any positive surgical margins or local failures require a total glansectomy.

Other treatment options for Ta/T1 lesions confined to glans include GR and laser therapy (CO_2 and Nd:YAG) as in Tis disease. However, the positive margin rate, revision rate, local recurrence rate and need for subsequent partial or total penile amputations is considerably higher when these approaches are used for Ta/T1 disease.[30]

Mohs Micrographic Surgery

A novel surgical technique described by Mohs, Mohs micrographic surgery, for Ta/T1 lesions aims to excise the lesion in thin slices with continuous histopathological evaluation of the slices till clear margins are achieved.[31] The technically demanding and time consuming technique, aimed to provide maximal tissue conservation, has failed to gain popularity because of high local recurrence rates, need of rigorous follow-up, high reoperation rates and technical complexities encountered.

Surgical Treatment of T2-T4 Disease

The standard treatment for T2 lesions involving corpus spongiosum or corpora cavernosa is partial penile amputation with tumor free margins. The degree of resection depends on location and size of the lesion but most guidelines agree that the standard margin of 2 cm is no longer mandatory. The amount of normal tissue to be excised as a margin depends, to a large extent, on the grade and stage of the lesion. Current recommendations advocate a 10 mm margin as adequate for grade 1 and 2 lesions and a margin of 15 mm for grade 3 lesions.[32] The urethral stump is traditionally kept 1-2 cm longer than the corporal stump in order to enable neourethral meatus creation. Recently, few modifications in surgical technique have been advocated to improve the sexual, functional and cosmetic outcomes following partial penectomy. Ventral phalloplasty, with removal of skin and dartos fascia from the penoscrotal junction, has been described to augment the length of the penile stump for better sexual function.[33] A novel technique has recently described the use of everted urethral stump to cover the corporal ends as a neo glans with reported improvements in cosmesis and glanular sensation for better sexual outcomes **(Figs. 6A to E)**.[34]

For selected T2 lesions limited to glans, total glansectomy with glanular reconstruction utilizing split thickness skin graft (STSG) offers maximal tissue preservation with optimal oncological and cosmetic outcomes. Intraoperative frozen section analysis of cut margins has been advocated in order to improve the oncological outcomes. For T3/T4 lesions, total penile amputation with perineal urethrostomy has been the most accepted surgical treatment. For locally advanced unresectable T4 tumors, role of neoadjuvant

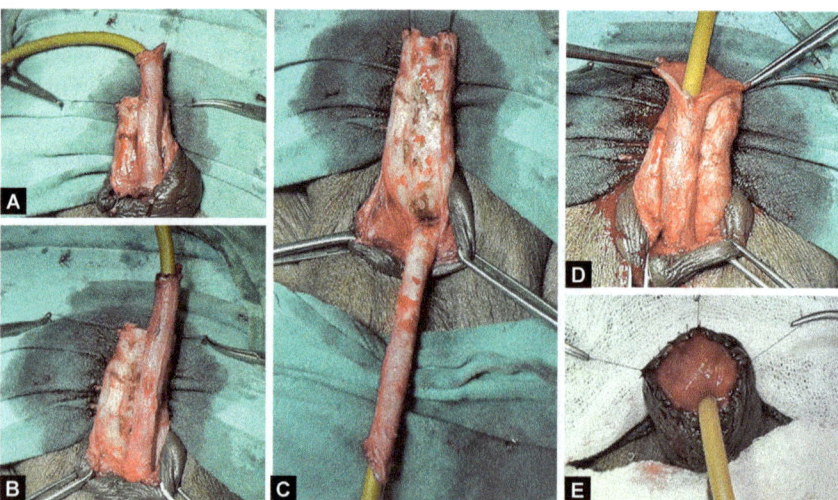

Figs. 6A to E: Urethral flap glanuloplasty. (A) Partial penectomy; (B) Urethral stump kept longer than usual; (C) Urethral dissection and mobilization up to penoscrotal junction; (D) Ventral urethral spatulation and advancement over corpora cavernosa; (E) Suture of urethral flap (neo glans) to skin.

chemotherapy has been explored with conflicting results in different studies. In lesions producing severe local symptoms, immediate surgical resection is the treatment of choice. Few recent studies have explored the role of complete penile reconstruction following total penectomy in carefully selected patients.[35]

Surgical Management of Regional Lymph Nodes

The most crucial factor affecting the prognosis and survival in penile cancer patients is the incidence and magnitude of inguinal lymph node involvement. A thorough assessment of inguinal lymph nodes by physical examination and relevant imaging modalities is critical in order to evaluate the presence and extent of inguinal and/or pelvic lymphadenopathy. Although physical examination offers reasonably high accuracy in detection of inguinal lymph nodes, certain clinical scenarios warrant use of cross-sectional imaging. These include conditions where physical examination may be difficult to perform, e.g., obese patients, prior surgery, radiation or chemotherapy. Although USG, CT and MRI all have been used for assessment of inguinal lymph nodes, the detection of sub-centimetric nodes remains a concern. Contrast enhanced MRI seems to be best suited for assessment in such patients as a supplement to physical examination.[18] Role of 18SDG-PET/CT has been evaluated in various studies regarding inguinal lymph node assessment. While PET/CT has high sensitivity and specificity in verifying the presence of metastases in palpable inguinal lymph nodes or detecting pelvic lymph nodes and distant metastases, its utility in detecting metastases in nonpalpable inguinal lymph nodes is hampered by poor sensitivity in picking up sub-centimetric lymph nodes.[21,22]

Dynamic Sentinel Node Biopsy

As discussed earlier, the concept of sentinel node biopsy, as originally propagated by Cabanas, is centered on the notion that initial landing site of lymphatic drainage from penile cancer is primarily to a particular zone located in the superomedial area of the superficial inguinal lymph nodes.[36] The technique of dynamic sentinel node biopsy (DSNB) is aimed to improve the accuracy of detection of inguinal lymph node metastases in patients with clinically normal groins.[13] DSNB involves injection of a vital dye such as isosulfan blue and Technetium-99m-labeled nanocolloid in the vicinity of the penile lesion. The dye helps in tracing out the lymphatic pathways leading to the sentinel node which is then identified by means of the gamma camera which picks up the concentrated radiotracer activity in the draining lymph node. In hands of experts, the reported sensitivity of DSNB has been as high as 90% in high volume centers.[37]

Surgical Treatment of Nonpalpable ILNs

In patients with nonpalpable inguinal nodes, the management is dictated by the stage, grade and status of LVI in the penile lesion. Low risk tumors (<5%

chances of ILN involvement), i.e., pTis, pTa, and pT1a and G1/G2 lesions without LVI, are best suited for surveillance with serial imaging and periodic physical examination.[38] For intermediate risk tumors (20-30% chances of ILN involvement), i.e., pT1 with LVI (pT1b), pT2-pT4, or G3/G4 lesions, and high risk tumors (pT2-pT4, G3/G4), an immediate bilateral prophylactic inguinal lymph node dissection (ILND) is advocated as long-term survival rates with this strategy are clearly superior to those with surveillance or radiotherapy.[39] A delayed ILND till nodes appear has been shown to have poorer results in this subset of patients.[40] In order to reduce the morbidity of the classical ILND, a more conservative and restricted approach to ILND has been utilized. This modified ILND involves limiting the dissection to femoral artery laterally and fossa ovalis caudally, preservation of fascia lata, sparing the saphenous vein, and omitting the transposition of sartorius muscle.[41] The outcome of this modified approach is minimal risk of lymphedema or lymphocele, reduced chances of skin flap necrosis and wound dehiscence and less chances of infection. However, frozen section examination of the nodes removed is required and in case of positive nodes, an ipsilateral radical ILND is recommended.

Surgical Treatment of Palpable ILNs

Presence of clinically palpable inguinal lymph nodes is a strong predictor of harboring metastases. Further imaging in form of 18F-PET/CT, USG or MRI is only indicated to know the status of pelvic LNs. Likewise, there is no role of DSNB in the setting of palpable inguinal nodes. The earlier practice of giving a course of antibiotics for 4-6 weeks to rule out infectious lymphadenopathy is no longer advisable. In equivocal cases, the contemporary recommendations of most of the guidelines is to go for USG-guided FNAC.[42]

The recommended treatment for clinically palpable inguinal nodes is a complete ILND in order to ensure complete surgical resection as well as accurate. The limits of dissection for a radical ILND are the sartorius laterally, adductor longus medially and the inguinal ligament superiorly. Both the superficial and the deep inguinal group of inguinal nodes are removed and long saphenous vein is ligated at saphenofemoral junction. Transposition of sartorius muscle forms an integral part of the radical ILND. The morbidity of radical ILND is considerable and the most common complications include flap necrosis, wound dehiscence, infection, lymphedema, hematoma, and lymphocele formation. A number of measures have been recommended to reduce the morbidity including use of meticulous dissection techniques, careful ligation/clipping of lymphatics, prophylactic antibiotics, use of compression stockings and sequential pneumatic compression devices, use of low molecular weight heparin, application of pressure dressings over the inguinal region and aggressive limb physiotherapy.

In the setting of unresectable disease, viz., large, multiple, matted and fixed inguinal nodes, a course of neoadjuvant chemotherapy followed by surgical resection in responders is recommended.[43] This subset of patients which exhibits good response to neoadjuvant chemotherapy and subsequently undergoes ILND has been shown to have significantly better long-term survival rates as compared to non-responders.[44]

Surgical Treatment of Pelvic LNs

Pelvic LND is recommended in patients who have ≥2 positive ILNs or extracapsular extension in any inguinal lymph node (pN3).[45] Usually an ipsilateral PLND, either together with ILND or at a separate session, is appropriate for unilateral ILN involvement since there is no crossover in the pelvic nodes. Thus, a bilateral PLND is required only if bilateral inguinal nodes are involved. The PLND entails removal of obturator, external iliac and internal iliac nodes and the anatomical extent is bounded by inguinal ligament distally, iliac bifurcation proximally, obturator nerve medially and ilioinguinal nerve laterally.

Endoscopic Surgical Approach to LND

In an era of minimally invasive techniques designed to reduce morbidity and hasten postoperative recovery, there have been a number of studies reporting the use of video endoscopy ILND (VEIL) and robot-assisted laparoscopic ILND with encouraging outcomes. The concept of endoscopic ILND was first propounded by Bishoff et al.[46] in animal models and subsequently in a patient with penile cancer and palpable inguinal nodes. The patient selection, surgical technique, steps and boundaries of dissection are essentially the same as in open approach.

Use of robotic assistance to perform VEIL was first described by Josephson and Sotelo et al. in patients with palpable and nonpalpable ILNs. The authors reported superior performance with improved dexterity due to the inherent advantages of robotic technology.[47] While the advent of endoscopic and robotic approaches undoubtedly has the potential of reducing the morbidity and patient discomfort, there is need for greater long-term data, gleaned from large, multicenter, prospective trials to confirm oncological outcomes before these minimally invasive surgical approaches can be validated as superior alternative techniques in the management of penile cancer.

MANAGEMENT OF ADVANCED OR METASTATIC PENILE CANCER (T4, N2-3, M1)

In patients with locally advanced disease, which includes regional lymph node involvement or unresectable bulky primary tumors, most of clinical guidelines recommend neoadjuvant chemotherapy, prior to radical surgery. The administration of neoadjuvant systemic therapy enables an opportune supply of chemotherapy to the systemic disease at an earlier stage, downstages the inguinal lymph nodes and makes them resectable, and aids future multimodal therapy. Many chemotherapy regimens used in the neoadjuvant setting have demonstrated modest activity with reported objective response rates (ORR) ranging from 15 to 50%, but majority of cases eventually relapse and none of the studies so far have reported any survival advantage.[48] Hence, management of advanced disease usually requires a multimodal approach. Currently, the preferred regimens for neoadjuvant chemotherapy include TIP (a combination of paclitaxel, cisplatin, and ifosfamide) or TPF (docetaxel, cisplatin, and 5-fluorouracil).[49] In the previous years, many small, single center, retrospective studies have reported outcomes with other regimens such as bleomycin, vincristine, methotrexate (BVM) and bleomycin, methotrexate, and cisplatin (BMP). As of today, these regimens are not recommended.

Adjuvant Chemotherapy

There is little data regarding the results of adjuvant chemotherapy following inguinal LND in patients with locoregionally advanced disease such as bulky nodes, pelvic node involvement, and extranodal disease. According to the EAU guidelines, adjuvant chemotherapy is indicated when the intent of treatment is curative.[20] Likewise, NCCN guidelines advocate administering four cycles of a combination of paclitaxel, cisplatin, and ifosfamide (TIP) in an adjuvant setting if the histopathology shows high-risk features and the patients did not receive any neoadjuvant chemotherapy.[19] Although the data is sparse, yet the few studies performed have reported a trend toward improved overall survival (OS) in patients who received multidrug adjuvant chemotherapy, especially in the setting of advanced disease like pelvic node involvement. The key to improving results of adjuvant chemotherapy in penile cancer lies in identifying the correct subset of patients likely to benefit from this therapy. There is recent data from few studies which indicates a role of biomarkers for patient selection in the adjuvant setting. A study from the Milan group demonstrated that the immunohistochemical expression of TP53 appeared to be associated with a shorter overall survival in patients who received docetaxel, cisplatin, and 5-fluorouracil (TPF) as adjuvant chemotherapy.[50]

Chemotherapy for Advanced Disease

There is a lack of consensus regarding the selection of first line chemotherapeutic agents for treatment of penile cancer with distant metastases. The main reason for this lies in the consistently dismal response rates, even in the short-term. Use of Cisplatin alone in this setting has shown poor efficacy with a partial response of 15% and a median OS of only 4.7 months.[51] Likewise, the response rates with multidrug regimens such as BMP have shown a median survival of only around 7 months.[48] A combination of cisplatinum and 5-fluorouracil has shown modest activity in the adjuvant setting in a few small retrospective studies. In a retrospective study on 25 patients, cisplatin plus 5-fluorouracil demonstrated an

ORR of 32% with median progression free survival (PFS) of 20 weeks and an OS of 8 months.[52] In general, cisplatin-based regimens have been shown to have better outcomes than noncisplatin-based regimens. Since taxanes were inducted for penile cancer chemotherapy, the outcomes of these regimens have improved.[49] Currently, the widely accepted first-line regimen for metastatic penile cancer consists of Paclitaxel plus ifosfamide plus cisplatin. A preferred alternative regimen consists of 5-FU plus cisplatin.[49,52] Small trials of intra-arterial chemotherapy in locally advanced cases of penile cancer, using cisplatin and gemcitabine, have failed to show any significant improvement in survival, despite a small clinical response.

Radiotherapy for Advanced Penile Cancer

There have been very few studies evaluating the role of radiotherapy for advanced penile carcinoma. There is weak evidence from single center studies to suggest that neoadjuvant radiotherapy for bulky but nonfixed inguinal nodes may enhance resectability of the nodal mass.[53] Use of radiotherapy as a palliative measure has been shown to be of help in alleviating pain from bony metastases and inguinal nodal masses.[53]

Targeted Therapy

Targeted therapy has been mainly used as a second-line treatment in metastatic penile cancer. The expression of epidermal growth factor receptor (EGFR) in penile carcinoma prompted the use of EGFR targeted monotherapy using anti-EGFR monoclonal antibodies, panitumumab and cetuximab.[54] A few recent studies have reported the use of tyrosine kinase inhibitors in advanced penile cancer. A phase 2 study by Italian investigators used dacomitinib in 28 patients with advanced penile cancer and reported an ORR of 32%.[55]

Immunotherapy and Immune Checkpoint Inhibitors

Immune checkpoint inhibitors have been shown to exhibit encouraging results in various cancers including virus-associated cancers such as squamous cell carcinomas of the head and neck, the cervix and the anus. A number of studies have demonstrated a high expression of PD-L1 in metastatic penile cancers, thus laying the grounds for use of immune-checkpoint inhibitors.[56] However, the clinical data is limited at present. A phase II trial in metastatic penile cancer patients (NCT02496208) comparing cabozantinib/nivolumab/ipilimumab to cabozantinib/nivolumab demonstrated a partial response in 50% of the patients (2/4) and a stable disease in the other 50% (2/4). Several key trials are currently underway to evaluate the role of immune checkpoint inhibitors, mainly nivolumab and pembrolizumab, in advanced penile cancer patients. This novel therapeutic approach has the potential to emerge as an important modality for advanced penile cancer patients.

Palliation in Advanced Penile Cancer

The palliative care in penile carcinoma patients is aimed to reduce pain, improve quality of life, optimize wound care, treat complications such as hypercalcemia, and minimize groin complications such as sepsis and hemorrhage. The modalities employed include multidrug chemotherapy, radiotherapy, hemipelvectomy in selected cases with unilateral gross disease or bony involvement, use of vascular stents for femoral vessel infiltration, and treatment of hypercalcemia.

5-year relative survival rates for penile cancer (Based on SEER database of men diagnosed with penile cancer between 2008 and 2014)
1. *Localized (confined to the penis):* 82%
2. *Regional (spread to adjacent structures or inguinal lymph nodes):* 48%
3. *Distant (Metastatic):* Not available
4. *Overall:* 67%

(*SEER = Surveillance, Epidemiology, and End Results)

FOLLOW-UP

The follow-up of penile cancer patients is crucial to pick up early recurrences or metastases. The follow-up protocol depends on the stage and grade of the primary lesion, status of the inguinal lymph nodes and the treatment modality chosen. Risk of inguinal node involvement in pathologically node negative patients is around 2–3% but increases to around 20% in patients with pathologically involved inguinal nodes. The patients need to be put on a stringent and frequent follow-up schedule consisting of thorough physical examination and selected investigations. A comparison of recommended follow-up schedules according to European Association of Urology (EAU) and NCCN guidelines is depicted in **Table 4**. Any patient who develops nodal recurrence or metastatic disease warrants a speedy salvage treatment.

CONCLUSION

Penile cancer is a lethal malignancy with a significantly high incidence in India and certain other regions of the world. It has a huge impact on the longevity and the quality of life of patients. Mutilating local surgical treatment has negative effects on the sexual function and self-esteem. Emerging recent data suggests that organ preserving approaches with much smaller surgical margins enable a better sexual function and quality of life and should be preferred in all feasible scenarios. A multidisciplinary approach involving oncologist, radiation oncologist, urologist, and a psychologist should be preferred. The involvement of inguinal lymph nodes is the single most important prognostic factor and treatment of inguinal nodes must be aggressive. In patients with involved lymph nodes, adjuvant therapy can improve outcomes. The advent of novel modalities such as DSNB and endoscopic and robotic inguinal LND

TABLE 4: EAU 2018 and NCCN 2018 guidelines for follow-up in penile cancer.

		Primary tumor				Lymph nodes			
		Penile-preserving treatment		Amputation (partial/total)		Surveillance		pN0		pN+
EAU guidelines 2018		Years 1–2	Years 3–5	Years 1–2	Years 3–5	Years 1–2	Years 3–5	Years 1–2	Years 3–5	Years 3–5
		Every 3 months	Every 6 months	Every 3 months	Every 1 year	Every 3 months	Every 6 months	Every 3 months	Every 1 year	Every 6 months
		Regular physician or self-examination. Repeat biopsy after topical or laser treatment for penile intraepithelial neoplasia		Regular physician or self-examination		Regular physician or self-examination		Regular physician or self-examination. Ultrasound with fine needle aspiration biopsy optional		Regular physician or self-examination. Ultrasound with fine needle aspiration cytology optional, computed tomography/magnetic resonance imaging optional

		Primary tumor				Lymph nodes			Imaging			
		Penile-preserving treatment		Amputation (partial/total)		Nx		N0, N1	N2, N3		Chest (CT or X-ray)	Abdominal/pelvic (CT or MRI)
NCCN guidelines 2018		Years 1–2	Years 3–5	Years 5–10	Years 1–2	Years 3–5	Years 1–2	Years 3–5	Every 3–6 months	Every 6–12 months		Years 1–2	Year 1	Year 2
		Every 3 months	Every 6 months	Every 12 months	Every 6 months	Every 12 months	Every 6 months	Every 12 months	Clinical examination	Years 3–5		Every 6 months	Every 3 months	Every 6 months
		Clinical examination			Clinical examination		Clinical examination						

(EAU: European Association of Urology; NCCN: National Comprehensive Cancer Network) techniques has resulted in reduced morbidity and improved psychosocial and oncological outcomes. The introduction of newer systemic therapies such as targeted therapy and immunotherapy has raised the hopes of finally offering a chance of lasting and effective oncological outcome for patients with advanced penile carcinoma.

REFERENCES

1. Christodoulidou M, Sahdev V, Houssein S, Muneer A. Epidemiology of penile cancer. Curr Probl Cancer. 2015;39(3):126-36.
2. Curado MP, Shin HR. Cancer incidence in five continents. Lyon: IARC Scientific Publications; 2007. pp. 160.
3. Favorito LA, Nardi AC, Ronalsa M, Zequi SC, Sampaio FJ, Glina S. Epidemiologic study on penile cancer in Brazil. Int Braz J Urol. 2008;34(5):587-93.
4. Maden C, Sherman KJ, Beckmann AM, Hislop TG, Teh CZ, Ashley RL, et al. History of circumcision, medical conditions, and sexual activity and risk of penile cancer. J Natl Cancer Inst. 1993;85(1):19-24.
5. Harish K, Ravi R. The role of tobacco in penile carcinoma. Br J Urol. 1995;75(3):375-7.
6. Tsen HF, Morgenstern H, Mack T, Peters RK. Risk factors for penile cancer: results of a population-based case-control study in Los Angeles County (United States). Cancer Causes control. 2001;12(3):267-77.
7. Madsen BS, van den Brule AJ, Jensen HL, Wohlfahrt J, Frisch M. Risk factors for squamous cell carcinoma of the penis—population-based case-control study in Denmark. Cancer Epidemiol Biomarkers Prev. 2008;17(10):2683-91.
8. Daling JR, Madeleine MM, Johnson LG, Schwartz SM, Shera KA, Wurscher MA, et al. Penile cancer: importance of circumcision, human papillomavirus and smoking in in situ and invasive disease. Int J Cancer. 2005;116(4):606-16.
9. Rubin MA, Kleter B, Zhou M, Ayala G, Cubilla AL, Quint WG, et al. Detection and typing of human papillomavirus DNA in penile carcinoma: evidence for multiple independent pathways of penile carcinogenesis. Am J Pathol. 2001;159(4):1211-8.
10. Narayana AS, Olney LE, oening SA, Weimar GW, Culp DA. Carcinoma of the penis: analysis of 219 cases. Cancer. 1982;49(10):2185-91.
11. Misra S, Chaturvedi A, Misra NC. Penile carcinoma: a challenge for the developing world. Lancet Oncol. 2004;5(4):240-7.
12. Cabanas RM. Anatomy and biopsy of sentinel lymph nodes. Urologic Clin North Am. 1992;19(2):267-76.
13. Leijte JA, Hughes B, Graafland NM, Kroon BK, Olmos RA, Nieweg OE, et al. Two-center evaluation of dynamic sentinel node biopsy for squamous cell carcinoma of the penis. J Clin Oncol. 2009;27(20):3325-9.
14. Leijte JA, Valdes Olmos RA, Nieweg OE, Horenblas S. Anatomical mapping of lymphatic drainage in penile carcinoma with SPECT-CT: implications for the extent of inguinal lymph node dissection. Eur Urol. 2008;54(4):885-90.
15. Horenblas S, Van Tinteren H, Delemarre JF, Moonen LM, Lustig V, Kröger R. Squamous cell carcinoma of the penis: accuracy of tumor, nodes and metastasis classification system, and role of lymphangiography, computerized tomography scan and fine needle aspiration cytology. J Urol. 1991;146(5):1279-83.
16. Solsona E, Algaba F, Horenblas S, Pizzocaro G, Windahl T. EAU Guidelines on Penile Cancer. Eur Urol. 2004;46(1):1-8.
17. Lont AP, Besnard AP, Gallee MP, van Tinteren H, Horenblas S. A comparison of physical examination and imaging in determining the extent of primary penile carcinoma. BJU Int. 2003;91(6):493-5.
18. Kayes O, Minhas S, Allen C, Hare C, Freeman A, Ralph D. The role of magnetic resonance imaging in the local staging of penile cancer. Eur Urol. 2007;51(5):1313-9.

19. National Comprehensive Cancer Network. (2018). NCCN penile cancer 2018. [online] Available from: https://www2.tri-kobe.org/nccn/guideline/urological/english/penile.pdf. [Last Accessed January, 2021].
20. European Association of Urology. (2018). EAU Guidelines Penile Cancer 2018. [online] Available from: https://uroweb.org/guideline/penile-cancer/. [Last Accessed January, 2021].
21. Souillac I, Rigaud J, Ansquer C, Marconnet L, Bouchot O. Prospective evaluation of (18) F-fluorodeoxyglucose positron emission tomography-computerized tomography to assess inguinal lymph node status in invasive squamous cell carcinoma of the penis. J Urol. 2012;187(2):493-7.
22. Graafland NM, Leijte JA, Olmos RA, Hoefnagel CA, Teertstra HJ, Horenblas S. Scanning with 18F-FDG-PET/CT for detection of pelvic nodal involvement in inguinal node-positive penile carcinoma. Eur Urol. 2009;56(2):339-45.
23. Zhu Y, Ye DW, Yao X, Zhang S, Dai B, Zhang H, et al. The value of squamous cell carcinoma antigen in the prognostic evaluation, treatment monitoring and follow-up of patients with penile cancer. J Urol. 2008;180(5):2019-23.
24. Velazquez EF, Barreto JE, et al. Limitations in the interpretation of biopsies in patients with penile squamous cell carcinoma. Int J Surg Pathol. 2004;12(2):139-46.
25. Slaton JW, Morgenstern N, Levy DA, Santos MW Jr, Tamboli P, Ro JY, et al. Tumor stage, vascular invasion and the percentage of poorly differentiated cancer: independent prognosticators for inguinal lymph node metastasis in penile squamous cancer. J Urol. 2001;165(4):1138-42.
26. Maiche AG, Pyrhonen S, Karkinen M. Histological grading of squamous cell carcinoma of the penis: a new scoring system. Br J Urol. 1991;67(5):522-6.
27. Brierley J, Gospodarowicz MK, Wittekind C. TNM Classification of Malignant Tumours, 8th edition. London: John Wiley & Sons, Inc.; 2016.
28. Alnajjar HM, Lam W, Bolgeri M, Rees RW, Perry MJ, Watkin NA. Treatment of carcinoma in situ of the glans penis with topical chemotherapy agents. Eur Urol. 2012;62(5):923-8.
29. Shabbir M, Muneer A, Kalsi J, Shukla CJ, Zacharakis E, Garaffa G, et al. Glans resurfacing for the treatment of carcinoma in situ of the penis: surgical technique and outcomes. Eur Urol. 2011;59(1):142-7.
30. Bandieramonte G, Colecchia M, Mariani L, Lo Vullo S, Pizzocaro G, Piva L, et al. Peniscopically controlled CO_2 laser excision for conservative treatment of in situ and T1 penile carcinoma: report on 224 patients. Eur Urol. 2008;54(4):875-82.
31. Shindel AW, Mann MW, Lev RY, Sengelmann R, Petersen J, Hruza GJ, et al. Mohs micrographic surgery for penile cancer: management and long-term follow-up. J Urol. 2007;178(5):1980-5.
32. Agrawal A, Pai D. The histological extent of the local spread of carcinoma of the penis and its therapeutic implications. BJU Int. 2000;85(3):299-301.
33. Wallen JJ, Baumgarten AS. Optimizing penile length in patients undergoing partial penectomy for penile cancer: novel application of the ventral phalloplasty oncoplastic technique. Int Braz J Urol. 2014;40(5):708-9.
34. Suarez-Ibarrola R, Heinze A, Reis G, Gratzke C, Miernik A. Urethral flap glanuloplasty after partial penectomy for penile carcinoma: Evaluation of urinary, sexual and quality of life outcomes. World J Urol. 2019;23:58-9.
35. Garaffa G, Raheem AA, Christopher NA, Ralph DJ. Total phallic reconstruction after penile amputation for carcinoma. BJU Int. 2009;104(6):852-6.
36. Cabanas RM. An approach for the treatment of penile carcinoma. Cancer. 1977;39(2):456-66.
37. Leijte JA, Kroon BK, Valdés Olmos RA, Nieweg OE, Horenblas S. Reliability and safety of current dynamic sentinel node biopsy for penile carcinoma. Eur Urol. 2007;52(1):170-7.
38. Leijte JA, Kirrander P, Antonini N, Windahl T, Horenblas S. Recurrence patterns of squamous cell carcinoma of the penis: recommendations for follow-up based on a two-centre analysis of 700 patients. Eur Urol. 2008;54(1):161-8.

39. Graafland NM, Lam W, Leijte JA, Yap T, Gallee MP, Corbishley C, et al. Prognostic factors for occult inguinal lymph node involvement in penile carcinoma and assessment of the high-risk EAU subgroup: a two-institution analysis of 342 clinically node-negative patients. Eur Urol. 2010;58(5):742-7.
40. McDougal WS. Preemptive lymphadenectomy markedly improves survival in patients with cancer of the penis who harbor occult metastases. J Urol. 2005;173(3):681.
41. Catalona WJ. Modified inguinal lymphadenectomy for carcinoma of the penis with preservation of saphenous veins: technique and preliminary results. J Urol. 1988;140(2):306-10.
42. Saisorn I, Lawrentschuk N, Leewansangtong S, Bolton DM. Fine-needle aspiration cytology predicts inguinal lymph node metastasis without antibiotic pretreatment in penile carcinoma. BJU Int. 2006;97(6):1225-8.
43. Leijte JA, Kerst JM, Bais E, Antonini N, Horenblas S. Neoadjuvant chemotherapy in advanced penile carcinoma. Eur Urol. 2007;52(2):488-94.
44. Pizzocaro G, Piva L. Adjuvant and neoadjuvant vincristine, bleomycin, and methotrexate for inguinal metastases from squamous cell carcinoma of the penis. Acta Oncologica. 1988;27(6b):823-4.
45. Liu JY, Li YH, Zhang ZL, Yao K, Ye YL, Xie D, et al. The risk factors for the presence of pelvic lymph node metastasis in penile squamous cell carcinoma patients with inguinal lymph node dissection. World J Urol. 2013;31(6):1519-24.
46. Bishoff JT, Teichman JM, Thompson IM. Endoscopic subcutaneous modified inguinal lymph node dissection (ESMIL) for squamous cell carcinoma of the penis. J Urol 2003;169(4):78.
47. Josephson DY, Jacobsohn KM, Giri S, Hassan N, Batra K, Shah SH, et al. Robotic-assisted endoscopic inguinal lymphadenectomy. Urology. 2009;73(1):167-71.
48. Corral DA, Sella A, Pettaway CA, Amato RJ, Jones DM, Ellerhorst J. Combination chemotherapy for metastatic or locally advanced genitourinary squamous cell carcinoma: a phase II study of methotrexate, cisplatin and bleomycin. J Urol. 1998;160(5):1770-4.
49. Pagliaro LC, Williams DL, Daliani D, Williams MB, Osai W, Kincaid M, et al. Neoadjuvant paclitaxel, ifosfamide, and cisplatin chemotherapy for metastatic penile cancer: a phase II study. J Clin Oncol. 2010;28(24):3851-7.
50. Necchi A, Lo Vullo S, Nicolai N, Raggi D, Giannatempo P, Colecchia M, et al. Prognostic Factors of Adjuvant Taxane, Cisplatin, and 5-Fluorouracil Chemotherapy for Patients With Penile Squamous Cell Carcinoma After Regional Lymphadenectomy. Clin Genitourin Cancer. 2016;14(6):518-23.
51. Gagliano RG, Blumenstein BA, Crawford ED, Stephens RL, Coltman CA Jr, Costanzi JJ. cis-Diamminedichloroplatinum in the treatment of advanced epidermoid carcinoma of the penis: a Southwest Oncology Group Study. J Urol. 1989;141(1):66-7.
52. Di Lorenzo G, Buonerba C, Federico P, Perdonà S, Aieta M, Rescigno P, et al. Cisplatin and 5-fluorouracil in inoperable, stage IV squamous cell carcinoma of the penis. BJU Int. 2012;110(11 Pt B):E661-6.
53. Ravi R, Chaturvedi HK, Sastry DV. Role of radiation therapy in the treatment of carcinoma of the penis. Br J Urol. 1994;74(5):646-51.
54. Gou HF, Li X, Qiu M, Cheng K, Li LH, Dong H, et al. Epidermal growth factor receptor (EGFR)-RAS signaling pathway in penile squamous cell carcinoma. PloS One. 2013;8(4):e62175.
55. Necchi A, Lo Vullo S, Perrone F, Raggi D, Giannatempo P, Calareso G, et al. First-line therapy with dacomitinib, an orally available pan-HER tyrosine kinase inhibitor, for locally advanced or metastatic penile squamous cell carcinoma: results of an open-label, single-arm, single-centre, phase 2 study. BJU Int. 2018;121(3):348-56.
56. Cocks M, Taheri D, Ball MW, Bezerra SM, Del Carmen Rodriguez M, Ricardo BFP, et al. Immune-checkpoint status in penile squamous cell carcinoma: a North American cohort. Hum Pathol. 2017;59:55-61.

CHAPTER 12
Microvascular Surgery

Arun Kumar Singh, Harsha Vardhan

INTRODUCTION

The development and refinement of microsurgery in the recent decades has ushered in the latest surgical revolution. Microsurgery has made possible feats that were difficult to imagine just a few decades ago. Changing faces from one person to another was possible only in fictional universe, but with the help of microsurgery, face transplant has become a reality. Just like asepsis and the advent of anesthesia, the impact of microsurgery has been revolutionary. It has had applications in all fields of surgery.

The Saga of Development: The Preparation

The invention of the microscope is credited to the father, son duo of Hans and Zacharias Janssen[1] in the late 16th century. Nylen[2] and Holmgren[3] brought the microscope into the operation theaters. Developments in other fields of medicine that laid the groundwork of microsurgery were the concept of asepsis by Lister and the demonstration of anesthesia by Morton. The work of Alexis Carrel on vascular repair, for which he was awarded the Nobel Prize, helped refine techniques, which were to become the cornerstone of microvascular surgery later. Discovery of heparin by McLean helped develop the specialty by improving the results.

The Saga of Development: A "Small" Stitch on Tissue, a Giant Leap in Surgery

The first use of a microscope for repair of a vessel was by Jacobson and Suarez[4] for the repair of carotid vessels in dogs. Malt and McKhann[5] performed the first arm replantation and Kleinert and Kasdan[6] did the first digital replantation in 1965. Transfer of the toe to the hand by Chen and Cobett[7] allowed restoration of function after loss of digits. The experimental work of others pioneers such as Guthrie, Snyder, Buncke,[8] etc. helped establish microsurgery as a promising specialty.

The Saga of Development: Advancing Frontiers

By 1960s the uses of microsurgery were expanding. Rapid development by maverick surgeons allowed the expansion of applications of microsurgery.

The modality was being used from head to toe, not just by Plastic Surgeons, but other specialties as well. Microscope was entering the operation theaters of various specialties. Harms[9] first reported the use of microscope in ocular surgery in 1953. Neurosurgeons had started using the microscope by late 1950s.[10] Silbar and Owen[11] used the microscope for performing vaso-vasostomy in 1970s, which became widely prevalent by the 1980s. Singh and Tahiliani,[12,13] have studied microsurgical experimental vaso-vasostomosis and fallopian tube anastomosis in experimental animals. Even dentistry has found applications with the microscope, with the first use being described in 1978 by Apotheker and Jako.[14] In Plastic Surgery, refinements in techniques allowed development of newer flaps. This completely changed the goals of treatment, from just providing wound cover to a functional and cosmetic restoration. The microsurgeon became an elite surgeon, providing solutions that the normal surgeon could not.

The Saga of Development: Microsurgery Everywhere

Currently microsurgery is performed by all surgical subspecialties. It is no longer a novelty but a necessary tool in the armamentarium of any worthy surgeon. The goals of surgery have radically changed with these techniques. Another change brought by the microsurgical revolution is in changing the mecca of surgery from the established centers of the West to the new beacons in the far-east. Centers in China, Taiwan and Japan have become the world leaders in microsurgical advancements, performing feats not envisaged by the rest of the world.[15]

PREPARATION

Masters of microsurgery maintain that microsurgery is not just a surgical field but a lifestyle choice. The first and foremost prerequisite for microsurgery is attitude. A clear, untroubled mind is a prerequisite for microsurgery. There is no place for shortcuts, gambits or disorderliness. The margin of error is miniscule and each mistake is magnified. A microsurgeon needs to be patient, meticulous, and honest in the appraisal of their own work.

Microsurgery can be equally rewarding and frustrating. Passion, persistence and patience are the hallmarks of a successful microsurgeon. No amount of remuneration is worth an umpteenth revision of a nonworking anastomosis at odd hours. Only a surgeon who has the motivation will succeed. This motivation is infrequently inherent. This zeal and passion is usually acquired. That is the importance of training institutes.

Asthenopia[16] or eye strain is normally associated with performing prolonged near vision tasks. However adding the additional cognitive load of operating using a microscope, increases the strain manifold.[17] Hence, it is important to give adequate rest to the eyes. Breaks from surgery may be taken before fatigue sets in. Recently major microscope manufacturers have

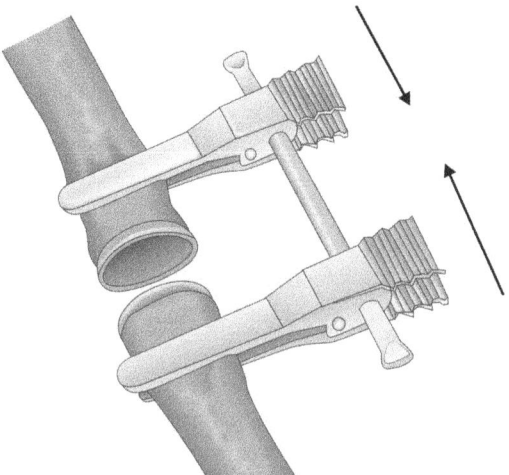

Fig. 1: Microvascular clamps bringing the two ends of the cut vessel in approximation.

utilized 3D technology to improve the ergonomics of surgery and reduce surgeon's fatigue.[18]

A microscope provides magnification, although few surgeons use binocular loupes as well. Specialized good quality instruments are mandatory.[19] A surgical set would routinely have a pair of fine forceps, a needle holder, a couple of scissors, a vessel dilator and a clamp applicator. These are very delicate instruments, and to be handled very carefully. The surgeon should personally take care of his instruments as even a small dent to the tip will make the instrument useless. Clamps are probably the most important piece of instrumentation for a microsurgeon. The clamps differ for artery and vein. They come in various grading depending on the pressure needed to occlude the vessels. A microsurgeon should have appropriate sets for optimum use and should avoid using a one size to fit all. Good vascular clamps not only occlude the vessels but also keep the cut ends in approximation **(Fig. 1)**. Clamps have refinements for carrying sutures,[20] and also for everting the back walls. Studies have also been done to eliminate the double clamp while during anastomosis, but such practices are rare.[21]

MECHANISM OF HEALING

Harashina et al.[22] found a pseudointima 5 days following anastomosis. This pseudointima disappears by 14 days giving rise to a new endothelium formation. Lidman and Daniel[23] performed microscopic examination post anastomosis of rat femoral vessels. They found that by 10 days the endothelial lining was restored in both arteries and veins. There was necrosis of the media at the site of anastomosis in the artery, but much more extensive in the veins. The adventitia regenerated in both types of vessels. There was compensatory hyperplasia of the intima, which provided the strength to the vessel. This hyperplasia was accompanied by dilatation of the vessel wall, which prevents stenosis at the site of anastomosis. Chaware et al.[24] used scanning electron microscopy to study initimal healing in conventional versus stented anastomosis.

PROCEDURE

The process of mastery of placing the suture is the critical step, which will determine the success of the anastomosis. The interested reader may refer to the videos and manual of microsurgery by Acland for a detailed description of the perfect technique.

Microsurgery is done in a calm, quiet atmosphere, with the surgeon and the staff comfortable. The surgeon is comfortably seated with the head in line of the microscope to prevent strain to the neck. Acland[25] performed electromyographic studies to assess the tremors in various muscle groups with different hand supports during microsurgery. He suggested that the elbow, forearm and the hands must be completely supported, before starting the procedure, in order to have the least tremors during microsurgery.

The ends are prepared. The adventia over the end of the vessel is stripped off. This is done to prevent the thrombogenic adventitia coming in contact with the platelet plug. The vasospasm is also reduced at the anastomosis site. A contrasting, nonreflective background helps ease the process. It is important not to perform the anastomosis in a dependent area, as all collections would collect at the repair site and impede the vision. A piece of gauze placed below the anastomosis prevents pooling of fluid at the anastomosis and makes the process easier.

Once the ends are prepared, the anastomosis starts. The smallest diameter suture with the finest possible needle is taken for anastomosis. Too small a thread will not have enough strength to hold the anastomosis and may lead to a catastrophic blowout. Too large sutures will result large punctures which are covered by platelet plugs. These platelet plugs may forms a thrombus, which occludes the vessel. The threshold for this occlusion is lower in vessels with lower flow, like veins as compared to higher flowing arteries. A similar process is followed for the number of sutures. The minimum sutures that provide strength and prevent perianastomotic leak are to be placed. Too many sutures damage the endothelium; too few sutures will result in leak and subsequent thrombus formation. Different techniques have been adopted, but the most commonly performed is loosely based on the work of Carrel.[26]

The "triangulation" technique[27] uses three stitches, which form the angles of the triangle, after which the sides can be sutured with ease **(Fig. 2)**. The reason to perform it in such a way is to prevent inadvertent inclusion of the posterior wall during the suturing. With the vessel ends secure in a clamp, two sutures are placed on either ends of the vessel wall, in a 10 o'clock and a 2 o'clock position. The threads are left long and hitched to the clamp. The

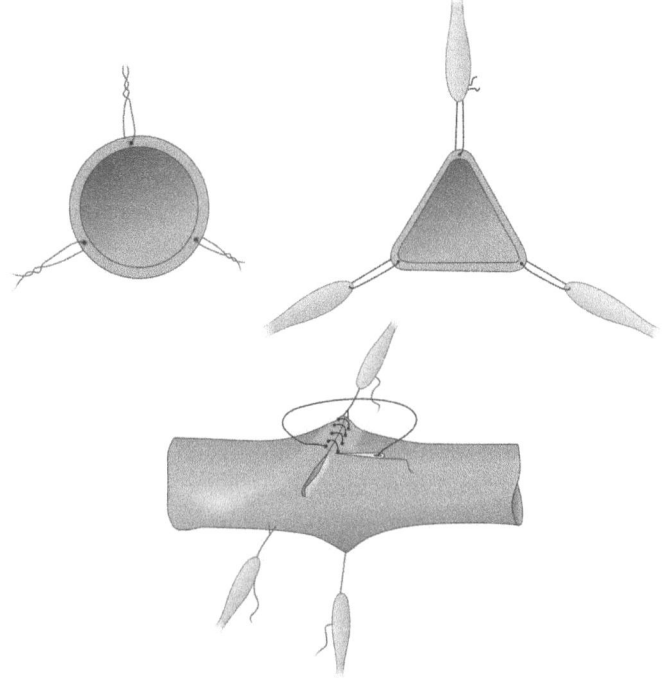

Fig. 2: "Triangulation" technique of vessel repair.

anterior wall is sutured. Once the repair is complete, the clamp is flipped and the posterior wall is approached. A suture is given at 6 o'clock position. This ensures universal placement of sutures. The posterior wall is then sutured. An alternative technique is there where two sutures may be given on either side at 3 and 9 o'clock positions, respectively.

In some instances operative space is limited and flipping the clamp may be difficult. Technique has been described to suture the posterior wall first, followed by anterior wall.[28]

The sutures may also be given in a continuous manner. The patency rates of the two techniques are comparable.[29] Continuous sutures are quicker to give and hence may reduce the ischemia time.[30,31]

The needle is inserted perpendicularly into the vessel wall, as that would minimize the trauma to the endothelium. The needle should be gently pushed into the wall and not pulled out roughly. It is imperative to remember that these are delicate tissues and must be handled with utmost respect. The vessel wall is never to be held within the jaws of the forceps. If required, the vessel should be held by the adventitia. Overcoming the tendency to hold the vessel wall is a habit that needs overcoming in the trainee microsurgeon.

At times there may be a discrepancy in the size of lumens of the anastomosing vessels, especially seen in flap surgery or when vein grafts are used. Small discrepancies can be corrected by taking halving bites to accommodate the extra tissue. In case of greater discrepancy, anastomosis is started from one side and the opposite side is closed in a zipper fashion. Alternatively end to side anastomosis can be performed.

Usually a microsurgeon will be able to immediately judge if the anastomosis is good or not. A prompt flow across the anastomosis is the best sign of a working anastomosis. Milking of vessels (Acland's test) can be performed to assess the patency. This however, is a traumatic test and can be harmful to the vessel itself. Flow in an artery can be judged by gently occluding the vessel partially. Spurts of blood flow will be seen in the lumen when the blood column flows against the occluding pressure. These clinical tests have their limitations. They are unable to detect partial occlusion.[32] More reliable tests assessment can be done using High Speed Video Recordings[33] or Fluorescein Angiography.[34]

Failure of anastomosis due to poor surgical technique will be evident within the first half hour. The anastomosis should be protected after the anastomosis, optimizing the ambient conditions for a positive outcome. Warmth, moisture and adequate analgesia are important in the immediate postoperative period.

Vasospasm is a difficult problem faced by the microsurgeon. Certain simple steps can prevent vascular spasm. One is respecting the tissues at all times. Gentle manipulation and atraumatic technique will reduce the chances of spasm. A warm, moist ambient atmosphere is required. Mechanical stripping of the adventitia is done to prevent postoperative spasm by denervating the smooth vessels around the anastomosis. Pharmacological agents also play a role in the prevention of spasm. The most commonly used drug is lignocaine.[35] The ideal dose of topical lignocaine is unclear, with studies suggesting 20% concentration as the most efficacious.[36] The systemic adverse effects at such doses remain to be assessed fully. Another commonly used drug is papaverine,[37] a phosphodiesterase inhibitor. Other agents have also been described for use in spasm such as calcium channel blockers, direct vasodilators like nitroglycerin and alpha antagonists.[36,38,39]

Postoperative Period

Postoperative monitoring of the microvascular procedure is probably the most important part of microsurgical practice.[40] Surgeons who do not have such luxuries strive to create a system for proper monitoring of flap. Well-trained nursing staffs, proper facilities for a microsurgical intensive care unit help in postoperative monitoring. Technological advances have helped in bringing the surgeon closer to the monitoring. Use of smart phones[41] allow the monitoring staff to transmit images, or even Doppler flow patterns to the senior surgeon at their comfort. Whatever the modality, the principle is the same. Early hours after surgery are the times where a problem is still correctable. Irreversible changes have not yet occurred in the tissue with salvage still a possibility. A microsurgeon with a high degree of suspicion and a keen eye will have an advantage at this stage.

If any problem is suspected, it is always preferred to explore. Bedside exploration of the anastomosis can be done cautiously. If a hematoma is present, decompression usually allows perfusion to be restored. If a thrombus is present the anastomosis needs to be revised. Embolectomy can be done to remove the thrombus. Embolectomy by itself has a limited role, as the thrombogenic foci will remain. It is conventionally done using a Fogarty catheter. A direct embolectomy by accessing from the anastomosis or a nearby side branch may help in reduce the trauma of a Fogarty catheter.[42,43] A revision of the anastomosis will be required, usually with a vein graft.

Advances have introduced the use of technology in the field of monitoring. Implantable Doppler probes[44] are available, which provide real time information about the anastomosis. By following the wave patterns, earlier detection of insult can be done. Noninvasive infrared monitoring can also be used for postoperative monitoring.[45]

OUTCOMES

Microsurgery has revolutionized the field of Plastic Surgery. Most major centers report a success rate of more than 95%.[46] Microsurgery can be safely performed in pediatrics[47] as well as aged individuals.[48] Other than the risks of surgery and anesthesia, outcomes do not differ in terms of success in this population. The old adage *Practice makes a man perfect* is true for microsurgery. The more a surgeon practices, the better he becomes. This also means the results are better in centers where microsurgery is routinely performed.[15,49] In addition to surgeon's skill, the setup also becomes more familiar with the needs of microsurgery.

Smoking habits may also affect the results following flap surgery. In a study in MD Anderson Cancer Center[50] on the effect of smoking on free flap surgery, the vascular thrombosis rates were similar to nonsmokers. However, these patients had significantly higher incidences of delayed wound healing and flap necrosis than nonsmokers. Complications reduced if the reconstruction was delayed or smoking was stopped for 4 weeks.

A group of patients who undergo free flap reconstruction is for *breast reconstruction*. Tamoxifen if used has found to have a significant increase in thrombosis. It is advised to stop Tamoxifen 4 weeks before microvascular surgery.[50]

COAGULATION AND MICROSURGERY

Microvascular surgery has intimate relationship with coagulation. However, hematological disorders are not a contraindication of microsurgery. A preoperative diagnosis of the disorder, aggressive hematological management with good collaboration with the hematologist, meticulous anastomosis, and high index of suspicion for postoperative complications are a prerequisite for success in these patients. Even then the failure of microsurgery is higher in such patients.[51] Wang et al. performed 58 free flaps in patients with hypercoagulable state. They reported a success rate of 80%, which was higher than their routine success rate. None of the flaps that they tried to salvage survived. They mention a role of late venous thrombosis in such patients.[52]

Anticoagulation agents are frequently prescribed following microsurgery. The benefit of such agents is doubtful,[53,54] stemming from the desire of the surgeon to do all possible, rather than any substantial evidence. It is for this reason surgeons are moving away from routine use of these agents. The use in salvage is much more common.

The most commonly used drug is Heparin and its derivatives. Heparin given topically at the anastomosis has shown to be of benefit in animal studies. However, these results have not been replicated in patients. Although used frequently, Heparin has not found to have improved patency rates.[55] Use of Heparin results in higher incidence of bleeding and hematoma.[56] This hematoma in addition to the hypovolemic effects can also physically compress the anastomosis and cause failure. Prompt removal of hematoma and decompression can prevent failure. Due to these problems routine use of Heparin is slowly being discontinued. Heparin at these doses has also not been found to be effective for prophylaxis of venous thromboembolism.[57] Low-molecular-weight heparin (LMWH) is also used as an alternative to Heparin. LMWH is not associated with the risk of bleeding and its subsequent complications.[58] The efficacy of this agent is however doubtful.

Low molecular weight dextran has also been studied in flap surgery.[59] It was found to not have any role as antithrombotic agents. Dextran also is associated with anaphylaxis and fluid overload especially in older individuals.[60] Antiplatelet agents such as Aspirin and clopidogrel have also been used following microsurgery. Aspirin did not improve the patency rate following anastomosis.[61] One agent that is being used for salvaging flaps post thrombosis is recombinant human tissue factor pathway inhibitor. Khouri et al. in their trial found that it was as efficacious as Heparin in preventing thrombosis and due to its low doses, there was less chance of complications associated with bleeding as compared to unfractionated Heparin.[53]

Thus, literature suggests that there is not much role of the abovementioned agents in improving vessel patency. However, combination therapy may have a better outcome. Chung et al. in their study found that a combination of heparin, aspirin and tirofiban (a glycoprotein 2b/3a receptor antagonist) improves patency following anastomosis.[62]

Hyperbaric oxygen therapy (HBOT) has been studied as an adjuvant to microsurgery. In a study by Shi et al.,[63] HBOT was found to have improved healing at the anastomosis site, especially in cases where there was a component of crush injury. There was some increase in the platelet count, which was not found to affect patency of the anastomosis. Adjuvant use of fibrin glue has also been described along with sutures.[64] This was found to have patency similar to suture only anastomosis, with lesser sutures being required for the anastomosis.

With refinement in microsurgical techniques and instrumentations, supermicrosurgery was possible. Supermicrosurgery involves repair of vessels less than 0.8 mm in diameter. This has had opened up new horizons which were closed to the previous generation of microsurgeons. Now even distal fingertip replantations are possible. Young age and small vessels are no longer a limitation for microsurgery.

APPLICATIONS OF MICROVASCULAR SURGERY

Microvascular surgery has many applications in the field of reconstructive surgery. Microsurgical tools are the workhorse for reconstruction following head and neck malignancy expiration. Both soft-tissue **(Figs. 3A to C)** and bony defects **(Figs. 4A to C)** are reconstructed in a single stage using microsurgical techniques. Microsurgical reconstruction is also the standard for breast reconstruction **(Figs. 5A to D)**. Soft-tissue defects in practically any part of the body can be covered using microsurgical tools **(Figs. 6A to E)**. Microsurgery also gives the surgeon ability to reattach amputated parts **(Figs. 7A to D)**. Thus the potential of microvascular surgery is limitless, depending upon the imagination and ingenuity of the surgeon.

Lymphatic Surgery

Lymphedema is another disease whose management is on the cusp of a revolution, thanks to the marvel of microsurgery. Classically surgery for lymphedema consisted of reductive procedures like those described by Charles

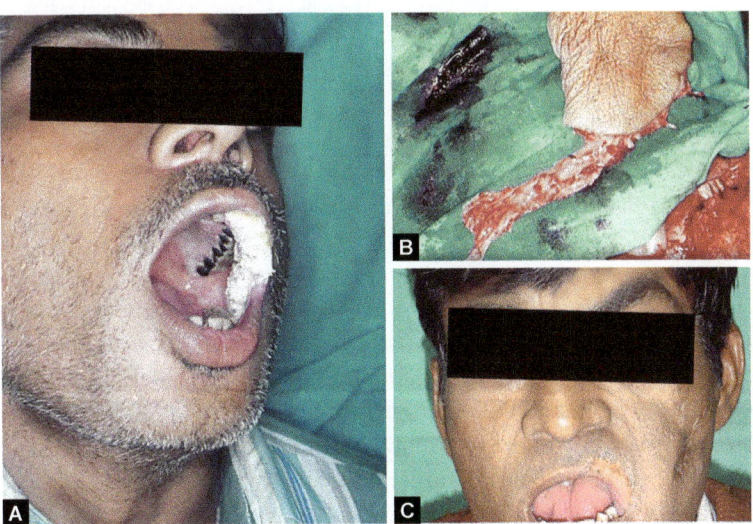

Figs. 3A to C: Free radial forearm flap for oral malignancy reconstruction.

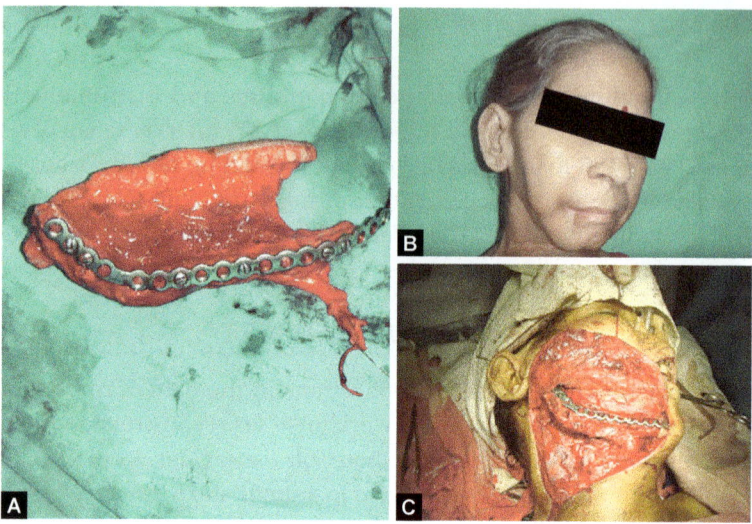

Figs. 4A to C: Free fibula osteocutaneous flap for mandible reconstruction. Skin paddle used for mucosa.

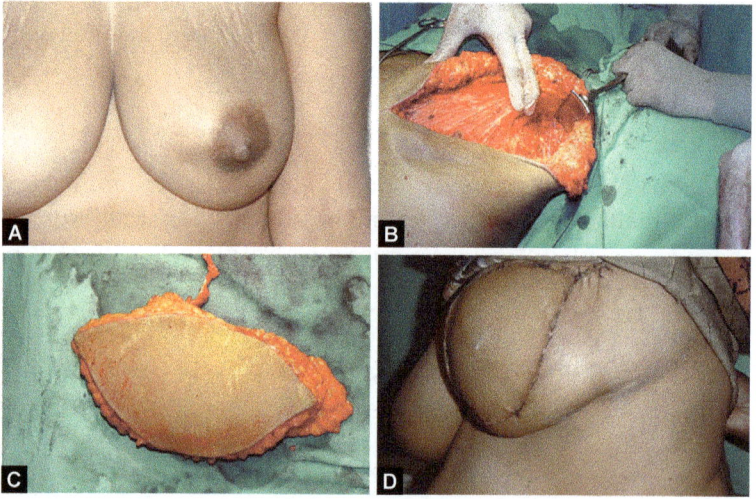

Figs. 5A to D: Breast reconstruction using deep inferior epigastric artery perforator (DIEP) flap.

and Homans. The result of such surgeries was usually disappointing, with recurrence being the rule. Liposuction was added to the armamentarium, which benefited a select group of patients. Microsurgical techniques are have added a new segment of management options. Physiological procedures can restore the continuity of the lymphatic channels. The initial procedures were the anastomosis between the lymph nodes and the veins. This was associated with high rates of failure due to the thrombogenic nature of the nodal tissue and also because of epithelialization at the anastomosis.

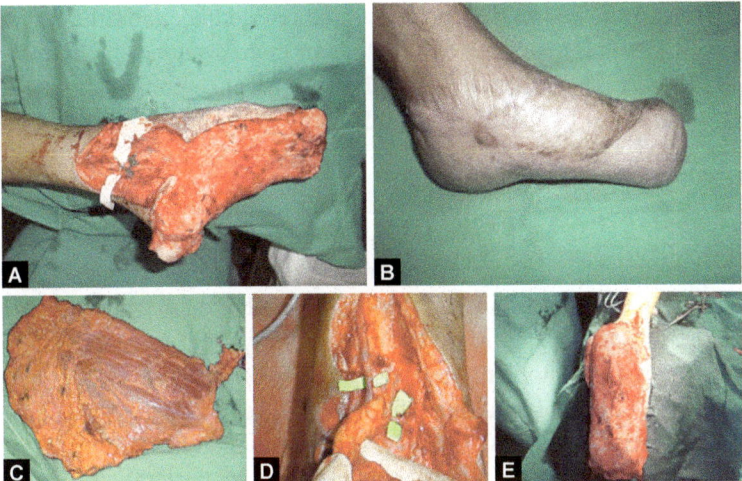

Figs. 6A to E: Free latissimus dorsi muscle flap with skin grafting for soft-tissue cover padding over sole of foot.

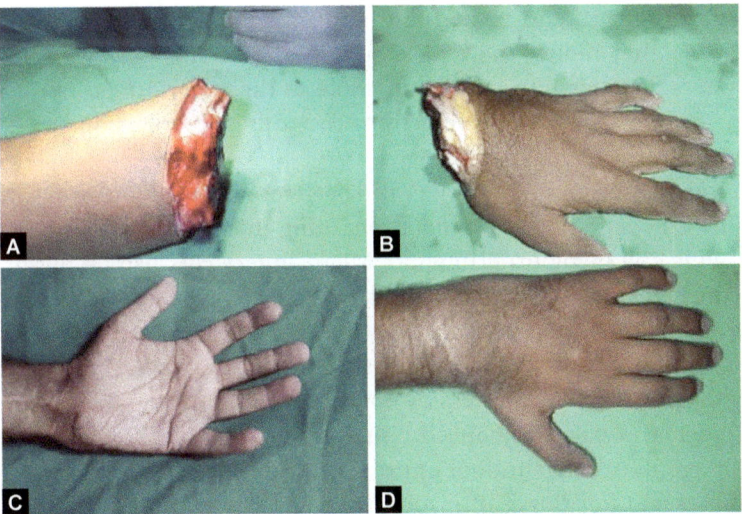

Figs. 7A to D: Replantation of an amputated hand.

Vascularized lymph node transfers provide definite, consistent reduction of lymphedema. In this procedure, lymph nodes along with surrounding soft-tissue is carried along a vascular pedicle and transferred to the site of lymphedema. Lymphatic channels are formed which carry the lymph into the node, which is then drained into the vessel. This has found application in reduction of lymphedema following cancer ablation of regional lymph nodes.

Lymphatic vessels for a long time were considered to be too fragile to be handled. With the advent of supermicrosurgery, lymphatics can be repaired. This has also been due to higher magnifications and addition of intraoperative fluorescein studies. These factors together enable the surgeon to visualize and repair lymphatic channels. Lymphaticovenous and lymphaticolymphatic anastomosis has revolutionized the management of lymphedema. Reconstruction of lymphatic channels using grafts can be done to bridge segmental defects.[65]

NEWER ADVANCES

Various newer advances have occurred in the field of microsurgery. With the refinement in techniques, improved surgical skill and finer instrumentation has helped to push the boundaries of microsurgery. The progeny of this union is *supermicrosurgery*. Replantations of tinier and tinier structure have become possible with time. Replantations of fingertips and ears have become common. Lymphatic surgery has revolutionized the management of lymphedema, with hope now in sight for these patients, who were probably the last of the untouchables of the previous generation of surgeons.

Coupling devices have been fashioned to reduce the time required for surgery. Venous couplers are routinely used in some centers. These are available for both end-to-end and end-to-side arrangement. Although expensive, they reduce the time required for anastomosis,[31] especially in beginners. Patency rates are comparable to those performed by sutures. Refinements are underway to reduce the cost of these couplers, and to expand their use in arterial anastomosis.

Laser assisted anastomosis has also been researched upon, with variable results. The experience and data regarding this is still sparse, with the technique still being experimental. Microsurgery can also be performed with the help of a robot.[66] Robotic Assisted Microsurgery (RAMS) can make microvascular anastomosis possible with greater precision and better dexterity than conventional suturing.[67] Robotic surgery helps to access the areas of the body that are difficult to access by open approach such as fallopian tubes[68] and brachial plexus.[69] Enhanced visual acuity and magnification gives an advantage over conventional approach. Accessories with robotics such as fluorescein imaging,[70] ultrasound sensing, laser probes and confocal microscopy.

REFERENCES

1. Tamai S. History of microsurgery from the beginning until the end of the 1970s. Microsurgery. 1993;14(1):6-13.
2. Nylen CO. The microscope in aural surgery, its first use and later development. Acta Otolaryngol. 1954;43(S116):226-40.
3. Holmgren J. Some experiences in the surgery of otosclerosis. Acta Otolaryngol. 1923;5:460-6.
4. Jacobson JH, Suarez EI. Microvascular surgery. Dis Chest. 1962;41:220-4.
5. Malt RA, Mckhann CF. Replantation of severed arms. J Am Med Assoc. 1964;189(10): 716-22.
6. Kleinert HE, Kasdan ML. Anastamosis of digital vessels. J Ky Med Assoc. 1965;63:106.

7. Cobbett JR. Free digital transfer. Report of a case of transfer of a great toe to replace an amputated thumb. J Bone Joint Surg Br. 1969;51(4):677-9.
8. Buncke HJ, Schulz WP. Total ear reimplantation in the rabbit utilising microminiature vascular anastomoses. Br J Plast Surg. 1966;19(C):15-22.
9. Roper-Hall MJ. Microsurgery in ophthalmology. Br J Ophthalmol. 1967;51(6):408-14.
10. Kriss TC, Kriss VM. History of the operating microscope: from magnifying glass to microneurosurgery. Neurosurgery. 1998:899-908.
11. Pastuszak AW, Wenker EP, Lipshultz LI. The History of Microsurgery in Urology. Urology. 2015.
12. Singh AK, Tahiliani ND. An evaluation of vas reanastomosis done by microsurgery: Ind J Plastic Surgery. 1998;16(1);221-5.
13. Singh AK, Tahiliani ND. Microsurgical tuboplasty following tubectomy (a study in dogs). Ind J Obstet Gynae. 1985;35(2):363-5.
14. Deepa D, Mehta D, Munjal V. Periodontal microsurgery: a must for perio-aesthetics. Indian J Oral Sci. 2014;5(3):103.
15. Sebastin SJ, Chung KC. A systematic review of the outcomes of replantation of distal digital amputation. Plast Reconstr Surg. 2011;128(3):723-37.
16. Maino DM, Chase C. Asthenopia: a technology induced visual impairment. Rev Optom Suppl. 2011;2:28-35.
17. Gowrisankaran S, Nahar NK, Hayes JR, Sheedy JE. Asthenopia and blink rate under visual and cognitive loads. Optom Vis Sci. 2012;89(1):97-104.
18. Mendez BM, Chiodo MV, Vandevender D, Patel PA. Heads-up 3D microscopy. Plast Reconstr Surg Glob Open. 2016;4(5):e717.
19. Acland RD. Instrumentation for microsurgery. Orthop Clin North Am. 1977;8(2):281-94.
20. Acland RD. Microvascular anastomosis: a device for holding stay sutures and a new vascular clamp. Surgery. 1974;75(2):185-7.
21. Park HC, Bahar Moni AS, Chang J, Cho SH, Park HS, Ahn SC. A microsurgical suture technique without the need for vascular clamps. J Hand Microsurg. 2014;6(2):102-5.
22. Harashina T, Fujino T, Watanabe S. The intimal healing of microvascular anastomoses. Plast Reconstr Surg. 1976;58(5):608-13.
23. Lidman D, Daniel RK. The normal healing process of microvascular anastomoses. Scand J Plast Reconstr Surg. 1981;15(2):103-10.
24. Chaware SM, Bhatnagar SK, Singh AK. A scanning electron microscopic evaluation of microsurgical anastomosis by conventional end to end and end to side anastomosis using 'temporary stent' technique of an experimental study. Ind J Plastic Surg. 2006;39(1):39-41.
25. Nissenbaum M, Meckler R, Acland R. Hand position in microsurgery. J Hand Surg Am. 1979;4(2):118-20.
26. Sood R, Bentz ML, Shestak KC, Browne EZ. Extremity replantation. Surg Clin North Am. 1991;71(2):317-29.
27. MacDonald JD. Learning to perform microvascular anastomosis. Skull Base. 2005;15(3):229-40.
28. Harris GD, Finseth F, Buncke HJ. Posterior-wall-first microvascular anastomotic technique. Br J Plast Surg. 1981;34:47-9.
29. Barros RSM de, Leal RA, Teixeira RK, Yamaki VN, Feijó DH, Gouveia EH, et al. Continuous versus interrupted suture technique in microvascular anastomosis in rats. Acta Cir Bras. 2017;32(9):691-6.
30. Man D, Acland RD. Continuous suture technique in microvascular end-to-end anastomosis. J Microsurg. 1981;2(4):238-43.
31. Umezawa H, Ogawa R, Nakamizo M, Yokoshima K, Hyakusoku H. A comparison of microsurgical venous anastomosis techniques. J Nippon Med Sch. 2015;82(1):14-20.
32. Krag C, Holck S. The value of the patency test in microvascular anastomosis—Correlation between observed patency and size of intraluminal thrombus: An experimental study in rats. Br J Plast Surg. 1981;34(1):64-6.

33. Zhu H, Zhu X, Zhang C, Zheng X. Patency test of vascular anastomosis with assistance of high-speed video recording in digit replantation. J Bone Jt Surg. 2018;100(9):729-34.
34. Holm C, Mayr M, Höfter E, Dornseifer U, Ninkovic M. Assessment of the patency of microvascular anastomoses using microscope-integrated near-infrared angiography: a preliminary study. Microsurgery. 2009;29(7):509-14.
35. Yu JT, Patel AJK, Malata CM. The use of topical vasodilators in microvascular surgery. J Plast Reconstr Aesthetic Surg. 2011;64(2):226-8.
36. Vargas CR, Iorio ML, Lee BT. A systematic review of topical vasodilators for the treatment of intraoperative vasospasm in reconstructive microsurgery. Plast Reconstr Surg. 2015;136(2):411-22.
37. Gherardini G, Gürlek A, Cromeens D, Joly GA, Wang BG, Evans GRD. Drug-induced vasodilation: in vitro and in vivo study on the effects of lidocaine and papaverine on rabbit carotid artery. Microsurgery. 1998;18(2):90-6.
38. Evans GR. Drug-induced vasodilation in an in vitro and in vivo study: the effects of nicardipine, papaverine, and lidocaine on the rabbit carotid artery. Plast Reconstr Surg. 1997;100(6):1475-81.
39. Ricci JA, Singhal D, Fukudome EY, Tobias AM, Lin SJ, Lee BT. Topical nitroglycerin for the treatment of intraoperative microsurgical vasospasm. Microsurgery. 2018;38(5):524-9.
40. Hee Hwang J, Mun GH. An evolution of communication in postoperative free flap monitoring. Plast Reconstr Surg. 2012;130(1):125-9.
41. Engel H, Huang JJ, Tsao CK, Lin CY, Chou PY, Brey EM, et al. Remote real-time monitoring of free flaps via smartphone photography and 3G wireless internet: a prospective study evidencing diagnostic accuracy. Microsurgery. 2011;31(8):589-95.
42. Hong KY, Chang LS, Chang H, Minn KW, Jin US. Direct thrombectomy as a salvage technique in free flap breast reconstruction. Microsurgery. 2017;37(5):402-5.
43. Schweitzer DL, Aguam AS, Wilder JR. Complications encountered during arterial embolectomy with the fogarty balloon catheter. Vasc Surg. 1976;10(3):144-56.
44. Swartz WM, Jones NF, Cherup L, Klein A. Direct monitoring of microvascular anastomoses with the 20-MHz ultrasonic Doppler probe: an experimental and clinical study. Plast Reconstr Surg. 1988;81(2):149-61.
45. Kagaya Y, Miyamoto S. A systematic review of near-infrared spectroscopy in flap monitoring: current basic and clinical evidence and prospects. J Plast Reconstr Aesthetic Surg. 2018;71(2):246-57.
46. Kwok AC, Agarwal JP. An analysis of free flap failure using the ACS NSQIP database. Does flap site and flap type matter? Microsurgery. 2017;37(6):531-8.
47. Izadpanah A, Moran SL. Pediatric microsurgery: a global overview. Clin Plast Surg. 2017;44(2):313-24.
48. Serletti JM, Higgins JP, Moran S, Orlando GS. Factors affecting outcome in free-tissue transfer in the elderly. Plast Reconstr Surg. 2000;106(1):66-70.
49. Hustedt JW, Bohl DD, Champagne L. The detrimental effect of decentralization in digital replantation in the United States: 15 years of evidence from the national inpatient sample. J Hand Surg Am. 2016;41(5):2-9.
50. Kelley BP, Valero V, Yi M, Kronowitz SJ. Tamoxifen increases the risk of microvascular flap complications in patients undergoing microvascular breast reconstruction. Plast Reconstr Surg. 2012;129(2):305-14.
51. Lin PY, Cabrera R, Chew KY, Kuo YR. The outcome of free tissue transfers in patients with hematological diseases: 20-year experiences in single microsurgical center. Microsurgery. 2014;34(7):505-10.
52. Wang TY, Serletti JM, Cuker A, McGrath J, Low DW, Kovach SJ, et al. Free tissue transfer in the hypercoagulable patient. Plast Reconstr Surg. 2012;129(2):443-53.
53. Kearns MC, Baker J, Myers S, Ghanem A. Towards standardization of training and practice of reconstructive microsurgery: an evidence-based recommendation for anastomosis thrombosis prophylaxis. Eur J Plast Surg. 2018;41(4):379-86.

54. Liu J, Shi Q, Yang S, Liu B, Guo B, Xu J. Does postoperative anticoagulation therapy lead to a higher success rate for microvascular free-tissue transfer in the head and neck? A systematic review and meta-analysis. J Reconstr Microsurg. 2018;34(02):87-94.
55. Chen CM, Ashjian P, Disa JJ, Cordeiro PG, Pusic AL, Mehrara BJ. Is the use of intraoperative heparin safe? Plast Reconstr Surg. 2008;121(3):49e-53e.
56. Numajiri T, Sowa Y, Nishino K, Arai A, Tsujikawa T, Ikebuchi K, et al. Use of systemic low-dose unfractionated heparin in microvascular head and neck reconstruction: influence in free-flap outcomes. J Plast Surg Hand Surg. 2016;50(3):135-41.
57. Bertolaccini C, Prazak A, Agarwal J, Goodwin I, Rockwell W, Pannucci C. Adequacy of fixed-dose heparin infusions for venous thromboembolism prevention after microsurgical procedures. J Reconstr Microsurg. 2018;34(09):729-34.
58. Davar D, Moore A, Gimbel M. Analysis of the use of low molecular weight heparin for thromboembolic complication chemoprophylaxis in microsurgical breast reconstruction. Plast Reconstr Surg. 2011;128:98.
59. Jayaprasad K, Mathew J, Thankappan K, Sharma M, Duraisamy S, Rajan S, et al. Safety and efficacy of low molecular weight dextran (dextran 40) in head and neck free flap reconstruction. J Reconstr Microsurg. 2013 22;29(07):443-8.
60. Jallali N. Dextrans in microsurgery: a review. Microsurgery. 2003;23(1):78-80.
61. Lighthall JG, Bell RA, Wax MK, Ghanem TA. Role of postoperative aspirin in free tissue transfer. Otolaryngol Neck Surg. 2011;145(2 Suppl):P143-P143.
62. Chung TL, Pumplin DW, Holton LH, Taylor JA, Rodriguez ED, Silverman RP. Prevention of microsurgical anastomotic thrombosis using aspirin, heparin, and the glycoprotein IIb/IIIa inhibitor tirofiban. Plast Reconstr Surg. 2007;120(5):1281-8.
63. Shi DY, Zhang F, Kryger Z, Komorowska-Timek E, Lineaweaver W, Buncke H. Effect of hyperbaric oxygen on microvascular anastomosis healing and patency in the rat. J Reconstr Microsurg. 1999;15(07):539-45.
64. Cho AB, Paulos RG, Bersani G, Iamaguchi RB, Torres LR, Wei TH, et al. A reinforcement of the sutured microvascular anastomosis with fibrin glue application: a retrospective comparative study with the standard conventional technique. Microsurgery. 2017;37(3):218-21.
65. Baumeister RG, Frick A. Die mikrochirurgische lymphgefäßtransplantation. Handchirurgie Mikrochirurgie Plast Chir. 2003;35(4):202-9.
66. Gudeloglu A, Brahmbhatt JV, Parekattil SJ. Robotic-assisted microsurgery for an elective microsurgical practice. Semin Plast Surg. 2014;28(1):11-9.
67. Siemionow M, Ozer K, Siemionow W, Lister G. Robotic assistance in microsurgery. J Reconstr Microsurg. 2000;16(8):643-9.
68. Degueldre M, Vandromme J, Huong PT, Cadière GB. Robotically assisted laparoscopic microsurgical tubal reanastomosis: a feasibility study. Fertil Steril. 2000;74(5):1020-3.
69. Garcia JC, Lebailly F, Mantovani G, Mendonca LA, Garcia J, Liverneaux P. Telerobotic manipulation of the brachial plexus. J Reconstr Microsurg. 2012;28(7):491-4.
70. Lenti LM, Spinoglio G, Marano A, Priora F, Ravazzoni F, Quarati R. Application of Fluorescence in Robotic General Surgery: Review of the Literature and State of the Art. World J Surg. 2013;37(12):2800-11.

CHAPTER 13

Inflammatory Breast Cancer

Vani Parmar, Garvit Chitkara

INTRODUCTION

Inflammatory breast cancer (IBC) is a rare variant of breast cancer seen in 2–4% of all breast cancers in the west.[1] It is an ever rarer entity in India, and even in the west seen more in African American women, although there is a reported rise in the incidence in white women. The incidence is higher in certain regions of Africa and in Egypt, where it is as high as 10% of all breast cancers. The primary IBC or true IBC must be distinguished with secondary IBC. The secondary IBC, are defined by the secondary changes in the breast or recurrence of breast cancer. IBC has a short rapid progression course unlike a secondary inflammatory progression of a previous noninflammatory cancer. IBC are aggressive tumor and have a poorer prognosis than noninflammatory breast cancer. However, combination of neoadjuvant chemotherapy, surgery and radiotherapy led to improvement in prognosis.

The diagnosis of IBC remains to be a clinicopathological one, characterized by presence of erythema and peau d'orange over at least one-third or more of the skin over breast [as defined by 2017 American Joint Committee on Cancer and the International Union for Cancer Control (AJCC-UICC) Tumor, Node, Metastasis (TNM) breast cancer staging system], with or without a lump, and presence of dermal lymphatic emboli in skin over breast being a pre-requisite to a diagnosis, and is designated as T4d. The history is usually short over a few months with a usual history of being previously misdiagnosed as acute mastitis not responding to antibiotics or anti-inflammatory drugs.[1] It is seen in relatively younger women as compared to all breast cancers in US, median age 59 versus 66 years. High body mass index (BMI) is considered one of the risk factors in IBC.[2-4] No specific genetic mutation has been discovered so far.

All of the following criteria must be met for the diagnosis of IBC as per a consensus statement in 2011:[5]
- Rapid onset of breast erythema, edema and/or peau d'orange, and/or warm breast, with or without an underlying palpable mass **(Figs. 1A and B)**
- Duration of history no more than 6 months
- Erythema occupying at least one-third of the breast
- Pathologic confirmation of invasive carcinoma

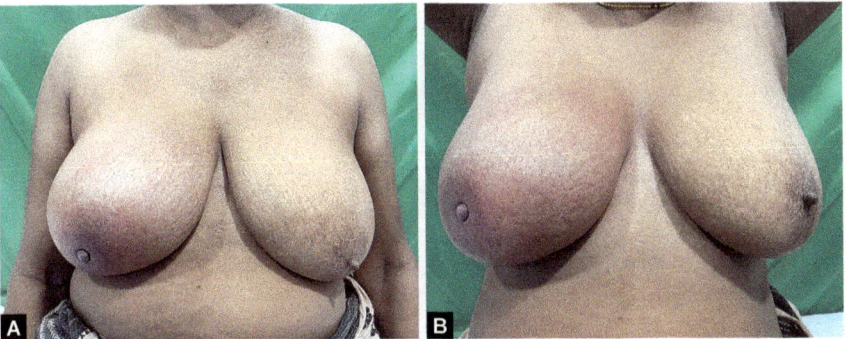

Figs. 1A and B: Clinical signs of inflammatory breast cancer.

SYMPTOMS AND SIGNS

The clinical symptoms mainly comprise of rapid onset of painful swelling and redness of breast, seen primarily as a progressive erythema, and edema of breast skin (orange peel) with or without a palpable lump, with no systemic symptoms. This may mislead as benign bacterial infection such as mastitis. Less than half of patients of IBC present with palpable breast lump. The redness seen classically with IBC is due to the presence of tumor emboli in dermal lymphatics and resultant lymphedema and not due to acute inflammation reaction. The diagnosis of breast cancer is often delayed as they mimic mastitis in clinical presentation, which failed to respond to antibiotics. It is associated mostly with significant adenopathy and higher incidence of advanced disease with distant metastases.[6,7] In other words, there is both a higher nodal burden and distant disease progression at a rapid rate in IBC.

The presence of dermal tumor emboli classifies it as T4d, unlike the signs of satellite nodules alone, peau d'orange and ulceration singularly which still classifies T4a-c. However, although required to clinch a clinical diagnosis, only tumor emboli in absence of all clinical signs is not labeled as inflammatory cancer. It is very important to clinically document the extent of erythema by a good clinical picture in addition to making a note of the same.

IMAGING

Imaging options are standard, including digital mammography and sonography.[8,9] The findings in a mammogram **(Figs. 2A and B)** may or may not show presence of associated lump, but classically shows skin thickening (84-93%) with parenchymal edema with trabecular thickening (62-81%) or architectural or trabecular distortion (37%) extending over a large area, with or without extensive microcalcification (47-56%), and axillary adenopathy (24%). The presence of diffuse dense background parenchyma due to edema can obscure an inflammatory lesion and may underestimate the extent of disease. Due to the breast skin thickening and difficulty in compression along

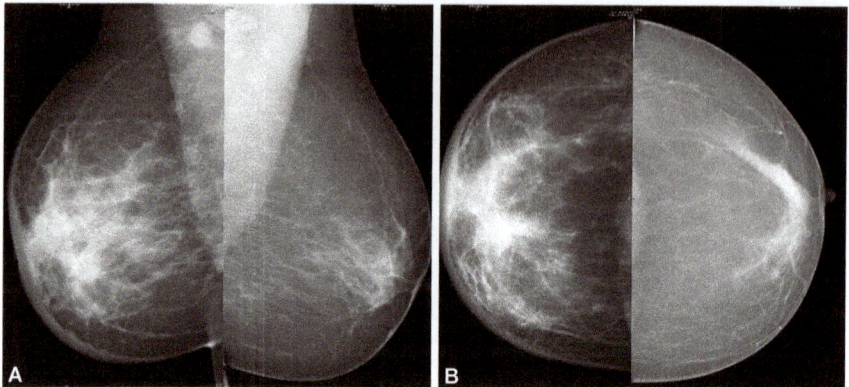

Figs. 2A and B: Bilateral mammograms showing right breast skin and parenchymal thickening with axillary adenopathy in suspected inflammatory breast cancer.

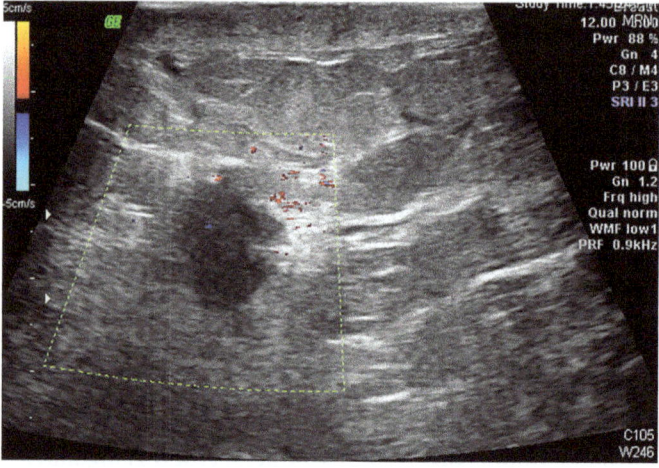

Fig. 3: Ultrasonography showing associated breast lesion.

with pain, it may sometimes be difficult to detect a mass lesion. Absence of a mass does not rule out breast cancer. A contralateral breast cancer is seen more often in IBC, anywhere between 0.9 and 5% of IBC patients as compared to 1.1% at 2 years for non-IBC patients.[10]

An ultrasound may be necessary to confirm presence or absence of a distinct lesion **(Fig. 3)** in parenchyma, and assist in guided core biopsy. While the sensitivity of a mammogram is only about 68%, ultrasound improves it to 92–94%. Ultrasound of the axillary lymph nodes shows suspicious or frankly malignant looking axillary lymph nodes. Magnetic resonance imaging (MRI) breast has higher sensitivity for detecting primary breast parenchymal lesions and skin abnormalities. The thickening of skin is seen in 90–100% of patients with IBC and it helps to differentiate patients with IBC from locally advanced (non-IBC) breast cancer. MRI provides accurate information regarding the extent of disease (locoregional staging), contralateral breast pathology, skin or

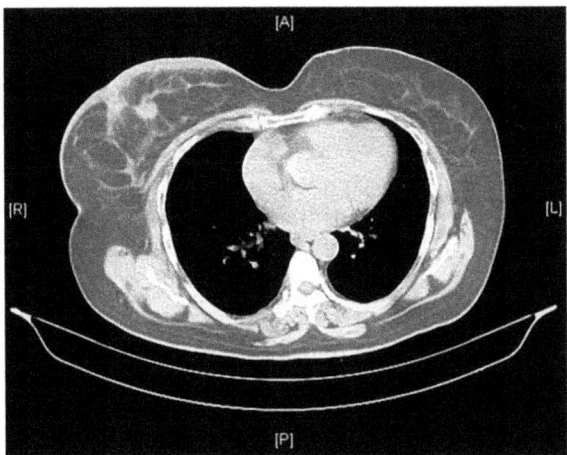

Fig. 4: CT scan confirming right breast lesion with parenchymal thickening and skin involvement with edema.

thoracic involvement, nodal metastases. In absence of intramammary lesions on conventional imaging (mammogram/ultrasound), MRI guided core biopsy can confirm the diagnosis in IBC.[11] The sensitivity of MRI to pick up a mass lesion is nearly 98% in these cases.

Workup for detection of distant metastases is usually recommended[12] in all and confirmative in view of high incidence of angioinvasion and distant progression in more than one-third of the disease at presentation. For evaluation of distant disease, computed tomography (CT) scans of chest, abdomen and pelvis along with a nuclide bone scan (FDG or F18 PET) is recommended. An additional positron emission test (PET) scan, although not a routine, may upstage disease especially with regards to nodal disease, as seen in a MD Anderson study wherein 10% had contralateral axillary lymph node metastases.[13] In addition to showing the ipsilateral breast lesion and edema **(Fig. 4)**, it can also pick up better a contralateral positive axillary node which could be the only site of distant metastasis in that patient. Effectively it results in upstaging, and improving progression-free survival in both lower and higher stage disease due to obvious reasons of stage migration.[14] Also it may be used to assess response to neoadjuvant therapy.[15]

PATHOLOGY

Inflammatory breast cancer has no specific diagnostic histopathological criteria and has no specific histological subtype. Mostly these are ductal carcinoma and have high histological grade. The presence of scattered tumor emboli and dermal lymphatic invasion are the key finding **(Fig. 5)**.[16]

There is also evidence to prove the highly angiogenic and angioinvasive character of IBC unlike noninflammatory breast cancer.[17] In SCID mice, implantation of the fat pad results in only satellite nodules with invasive breast

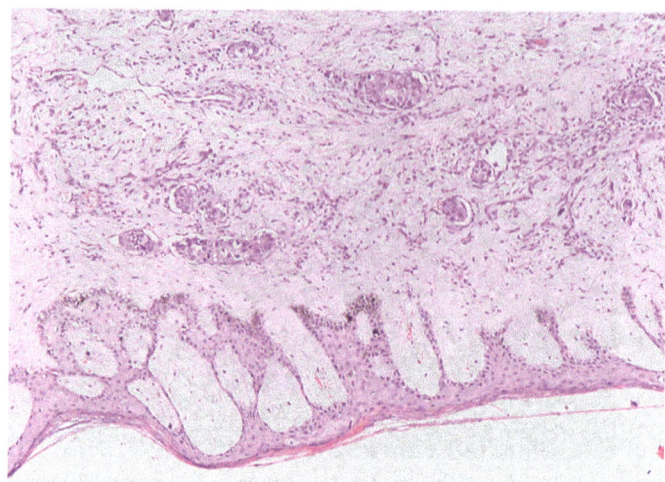

Fig. 5: Dermal lymphatic tumor emboli in background of parenchymal edema and skin thickening.
Courtesy: Dr Tanuja Shet, Professor and Consultant Pathologist, Tata Memorial Centre.

cancer cells, whereas, the inflammatory cancer cells result in rapid growth of the cancer cells inside lymphatics and blood vessels with rapidly progressing skin redness or "erythema".[18]

All molecular subtype including hormone receptor (HR) positive, human epidermal growth factor receptor 2 (HER 2) positive and triple negative cancer (TNBC) exist in IBC, however, the proportion of these subtype are different.[19] The incidence of HR positive subtype is lower in IBC (30% in IBC vs. 60–80% in non-IBC), and also incidence rate of both the HER 2 positive and TNBC subtypes are higher in IBC (Her 2 positive: 40% in IBC vs. 25% in non-IBC; TNBC: 30% in IBC vs. 10–15% in non-IBC).[19,20] All the molecular subtypes are more aggressive in IBC than in non-IBC, with poorer disease free survival and overall survival.[21]

GENETICS IN INFLAMMATORY BREAST CANCER

No specific genetic mutation has been discovered so far. However an association has been noted with p53, angiogenesis and angioinvasion, and cytokines. Although called as "inflammatory", there is no true inflammation in these tumors, rather a presence of tumor emboli in lymphatics and blood vessels.

Half the IBCs show loss of heterozygosity (LOH) with commonly lost alleles at sites 3p, 6p, 8p, 11q, 13q, and 17q,[22] which may have phenotypic and prognostic importance.[23] Mutations in p53 tumor suppressor gene have been reported in 20–50% of human breast cancers,[24,25] more often seen in patients with familial/hereditary breast cancer syndromes (such as the familial breast and ovarian cancer and Li-Fraumeni syndromes) than in those with sporadic breast cancer. Those with p53 mutation and/or p53 protein overexpression in the nucleus had a 8.6-fold increased risk of death. Also, if associated with ER negative disease, there was a 17.9-fold increase in risk of death as against those that had only a p53 nuclear overexpression. There is an overexpression of RhoC GTPase gene in preclinical models with IBC cell lines SUM149, and loss of WISP3 gene/LIBC. WISP3 acts as a tumor suppressor gene and its loss increases invasiveness and metastatic potential of breast cancer.

INFLAMMATORY CYTOKINES AND THEIR SIGNIFICANCE IN INFLAMMATORY BREAST CANCER

Inflammation in IBC is implied by tumor cell invasion of dermal lymphatics. In the tumor microenvironment, a variety of inflammatory cells, immune cells, matrix cells and cancer cells and the bioactive molecules produced by these cells interact with each other, forming a complex signal transduction network to regulate IBC formation, development and progression.[26] The aberrant expressions of inflammatory factors and immune factors may promote carcinogenesis, tumor cell proliferation, migration, invasion and metastasis.

The actual cytokines are only marginally raised, mostly IL-1 and IL-2, in addition to gamma interferon. There is also evidence of their vascularity and angioinvasive nature as evidenced by an increase in VEGF, FGF, IL6 and IL8, also linked to an overexpression of RhoC GTPase gene.[27,28] In addition the VEGF receptor-3 is expressed in lymphatics, has a role in lymphatic development, and is activated by binding to VEGF-C and VEGF-D. It plays a major role in lymphangiogenesis and onset of distant metastases.

DIFFERENTIAL DIAGNOSIS

The most common differential is an acute breast abscess and is the initial diagnosis in most cases. A failure to respond to antibiotics and no purulent discharge on attempted incision and drainage should immediately suspect an IBC. In addition there are never associated systemic symptoms of fever or leukocytosis.

Other differentials are duct ectasia and rarely other malignancies such as lymphoma and leukemia which may mimic IBC by similar clinical appearance but will not show tumor emboli. The hematological profile in such cases will confirm a disorder of the hemato-lymphatic system.

TREATMENT

In the past, IBC was treated by surgery and/or radiotherapy and 5-year overall survival were <5%. The combination of surgery and radiotherapy has improved overall survival. The induction of systemic chemotherapy has showed additional survival benefit. Now, the trimodal therapy including chemotherapy, surgery and radiotherapy has become the standard of care in the management of IBC. In metastatic disease, treatment is chemotherapy with/without target therapy. Surgery and radiotherapy are used only to control palliative symptoms.

Neoadjuvant/Adjuvant Therapy

Once diagnosis is confirmed, treatment is always a multimodality therapy in IBC. Neoadjuvant systemic chemotherapy followed by locoregional treatment is standard for non-metastatic IBC (Level IB evidence). Routinely, anthracycline- and taxane-based chemotherapy regimens are typically recommended as in other invasive breast carcinomas. Her 2 neu is overexpressed in approximately 40% of IBC patients and these patients get benefits from anti HER 2 neu directed therapy. It requires addition of weekly trastuzumab concurrent with paclitaxel, and later maintenance trastuzumab in adjuvant setting.

In the NOAH trial,[29] a pivotal trial that demonstrated the benefit of the anti-HER2 agent trastuzumab in the neoadjuvant setting, in IBC. For HER2-positive disease, dual anti-HER2-directed therapy with pertuzumab and trastuzumab is recommended. In the NeoSphere trial, dual anti-HER2 blockade was studied, in which 7% of patients had IBC, and the combination of pertuzumab and trastuzumab with chemotherapy raised the pCR rate to 45.8%.[30] The TRYPHAENA trial tests a non-anthracycline-containing regimen, consisting of a taxane, carboplatin, trastuzumab, and pertuzumab (TCHP) in which 6% of patients had IBC, and carboplatin raised the pCR rate to 64%.[31] A standard 1-year anti-HER2 therapy should be trastuzumab and pertuzumab recently published results from the APHINITY trial that showed a modest reduction in disease recurrence events (7.1% compared with 8.7%, hazard ratio 0.81; p = 0.045), with taxane/trastuzumab and addition of pertuzumab in the adjuvant setting.[32]

The hormone receptor positive cancers are treated in a similar fashion with adjuvant endocrine therapy as in non-inflammatory breast cancers. Premenopausal women are advised tamoxifen with or without ovarian suppression, while postmenopausal women receive aromatase inhibitors. Use of full course of trastuzumab with or without pertuzumab is preferred as there may be an element of resistance to hormone therapy due to the HER2 overexpression.

Locoregional Treatment for Inflammatory Breast Cancer—Surgery

Inflammatory breast cancer is an aggressive form of breast cancer and has to be addressed as a locally advanced breast cancer, when no distant metastases are identified. Systemic therapy is a mandatory requisite before considering surgery. This is always followed by radiation therapy.

Neoadjuvant chemotherapy has improved the overall survival of this aggressive disease from a dismal 4% when no systemic therapy was offered to nearly 46% 5 year OS and DFS of 40% in the 1990s as neoadjuvant systemic therapy was routinely offered. The debate for need of locoregional surgery was also laid to rest as no surgery yielded an inferior OS of 36% and DFS of 21%.[33]

The extent of surgery, irrespective of extent of response to neoadjuvant systemic therapy is always a modified radical mastectomy with axillary clearance. Again, surgery mandates a clear margin and is attempted only if a complete resection is possible.[34] A skin sparing mastectomy or breast conservation is absolutely contraindicated due to high failure rate with poor outcome.

Evidence from a case series indicated that mastectomy improves local control, relapse-free survival, and cancer related survival in IBC.[35,36] Safety of conservation is not clear in these locally aggressive and systemically progressive diseases and should not be offered.

Similarly, due to a higher frequency of nodal disease in IBC, axillary staging procedures are to be avoided, even if node negative after systemic treatment. There is no role of sentinel node biopsy or axillary staging, or any limited surgical addressal of axilla.[37]

As far as reconstructive procedures are concerned, since postmastectomy radiation therapy is mandatory, breast reconstruction may sometimes be delayed after radiation completion. This is more for ensuring early RT rather than a contraindication for whole breast reconstruction by free flap or any effect of radiation on the flap itself. Small studies[38] have shown comparable outcomes of early versus late breast reconstruction and no impact of any apparent delay in radiation delivery. A delay is at times suggested to ensure adequate radiation doses to chest wall with or without internal mammary chain irradiation as necessary,[39] and to supraclavicular fossa. A concurrent whole breast reconstruction is preferred also due to a positive impact on quality of life and economically better as a single surgical intervention, if logistically feasible. In metastatic disease, surgery may be indicated in uncontrolled hemorrhage.

Locoregional Radiation Therapy

Radiation therapy is mandated in all patients with inflammatory breast cancer with direct impact on locoregional control, although a definite survival benefit has not been proven. Postmastectomy, a standard fractionation of 50 Gy in 25 fractions covering chest wall and supraclavicular fossa with or without internal mammary chain of LNs, with a 10 Gy boost to chest wall.[40] Hyperfractionation protocols have also been suggested and tried in small populations with a total dose of 66 Gy (50 Gy plus 16 Gy in 8 fractions boost) with reported improvement in locoregional disease control.[41,42] There may be a slight higher incidence of toxicity due to the higher doses. Preoperative radiotherapy trials have shown higher complications and risk of postoperative complications in dose dependent manner. Use of concomitant chemotherapy is not indicated in IBC.

FOLLOW-UP AND PROGNOSIS

The follow-up protocols are similar to any type of breast cancer, with the knowledge and alertness on the fact that these are cancers with poor prognosis and higher relapse rates. With the increasing use of targeted therapies the outcomes have improved significantly in the HER2 expression IBC.[43,44] However, the triple negative and hormone receptor positive HER2 negative subset of IBC still do worse comparatively.[45,46] Overall, the inflammatory breast cancers do far worse than noninflammatory breast cancer as also supported by SEER database, with 2 year breast cancer specific survival rate of 84% versus 91%, HR 1.43, 95% CI 1.10-1.86.[47]

CONCLUSION

Inflammatory breast cancer continues to be a rare clinicopathological entity, with an aggressive course of progression, characterized by angioinvasion and tumor emboli in lymphatics. The treatment is always multimodality as there is still no specific targeted treatment for IBC, only for the identified receptors, as in case of noninflammatory breast cancers. The outcomes are better if early installation of systemic chemotherapy is followed before considering surgical treatment, which in most cases is with radical intent followed by radiation therapy. Research is continuing at molecular levels to find ways to improve outcomes in this relatively poor outcome disease condition.

REFERENCES

1. Hance KW, Anderson WF, Devesa SS, Young HA, Levine PH. Trends in inflammatory breast carcinoma incidence and survival: the surveillance, epidemiology, and end results program at the National Cancer Institute. J Natl Cancer Inst. 2005;97(13):966-75.
2. Chang S, Buzdar AU, Hursting SD. Inflammatory breast cancer and body mass index. J Clin Oncol. 1998;16:3731-5.
3. van den Brandt PA, Spiegelman D, Yaun SS, Adami HO, Beeson L, Folsom AR, et al. Pooled analysis of prospective cohort studies on height, weight, and breast cancer risk. Am J Epidemiol. 2000;152:514-27.
4. Fouad TM, Ueno NT, Yu RK, Ensor JE, Alvarez RH, Krishnamurthy S, et al. Distinct epidemiological profiles associated with inflammatory breast cancer (IBC): a comprehensive analysis of the IBC registry at The University of Texas MD Anderson Cancer Center. PLoS One. 2018;13(9):e0204372.
5. Dawood S, Merajver SD, Viens P, Vermeulen PB, Swain SM, Buchholz TA, et al. International expert panel on inflammatory breast cancer: consensus statement for standardized diagnosis and treatment. Ann Oncol. 2011;22(3):515-23.
6. Chang S, Parker SL, Pham T, Buzdar AU, Hursting SD. Inflammatory breast carcinoma incidence and survival: the surveillance, epidemiology, and end results program of the National Cancer Institute, 1975-1992. Cancer. 1998;82(12):2366-72.
7. Matro JM, Li T, Cristofanilli M, Hughes ME, Ottesen RA, Weeks JC, Wong YN. Inflammatory breast cancer management in the national comprehensive cancer network: the disease, recurrence pattern, and outcome. Clin Breast Cancer. 2015;15(1):1-7.

8. Yang WT, Le-Petross HT, Macapinlac H, Carkaci S, Gonzalez-Angulo AM, Dawood S, et al. Inflammatory breast cancer: PET/CT, MRI, mammography, and sonography findings. Breast Cancer Res Treat. 2008;109:417-26.
9. Günhan-Bilgen I, Üstün EE, Memiş A. Inflammatory breast carcinoma: mammographic, ultrasonographic, clinical, and pathological findings in 142 cases. Radiology. 2002;223:829-38.
10. Schairer C, Brown LM, Mai PL. Inflammatory breast cancer: high risk of contralateral breast cancer compared to comparably staged non-inflammatory breast cancer. Breast Cancer Res Treat. 2011;129:117-24.
11. Ueno NT, Espinosa Fernandez JR, Cristofanilli M, Overmoyer B, Rea D, Berdichevski F, et al. International Consensus on the Clinical Management of Inflammatory Breast Cancer from the Morgan Welch Inflammatory Breast Cancer Research Program 10th Anniversary Conference. J Cancer. 2018;9(8):1437-47.
12. Groheux D, Giacchetti S, Delord M, Hindie E, Vercellino L, Cuvier C, et al. 18F-FDG PET/CT in staging patients with locally advanced or inflammatory breast cancer: comparison to conventional staging. J Nucl Med. 2013;54:5-11.
13. Woodward WA, Koav E, Tajkar V. Radiation therapy for inflammatory breast cancer: technical considerations and diverse clinical scenarios. Breast Can Manag. 2013;3(1):1-9.
14. Champion L, Lerebours F, Cherel P, Edeline V, Giraudet AL, Wartski M, et al. (18)F-FDG PET/CT imaging versus dynamic contrast-enhanced CT for staging and prognosis of inflammatory breast cancer. Eur J Nucl Med Mol Imaging. 2013;40(8):1206-13.
15. Champion L, Lerebours F, Alberini JL, Fourme E, Gontier E, Bertrand F, et al. 18F-FDG PET/CT to predict response to neoadjuvant chemotherapy and prognosis in inflammatory breast cancer. J Nucl Med. 2015;56(9):1315-21.
16. Robbins GF, Shah J, Rosen P, Chu F, Taylor J. Inflammatory carcinoma of the breast. Surg Clin North Am. 1974;54(4):801-10.
17. Colpaert CG, Vermeulen PB, Benoy I, Soubry A, van Roy F, van Beest P, et al. Inflammatory breast cancer shows angiogenesis with high endothelial proliferation rate and strong E-cadherin expression. Br J Cancer. 2003;88(5):718-25.
18. Alpaugh ML, Tomlinson JS, Shao ZM, Barsky SH. A novel human xenograft model of inflammatory breast cancer. Cancer Res. 1999;59(20):5079-84.
19. Masuda H, Brewer TM, Liu DD, Iwamoto T, Shen Y, Hsu L, et al. Long-term treatment efficacy in primary inflammatory breast cancer by hormonal receptor- and HER2-defined subtypes. Ann Oncol. 2014;25:384-91.
20. Kertmen N, Babacan T, Keskin O, Solak M, Sarici F, Akin S, et al. Molecular subtypes in patients with inflammatory breast cancer; a single center experience. J BUON. 2015;20:35-9.
21. Masuda H, Baggerly KA, Wang Y, Iwamoto T, Brewer T, Pusztai L, et al. Comparison of molecular subtype distribution in triple- negative inflammatory and noninflammatory breast cancers. Breast Cancer Res. 203;15:R112.
22. Lerebours F, Bertheau P, Bieche I, Driouch K, De The H, Hacene K, et al. Evidence of chromosome regions and gene involvement in inflammatory breast cancer. Int J Cancer. 2002;102(6):618-22.
23. Moll UM, Riou G, Levine AJ. Two distinct mechanisms alter p53 in breast cancer: mutation and nuclear exclusion. Proc Natl Acad Sci USA. 1992;89(15):7262-6.
24. Davidoff AM, Humphrey PA, Iglehart JD, Marks JR. Genetic basis for p53 overexpression in human breast cancer. Proc Natl Acad Sci USA. 1991;88 (11):5006-10.
25. Riou G, Lê MG, Travagli JP, Levine AJ, Moll UM. Poor prognosis of p53 gene mutation and nuclear overexpression of p53 protein in inflammatory breast carcinoma. J Natl Cancer Inst. 1993;85(21):1765-7.
26. Huang A, Cao S, Tang L. The tumor microenvironment and inflammatory breast cancer J Cancer. 2017;8(10):1884-91.

27. van Golen KL, Wu ZF, Qiao XT, Bao LW, Merajver SD. RhoC GTPase, a novel transforming oncogene for human mammary epithelial cells that partially recapitulates the inflammatory breast cancer phenotype. Cancer Res. 2000;60(20):5832-8.
28. van Golen KL, Wu ZF, Qiao XT, Bao L, Merajver SD. RhoC GTPase overexpression modulates induction of angiogenic factors in breast cells. Neoplasia. 2000;2(5):418-25.
29. Gianni L, Eiermann W, Semiglazov V, Lluch A, Tjulandin S, Zambetti M, et al. Neoadjuvant and adjuvant trastuzumab in patients with HER2-positive locally advanced breast cancer (NOAH): follow-up of a randomised controlled superiority trial with a parallel HER2-negative cohort. Lancet Oncol. 2014;15:640-7.
30. Gianni L, Pienkowski T, Im YH, Roman L, Tseng LM, Liu MC, et al. Efficacy and safety of neoadjuvant pertuzumab and trastuzumab in women with locally advanced, inflammatory, or early HER2-positive breast cancer (NeoSphere): a randomised multicentre, open-label, phase 2 trial. Lancet Oncol. 2012;13:25-32.
31. Schneeweiss A, Chia S, Hickish T, Harvey V, Eniu A, Hegg R, et al. Pertuzumab plus trastuzumab in combination with standard neoadjuvant anthracycline-containing and anthracycline-free chemotherapy regimens in patients with HER2-positive early breast cancer: a randomized phase II cardiac safety study (TRYPHAENA). Ann Oncol. 2013;24(9):2278-84.
32. von Minckwitz G, Procter M, de Azambuja E, Zardavas D, Benyunes M, Viale G, et al. Adjuvant Pertuzumab and Trastuzumab in Early HER2-Positive Breast Cancer. N Engl J Med. 2017;377(2):122-31.
33. Singletary SE. Surgical management of inflammatory breast cancer. Semin Oncol. 2008;35:72-7.
34. Curcio LD, Rupp E, Williams WL, Chu DZ, Clarke K, Odom-Maryon T, et al. Beyond palliative mastectomy in inflammatory breast cancer--a reassessment of margin status. Ann Surg Oncol. 1999;6(3):249-54.
35. Perez CA, Fields JN, Fracasso PM, Philpott G, Soares RL Jr, Taylor ME, et al. Management of locally advanced carcinoma of the breast. II. Inflammatory carcinoma. Cancer. 1994;74:466-76.
36. Panades M, Olivotto IA, Speers CH, Shenkier T, Olivotto TA, Weir L, et al. Evolving treatment strategies for inflammatory breast cancer: a population-based survival analysis. J Clin Oncol. 2005;23(9):1941-50.
37. Stearns V, Ewing CA, Slack R, Penannen MF, Hayes DF, Tsangaris TN. Sentinel lymphadenectomy after neoadjuvant chemotherapy for breast cancer may reliably represent the axilla except for inflammatory breast cancer. Ann Surg Oncol. 2002;9(3):235-42.
38. Chin PL, Andersen JS, Somlo G, Chu DZ, Schwarz RE, Ellenhorn JD. Esthetic reconstruction after mastectomy for inflammatory breast cancer: is it worthwhile? J Am Coll Surg. 2000;190 (3):304-9.
39. Motwani SB, Strom EA, Schechter NR, Butler CE, Lee GK, Langstein HN, et al. The impact of immediate breast reconstruction on the technical delivery of postmastectomy radiotherapy. Int J Radiat Oncol Biol Phys. 2006;66(1):76-82.
40. Liauw SL, Benda RK, Morris CG, Mendenhall NP. Inflammatory breast carcinoma: outcomes with trimodality therapy for nonmetastatic disease. Cancer. 2004;100(5):920-8.
41. Liao Z, Strom EA, Buzdar AU, Singletary SE, Hunt K, Allen PK, et al. Locoregional irradiation for inflammatory breast cancer: effectiveness of dose escalation in decreasing recurrence. Int J Radiat Oncol Biol Phys. 2000;47(5):1191-200.
42. Bristol IJ, Woodward WA, Strom EA, Cristofanilli M, Domain D, Singletary SE, et al. Locoregional treatment outcomes after multimodality management of inflammatory breast cancer. Int J Radiat Oncol Biol Phys. 2008;72(2):474-84.
43. Liu J, Chen K, Jiang W, Mao K, Li S, Kim MJ, et al. Chemotherapy response and survival of inflammatory breast cancer by hormone receptor- and HER2-defined molecular

subtypes approximation: an analysis from the National Cancer Database. J Cancer Res Clin Oncol. 2017;143(1):161-8.
44. Harris EE, Schultz D, Bertsch H, Fox K, Glick J, Solin LJ. Ten-year outcome after combined modality therapy for inflammatory breast cancer. Int J Radiat Oncol Biol Phys. 2003;55(5):1200-8.
45. Li J, Gonzalez-Angulo AM, Allen PK, Yu TK, Woodward WA, Ueno NT, et al. Triple-negative subtype predicts poor overall survival and high locoregional relapse in inflammatory breast cancer. Oncologist. 2011;16(12):1675-83.
46. Zell JA, Tsang WY, Taylor TH, Mehta RS, Anton-Culver H. Prognostic impact of human epidermal growth factor-like receptor 2 and hormone receptor status in inflammatory breast cancer (IBC): analysis of 2,014 IBC patient cases from the California Cancer Registry. Breast Cancer Res. 2009;11(1):R9.
47. Dawood S, Ueno NT, Valero V, Woodward WA, Buchholz TA, Hortobagyi GN, et al. Differences in survival among women with stage III inflammatory and non-inflammatory locally advanced breast cancer appear early: a large population-based study. Cancer. 2011;117(9):1819-26.

CHAPTER 14

Phyllodes Tumors of the Breast

Chintamani, Megha Tandon

INTRODUCTION

The phyllodes are relatively rare group of tumors that are heterogeneous and complex in their presentation and behavior.[1,2] They were described for the first time in 1838 by a German physician Johannes Muller, and he called them as cystosarcoma phyllodes, term based on the Latin *Phyllodium* or "*leaf like*" essentially relating to its microscopic appearance.[3] The clinical course, outcome, and management of these tumors depend on the histological type. While the benign type has very benign and indolent course like other benign breast lumps, the malignant phyllodes may be very aggressive both in its local presentation and distant spread. The tumor when malignant has a sarcoma like behavior and may be associated with frequent local recurrences. World Health Organization (WHO) adopted the nomenclature as Phyllodes in 1981. The tumors have further been classified as benign, malignant and borderline malignant based on their histological features.[4]

Diagnosis of these tumors poses a distinct challenge as benign tumors may present and behave like fibro-adenoma and the malignant tumors need to be distinguished from primary breast sarcomas or some aggressive forms of mixed tumors such as carcinosarcomas or spindle cell metaplastic carcinomas. There are only few distinguishing characteristics on radiology and even core needle biopsy may not be very useful. The treatment also varies according to the histology and ranges from wide local excision to mastectomy. Chemotherapy in the adjuvant setting still remains a matter of debate. Radiation therapy, used for malignant or recurrent phyllodes tumor (PT) has shown controversial results in small series.

EPIDEMIOLOGY

Phyllodes tumor is most common in women in their forties but can occur at any age. Median age of presentation is 45 years with an age range 9–93 years.[2,5] Women with Li-Fraumeni syndrome, p53 germline mutation, are at an increased risk for developing malignant PT. There is some evidence suggesting that there is increased risk for East Asians and for Latina women born in Central or South America but living in the United States.[5-7] Only a few cases have been reported in men which have invariably been associated with gynecomastia.[8,9] Most PT is benign, but about 1 out of 4 of these tumors may be malignant.

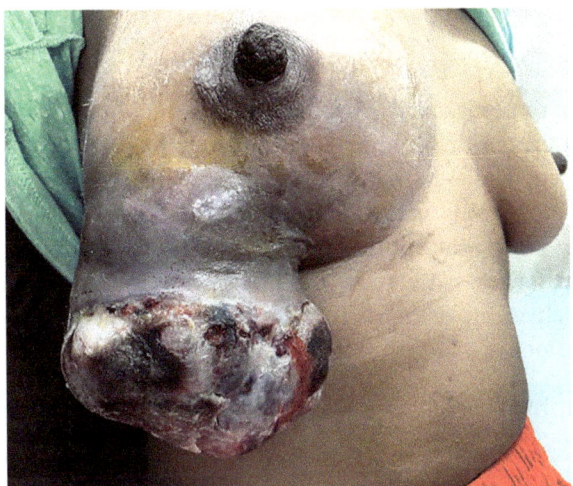

Fig. 1: The recurrence of the phyllodes tumor may be associated with grade progression as in this 25-year-old female with de-differentiation in the recurrent phyllodes that has now presented with a poorer grade and a more aggressive biology.

CLINICAL PRESENTATION (FIG. 1)

The most common symptom at the time of presentation is a rapidly growing mass in the breast. Dilated veins and a blue discoloration can also be observed with large tumors. Nipple retraction and skin ulcerations are uncommon. Skin ulcers can be seen with large tumors and are usually caused by ischemia due to over stretching of skin rather than direct infiltration as is the case with breast carcinomas. Bilateral involvement is rare, with an occurrence rate of 1.6%.[8] The mean tumor size ranges between 5.2 and 7.3 cm although tumors up to 50 cm have been reported in the literature.[10-15] Chest wall infiltration is very rare even with malignant lumps and axillary lymphadenopathy may be present in around 10–20% of cases and these lymph nodes are mostly reactive. The tumor spreads mostly by hematogenous route such as any sarcoma and routine axillary dissection is not recommended.

Distant metastases (DM) occur mainly with malignant and borderline PT. However, metastatic spread in the benign type of PT has been described.[11,12] The incidence of metastatic disease among patients with malignant type is estimated to be approximately 20–25%.[2,3] The spread is mostly to lungs, liver, bones and brain, although other unusual sites have also been described. A metastatic PT carries a poorer prognosis with an average survival of less than 2 years.[2,12-14]

DIAGNOSIS

Since the most common presentation is lump in the breast, triple assessment is the bottom line which includes clinical, radiological and histopathological evaluation.

Radiology

Ultrasonography/Elastography/Color Doppler of the Breast

Ultrasound of the breast shows well-defined, sometime capsulated, smooth multi-lobulated hypoechoic masses that may be indistinguishable from fibroadenoma of the breast. In a recent studies, use of shear wave elastography along with color Doppler has been found to be useful for distinguishing between fibroadenoma and PT.[15,16] Ultrasound of axilla is now routinely recommended for assessment of axilla and for the primary a guided core needle biopsy may help improve the yield and one may needle only the non-necrotic parts of the tumor.[17]

Mammography/MRI of the Breast

Around 20% of non-palpable phyllodes may be picked up on mammography and typically appear as nonspecific, large, round, or oval masses with well-circumscribed margins. Coarse macrocalcifications are mostly seen but malignant calcifications can also be appreciated in few cases. Magnetic resonance imaging (MRI) that is generally considered a problem solving tool in the event of equivocal diagnosis but is not very specific in making a diagnosis of PTs. Although MRI may not distinguish between benign and malignant lesions accurately but can help in the planning of surgical treatment. These tumors have higher signal intensities than normal breast parenchyma on T1-weighted images and lower or equal signal intensity on T2-weighted images on MRI and may have some correlation with histopathology.[18] There are no prospective trials to confirm but it has been observed that T1 weighted images with high intensity and T2 images with low intensity along with rapid enhancement can help in making the diagnosis of malignant phyllodes.[19]

Histopathology

This forms the cornerstone of making a diagnosis of phyllodes. Majority, i.e., up to 75% are benign. Microscopic examination of both epithelial and stromal components is mandatory in making a diagnosis. The prognosis, however, depends on the biology of the tumor that is determined by the stromal part.[11] Broadly, diagnosis of PT is made when the fibroepithelial architecture shows an increased intracanalicular pattern with dilated cystic spaces having leaf-like fronds protruding, giving it a staghorn appearance along with hypercellularity of the stroma.

The division of these tumors by WHO is shown in **Table 1** as adapted from the WHO classification book 2012.

Grading of Phyllodes Tumor[20,21]

Benign Phyllodes Tumor

There is increased stromal cellularity when compared to fibroadenomas and may have minimal nuclear atypia, pushing borders, and mitoses of less

TABLE 1: Histological grading of phyllodes tumors.[20,21]

	Benign phyllodes	Borderline phyllodes	Malignant phyllodes
Border	Well defined	May be focally permeative	Permeative
Stromal cellularity	Usually mild, may be non-uniform or diffuse	Usually moderate, may be non-uniform or diffuse	Marked
Stromal atypia	Mild or none	Mild or moderate	Marked
Mitotic activity	<5 per 10 high power fields (HPFs)	5–9/10 HPF	Abundant >10/HPF
Stromal overgrowth	Absent	Absent or focal	Present
Mitotic stromal activity	Absent	Absent	May be present

Source: Adapted from WHO Classification Book, 2012.

than 4/10 high-power fields. The most important distinguishing feature from fibroadenoma is however an excessive intracanalicular growth pattern along with increased stromal cellularity. Getting back to the basics, the typical leaf-like pattern of phyllodes is not seen in fibroadenoma. If at all present, this is usually focal and underdeveloped in fibroadenomas. It is important to note that there may be some focal areas resembling fibroadenoma in a case of PT. Therefore inspite of so many characteristics, it is a challenge even for an experienced histopathologist to differentiate a benign phyllodes from a fibroadenoma, especially if one has to do so simply based on a core needle biopsy.[20,21]

Although there are reports in literature regarding the evolution of phyllodes from fibroadenomas but there is not enough proof of the mechanism. Most criteria to stratify these tumors are subjective such as degree of stromal hypercellularity, atypia, etc., and may actually add to the difficulty at grading them.[21-23]

The stromal cellularity must be assessed in most cellular areas and is categorized into mild if the increase in cellularity is almost twice the normal perilobular stroma and there are rarely or almost never stromal nuclei touching each other. This must be assessed in the most cellular areas. There are studies that suggest that stromal cellularity is mild if there is at least 50% increase in stroma when compared with a typical fibroadenoma. Some studies define increased stromal activity in terms of stromal nuclear overcrowding or overlapping.[21-25]

Borderline Phyllodes Tumor

As the term indicates, these are a group of tumors that have characteristics between benign and malignant phyllodes, and are roughly around 12–26% of all the phyllodes. These have local recurrence rates of around 14–25% almost similar to the benign variety. The accepted rates of mitoses (mitotic figures) are 5–9% per 10 high power fields.[21-24]

Malignant Phyllodes Tumor

These tumors show marked stromal cellularity and atypia with permeative margins, and mitotic activity of at least 10 or more than 10 per 10 high power fields. The overgrowth of stroma, which is defined as the presence of stroma without epithelium in at least one low-power field with a 4X microscope objective, identified. It is important to note that presence of heterologous element such as liposarcoma, chondrosarcoma or osteosarcoma confirms the suspicion of malignant phyllodes irrespective of whether other histological parameters of malignant phyllodes are present or not.[21,25-27]

There have been many studies to predict and determine the clinical behavior of these tumors, the important one being the AMOS (age, mitoses, overgrowth, and surgical margins). In most studies, the margins were considered the most consistent and reliable predictors of outcome. A nomogram has been designed to help predict the outcome in order to counsel the patients and also help in prognosticating the disease in terms of local recurrence.[23]

Like in other cancers, there can be de-differentiation and grade progression with each recurrence making the outcome worse each time. There are also reports of reduced stromal-epithelial interdependency as a factor.[21-24]

MOLECULAR AND GENETIC FEATURES AND THEIR ROLE IN THE DEVELOPMENT AND BIOLOGY OF PHYLLODES

What genetic changes lead to development of phyllodes and whether there is any correlation of histological grade with the tumor biology and behavior of these tumors continues to be an enigma. There are many hypotheses to explain these issues:

1. *Based on the interaction between epithelial and stromal components:* This continues to be the most favored concept and is based on the hypothesis that most stromal growth happens close to the epithelial compartment and is perhaps dependent on the epithelial component.[28] There are observations that support this hypothesis such as finding of stromal expression of beta-catenin and also some insulin-like growth factors (IGF-1 and II). Also, the activation of the *murine Int-1* gene (also called as *Wnt* gene) especially the Wnt5a whose overexpression has been shown to increase the stromal overgrowth is associated with benign or borderline phyllodes. Expression of biomarkers such as CXCR4, a molecule related to the epithelial and stromal interaction has been found to be overexpressed in tumors with more stromal growth and higher grade tumors.[29-32]

2. *Biomarkers associated with phyllodes:* Besides the histological features, there are a large number of biomarkers that have been studied such as Ki-67, p53 and DNA topoisomerase 2, etc., to differentiate between benign and malignant phyllodes. Proliferation markers especially the Ki-67 (labeling index) has been found to extremely useful in this regard. Increased expression of p53 has also been observed in malignant phyllodes as opposed to benign tumors and also fibroadenomas. These biomarkers can therefore help in distinguishing a benign from malignant phyllodes.[33-36]

Molecular Classification of Phyllodes

There has been a general effort but no definite and objective classification exists as there are chromosomal aberrations specific to phyllodes have been found. Based on genomic alterations they have been divided in to low grade (benign) and high grade (that can be benign or malignant). The high-grade and borderline phyllodes were found to have Iq gain, 13q loss, p53, Rb1, NF-1 mutations and *EGFR, IGFR* gene amplifications as compared to low-grade tumors showing no such alterations.[37,38] There have been other classifications based on gene expression where the malignant phyllodes were found to be associated with claudin low and basal-like appearance along with cancer stem related biology as in metaplastic carcinomas.[39]

Phyllodes and Hormone Receptor Expression

The hormonal receptor expression especially ER and PR is essentially are the features of carcinomas arising out of ductal epithelial cells and there is an inverse relationship of expression of these receptors with the tumor grade. There is, however, an observation that ER-alpha expression is confined to predominantly epithelial with no stromal component, while ER-beta expression may show positivity in both stromal and epithelial components. There may be expression of epidermal growth factors and Her2 neu expression has been observed in some tumors.[40-46] Inspite of these observations, the role of hormone therapy in these tumors is not clear except for a recent observation with MED12 mutations. Similarly, the expression of androgen receptors has been observed to be low and insignificant in these tumors.[47,48]

MANAGEMENT

Surgery

Phyllode is considered essentially a surgical disease and excision with wide margins that are recommended by most studies to be more than 1 cm is the standard of care. There are studies, however to suggest that it may not be mandatory in all cases and one may get away with no tumor.[49] Very large and malignant tumors may require mastectomy. While it may be argued that the clear margin lies one cell away, one should not get carried away as these tumors have a tendency to recur frequently. In addition, one needs to take in to account issues such as multifocality, technical issues relating to fixation and inking of specimen (seepage of ink) affecting the accuracy of histological diagnosis. There may also be other factors such as sampling and issues while sectioning the fixed tissue. Although there are these issues that may appear confusing, there are studies to recommend wider margins and also to treat them as sarcomas in this regard. These studies have looked in to the correlation between margins and outcome in terms of recurrence free survival and disease free.[16,48,50-53]

There are other studies, however, that observed no correlation between wider surgical margins and extent of excision with disease-free survival.[1,48,54] This being said, the minimum recommended margin and the practice that is followed at most centers is to have at least a margin of >1 cm. In cases where enucleation has been done for benign or borderline phyllodes, the practice is to revise and re-excise margins. There are studies that have reported their observations on the benefits of re-excision of inadequate margins. They observed that only tumor size and mitotic activity were independent prognostic markers for local recurrence while the surgical technique and margins were not found to be significant. This is essentially to highlight that while most centers would follow the policy of observation for benign phyllodes that has been enucleated or excised with inadequate margins, most would recommend re-excision of margins for all malignant and borderline phyllodes.[55]

While wait and watch policy is widely adopted for benign PT enucleated during surgery, for borderline and malignant phyllodes tumors most centers have the policy for going in again for re-excision of the margins. This was therefore recommended that wide margins must be the goal in all small tumor that are less than 5 cm and with high mitotic activity (>10 mitoses/10 high power fields) because there is a very high local recurrence rate in this very distinct group (55.6%) as these tumors constituted a distinct group associated with a significant (55.6%) local recurrence rate.[55]

A positive margin in some studies have been taken as tumor on the ink like in other breast cancers but it is recommended that we must achieve to get a clear margin of more than 1 cm in view of various factors and confounding factors discussed earlier.[56,57] There is certainly no indication for addressal of axilla in the form of sentinel node biopsy/sampling or dissection as the lymph nodes are rarely involved in phyllodes. Recommended management of a *phyllodes tumor* is therefore wide local excision with a three-dimensional clearance with minimum 1 cm margin and no sentinel node biopsy.[52,53,58,59]

Mastectomy and wide local excision (with >1 cm margins) for malignant phyllodes have been found to be comparable in terms of overall survival and recurrence in studies with a large database. As local recurrence is a challenge especially in malignant and borderline phyllodes, patient should be offered breast conservation surgery, if oncologically and in terms of cosmesis, satisfactory outcome could be achieved.[17] It may be crucial therefore to differentiate these tumors from metaplastic carcinoma where there is indeed a role of sentinel node biopsy and also chemotherapy both in the neoadjuvant and adjuvant settings.

Radiotherapy

There is no defined role of radiations in these tumors while the SEER database may show an increased use of radiations in these tumors.[17] There are studies to suggest a reduction in local recurrence rates in larger malignant tumors with the use of radiotherapy. It has also been observed that those undergoing axillary staging/dissection are more likely to receive radiotherapy.[16] There are, however, now a large number of studies that although found no survival benefit, disease-free survival but observed reduced local recurrence rates following both mastectomy and/or lumpectomy for malignant phyllodes.[60,61]

Hormone Therapy

There is definite role as mentioned earlier as no defined benefit could be demonstrated and this therapy is yet a part of the management protocol for these tumors.[62]

Chemotherapy

There is no level-I evidence to support the role of chemotherapy in these tumors and the role of chemotherapy in adjuvant setting remains controversial. Combination of cisplatin, etoposide and ifosfamide along with doxorubicin have been shown to be effective in some case series. Recurrent or large malignant tumors (more than 5 cm) have been found to be the scenarios where it may be beneficial. These decisions should, however, be taken in multidisciplinary teams (MDTs) and are decided on case to case basis.[63,64]

Management of Distant Metastases in Phyllodes

Metastatic phyllodes carry a poor prognosis with less than 2 years average survival after diagnosis. There is a limited role of surgery, radiotherapy and chemotherapy in these tumors. There are reports of resection or radiation treatment of isolated distant metastasis and there is of course no role of hormone therapy in this setting. The limited options in this scenario include using novel combination of docetaxel, gemcitabine, pazopanib or trabectedin Chemotherapy with doxorubicin and ifosfamide may be useful. The search for the relevant molecular targets and the drugs to hit them is still on.[65,66]

The management of metastatic phyllodes is similar to the management of soft-tissue sarcomas in metastatic setting. The recommendations of National Comprehensive Cancer Network (NCCN) are to manage on the basis of the algorithmic approach as defined for metastatic soft-tissue sarcomas.[59]

CONCLUSION

Phyllodes tumors continue to be an enigma in terms of their diagnosis, staging, biological behavior, grading, classification, and management. In view of similar outcomes, it may not be very important to distinguish benign phyllodes from fibroadenomas. In situations where a clear diagnostic distinction cannot be made, one may use the term fibroepithelial lesion. The diagnosis of malignant phyllodes is made when there is marked hypercellularity, atypia, increased mitoses (*equal or more than 10 per 10 high power fields*), stromal overgrowth and permeative tumor borders, etc. The presence of malignant heterologous component automatically categorizes the tumor as malignant regardless of other histological features. Management of benign phyllodes may not be very aggressive especially in cases where they have been enucleated without clear margins previously. But the bottom line in the management of malignant or recurrent phyllodes is R0 margins (*no tumor on ink*). There is a general consensus to achieve at least 1 cm clear margin of resection, but there is no robust evidence to support this. There is a limited or no defined role of adjuvant radiotherapy for borderline or malignant tumors. There is no role of axillary lymph node dissection in these tumors.

REFERENCES

1. Jang JH, Choi MY, Lee SK, Kim S, Kim J, Lee J, et al. Clinicopathologic risk factors for the local recurrence of phyllodes tumors of the breast. Ann Surg Oncol. 2012;19:2612-7.
2. Bernstein L, Deapen D, Ross RK. The descriptive epidemiology of malignant cystosarcoma phyllodes tumors of the breast. Cancer. 1993;71:3020-4.
3. Gradishar WJ, Anderson BO, Balassanian R, Blair SL, Burstein HJ, Cyr A, et al. Breast Cancer, Version 1.2016. J Natl Compr Canc Netw. 2015;13:1475-85.
4. Birch JM, Alston RD, McNally RJ, Evans DG, Kelsey AM, Harris M, et al. Relative frequency and morphology of cancers in carriers of germline TP53 mutations. Oncogene. 2001;20:4621-8.
5. Mituś J, Reinfuss M, Mituś JW, Jakubowicz J, Blecharz P, Wysocki WM, et al. Malignant phyllodes tumour of the breast: treatment and prognosis. Breast J. 2014;20:639-44.
6. Reinfuss M, Mituś J, Smolak K, Stelmach A. Malignant phyllodes tumours of the breast: a clinical and pathological analysis of 55 cases. Eur J Cancer. 1993;29A:1252-6.
7. Sedgwick EL, Ebuoma L, Hamame A, Phalak K, Ruiz-Flores L, Ortiz-Perez T, et al. BI-RADS update for breast cancer caregivers. Breast Cancer Res Treat. 2015;150:243-54.
8. Oken MM, Creech RH, Tormey DC, Horton J, Davis TE, McFadden ET, et al. Toxicity and response criteria of the Eastern Cooperative Oncology Group. Am J Clin Oncol. 1982;5:649-55.
9. Ma XB, Zheng Y, Yuan HP, Jiang J, Wang YP. CD43 expression in diffuse large B-cell lymphoma, not otherwise specified: CD43 is a marker of adverse prognosis. Hum Pathol. 2015;46:593-9.
10. Lakhani SR, Ellis IO, Schnitt SJ, Tan PH, van de Vijver MJ. IARC WHO Classification of Tumours. In: WHO classification of tumours of the breast, 4th edition. Lyon: IARC Press; 2012.
11. Wu DI, Zhang H, Guo L, Yan XU, Fan Z. Invasive ductal carcinoma within borderline phyllodes tumor with lymph node metastases: a case report and review of the literature. Oncol Lett. 2016;11:2502-6.

12. Bellocq JP, Magro G. Fibroepithelial tumours (Tumours of the Breast). In: Tavassoli FA, Devilee P (Eds). Pathology and Genetics: Tumours of the Breast and Female Genital Organs (World Health Organization Classification of Tumours). Lyon, France: IARC Press; 2003. pp. 99-103.
13. Barth RJ Jr, Wells WA, Mitchell SE, Cole BF. A prospective, multi-institutional study of adjuvant radiotherapy after resection of malignant phyllodes tumors. Ann Surg Oncol. 2009;16:2288-94.
14. Kim GR, Choi JS, Han BK, Ko EY, Ko ES, Hahn SY. Combination of shear-wave elastography and color Doppler: Feasible method to avoid unnecessary breast excision of fibroepithelial lesions diagnosed by core needle biopsy. PLOS One. 2017;12(5):e0175380.
15. Li TT, Kang CS, Li HZ, Xue JP, Yang QM, Lyu J. Value of shear wave elastrography image classification in the diagnosis of breast masses. Zhonghua Zhong Liu Za Zhi. 2019;41(7):540-5.
16. Macdonald OK, Lee CM, Tward JD, Chappel CD, Gaffney DK. Malignant phyllodes tumor of the female breast: association of primary therapy with cause-specific survival from the Surveillance, Epidemiology, and End Results (SEER) program. Cancer. 2006;107:2127-33.
17. Guo Y, Cai YQ, Cai ZL, Gao YG, An NY, Ma L, et al. Differentiation of clinically benign and malignant breast lesions using diffusion-weighted imaging. J Magn Reson Imaging. 2002;16:172-8.
18. Wedegartner U, Bick U, Wortler K, Rummeny E, Bongartz G. Differentiation between benign and malignant findings on MR-mammography: usefulness of morphological criteria. Eur Radiol. 2001;11:1645-50.
19. Jara-Lazaro AR, Akhilesh M, Thike AA, Lui PC-W, Tse GMK, Tan PH. Predictors of phyllodes tumours on core biopsy specimens of fibroepithelial neoplasms. Histopathology. 2010;57:220-32.
20. Strode M, Khoury T, Mangieri C, Takabe K. Update on the diagnosis and management of malignant phyllodes tumors of the breast. Breast. 2017;33:91-6.
21. Lee AH, Hodi Z, Ellis IO, Elston CW. Histological features useful in the distinction of phyllodes tumour and fibroadenoma on needle core biopsy of the breast. Histopathology. 2007;51(3):336-44.
22. Tan PH, Thike AA, Tan WJ, Thu MM, Busmanis I, Li H, et al. Predicting clinical behaviour of breast phyllodes tumours: a nomogram based on histological criteria and surgical margins. J Clin Pathol. 2012;65:69-76.
23. Jacobs TW, Chen YY, Guinee DG Jr, Holden JA, Cha I, Bauermeister DE, et al. Fibroepithelial lesions with cellular stroma on breast core needle biopsy: Are there predictors of outcome on surgical excision? Am J Clin Pathol. 2005;124:342-54.
24. Yasir S, Gamez R, Jenkins S, Visscher DW, Nassar A. Significant histologic features differentiating cellular fibroadenoma from phyllodes tumor on core needle biopsy specimens. Am J Clin Pathol. 2014;142(3):362-9.
25. Chia Y, Thike AA, Cheok PY, Yong-Zheng Chong L, Man-Kit Tse G, Tan PH. Stromal keratin expression in phyllodes tumours of the breast: a comparison with other spindle cell breast lesions. J Clin Pathol. 2012;65:339-47.
26. Rakha EA, Tan PH, Shaaban A, Tse GMK, Esteller FC, van Deurzen CH, et al. Do primary mammary osteosarcoma and chondrosarcoma exist? A review of a large multi-institutional series of malignant matrix-producing breast tumours. Breast. 2013;22:13-8.
27. Sawhney N, Garrahan N, Douglas-Jones AG, Williams ED. Epithelial–stromal interactions in tumors: a morphologic study of fibroepithelial tumors of the breast. Cancer. 1992;70:2115-20.
28. Lacroix-Triki M, Geyer FC, Lambros MB, Savage K, Ellis IO, Lee AH, et al. β-catenin/Wnt signalling pathway in fibromatosis, metaplastic carcinomas and phyllodes tumours of the breast. Mod Pathol. 2010;23:1438-48.

29. Sawyer EJ, Hanby AM, Rowan AJ, Gillett CE, Thomas RE, Poulsom R, et al. The Wnt pathway, epithelial–stromal interactions, and malignant progression in phyllodes tumours. J Pathol. 2002;196:437-44.
30. Sawyer EJ, Hanby AM, Poulsom R, Jeffery R, Gillett CE, Ellis IO, et al. Beta-catenin abnormalities and associated insulin-like growth factor overexpression are important in phyllodes tumours and fibroadenomas of the breast. J Pathol. 2003;200:627-32.
31. Tsang JYS, Mendoza P, Lam CCF, Yu AM, Putti TC, Karim RZ, et al. Involvement of α- and β-catenins and E-cadherin in the development of mammary phyllodes tumours. Histopathology. 2012;61:667-74.
32. Yerushalmi R, Woods R, Ravdin PM, Hayes MM, Gelmon KA. Ki67 in breast cancer: Prognostic and predictive potential. Lancet Oncol. 2010;11:174-83.
33. Lin CK, Tsai WC, Lin YC, Yu JC. Biomarkers distinguishing mammary fibroepithelial neoplasms: a tissue microarray study. Appl Immunohistochem Mol Morphol. 2014;22:433-41.
34. Went P, Dirnhofer S, Schöpf D, Moch H, Spizzo G. Expression and prognostic significance of EpCAM. J Cancer Mol. 2008;3:169-74.
35. Martowicz A, Spizzo G, Gastl G, Untergasser G. Phenotype-dependent effects of EpCAM expression on growth and invasion of human breast cancer cell lines. BMC Cancer. 2012;12:501.
36. Laé M, Vincent-Salomon A, Savignoni A, Huon I, Fréneaux P, Sigal-Zafrani B, et al. Phyllodes tumors of the breast segregate in two groups according to genetic criteria. Mod Pathol. 2007;20:435-44.
37. Tan J, Ong CK, Lim WK, Ng CC, Thike AA, Ng LM, et al. Genomic landscapes of breast fibroepithelial tumours. Nat Genet. 2015;47(11):1341-5.
38. Vidal M, Peg V, Galvan P, Tres A, Cortes J, Ramon Y, et al. Gene expression based classifications of fibroadenomas and phyllodes tumours of the breast. Mol Oncol. 2015;9(6)1081-90.
39. Rao BR, Meyer JS, Fry CG. Most cystosarcoma phyllodes and fibroadenomas have progesterone receptor but lack estrogen receptor: stromal localization of progesterone receptor. Cancer. 1981;47:2016-21.
40. Mechtersheimer G, Krüger KH, Born IA, Möller P. Antigenic profile of mammary fibroadenoma and cystosarcoma phyllodes. A study using antibodies to estrogen- and progesterone receptors and to a panel of cell surface molecules. Pathol Res Pract. 1990;186:427-38.
41. Singh Y, Hatano T, Uemura Y, Shikata N, Senzaki H, Hioki K, et al. Immunohistochemical profile of phyllodes tumors of the breast. Oncol Rep. 1996;3:677-81.
42. Shpitz B, Bomstein Y, Sternberg A, Klein E, Tiomkin V, Kaufman A, et al. Immunoreactivity of p53, Ki-67, and c-erbB-2 in phyllodes tumors of the breast in correlation with clinical and morphologic features. J Surg Oncol. 2002;79:86-92.
43. Tse GMK, Lee CS, Kung FYL, Scolyer RA, Law BK, Lau TS, et al. Hormonal receptors expression in epithelial cells of mammary phyllodes tumors correlates with pathologic grade of the tumor: a multicenter study of 143 cases. Am J Clin Pathol. 2002;118:522-6.
44. Sapino A, Bosco M, Cassoni P, Castellano I, Arisio R, Cserni G, et al. Estrogen receptor-beta is expressed in stromal cells of fibroadenoma and phyllodes tumors of the breast. Mod Pathol. 2006;19:599-606.
45. Kim YH, Kim GE, Lee JS, Lee JH, Nam JH, Choi C, et al. Hormone receptors expression in phyllodes tumors of the breast. Anal Quant Cytol Histol. 2012;34:41-8.
46. Lim WK, Ong CK, Tan J, Thike AA, Ng CC, Rajasegaran V, et al. Exome sequencing identifies highly recurrent MED12 somatic mutations in breast fibroadenoma. Nat Genet. 2014;46:877-80.
47. Cani AK, Hovelson DH, McDaniel AS, Sadis S, Haller MJ, Yadati V, et al. Next-gen sequencing exposes frequent MED12 mutations and actionable therapeutic targets in phyllodes tumors. Mol Cancer Res. 2015;13:613-9.

48. Yom CK, Han W, Kim SW, Park SY, Park IA, Noh DY. Reappraisal of conventional risk stratification for local recurrence based on clinical outcomes in 285 resected phyllodes tumors of the breast. Ann Surg Oncol. 2015;22:2912-8.
49. Barth RJ. Histologic features predict local recurrence after breast conserving therapy of phyllodes tumors. Breast Cancer Res Treat. 1999;57:291-5.
50. Mangi AA, Smith BL, Gadd MA, Tanabe KK, Ott MJ, Souba WW. Surgical management of phyllodes tumors. Arch Surg. 1999;134:487-93.
51. Wood WC. Close/positive margins after breast-conserving therapy: additional resection or no resection? Breast. 2013;22(Suppl 2):S115-7.
52. Geisler DP, Boyle MJ, Malnar KF, McGee JM, Nolen MC, Fortner SM, et al. Phyllodes tumors of the breast: a review of 32 cases. Am Surg. 2000;66:360-6.
53. Kapiris I, Nasiri N, A'Hern R, Healy V, Gui GP. Outcome and predictive factors of local recurrence and distant metastases following primary surgical treatment of high-grade malignant phyllodes tumours of the breast. Eur J Surg Oncol. 2001;27:723-30.
54. Onkendi EO, Jimenez RE, Spears GM, Harmsen WS, Ballman KV, Hieken TJ. Surgical treatment of borderline and malignant phyllodes tumors: the effect of the extent of resection and tumor characteristics on patient outcome. Ann Surg Oncol. 2014;23:3304-9.
55. Lin CC, Chang HW, Lin CY, Chiu CF, Yeh SP. The clinical features and prognosis of phyllodes tumors: a single institution experience in Taiwan. Int J Clin Oncol. 2013;18:614-20.
56. Kim S, Kim JY, Kim DH, Jung WH, Koo JS. Analysis of phyllodes tumor recurrence according to the histologic grade. Breast Cancer Res Treat. 2013;141:353-63.
57. Teo JY, Cheong CS-J, Wong CY. Low local recurrence rates in young Asian patients with phyllodes tumours: less is more. ANZ J Surg. 2012;82:325-8.
58. Fajdić J, Gotovac N, Hrgović Z, Kristek J, Horvat V, Kaufmann M. Phyllodes tumors of the breast diagnostic and therapeutic dilemmas. Onkologie. 2007;30:113-8.
59. National Comprehensive Cancer Network (NCCN). Clinical Practice Guidelines in Oncology. Available from: https://www.nccn.org/professionals/physician_gls/pdf/aml.pdf [Last Accessed December, 2020].
60. Gnerlich JL, Williams RT, Yao K, Jaskowiak N, Kulkarni SA. Utilization of radiotherapy for malignant phyllodes tumors: analysis of the National Cancer Data Base. Ann Surg Oncol. 2014; 21(4):1222-30.
61. Belkacémi Y, Bousquet G, Marsiglia H, Ray-Coquard I, Magné N, Malard Yetal. Phyllodes tumor of the breast. Int J Radiat Oncol Biol Phys. 2008;70(2):492-500.
62. Lim SZ, Ong KW, Tan BK, Selvarajan S, Tan PH. Sarcoma of the breast: an update on a rare entity. J Clin Pathol. 2016;69:373-81.
63. Judson I, van der Graaf WT. Sarcoma: Olaratumab—really a breakthrough for soft-tissue sarcomas? Nat Rev Clin Oncol. 2016;13:534-6.
64. Burton GV, Hart LL, Leight GS Jr, Iglehart JD, McCarty KS, Jr, Cox EB. Cystosarcoma phyllodes. Effective therapy with cisplatin and etoposide chemotherapy. Cancer. 1989;63(11):2088-92.
65. Hawkins RE, Schofield JB, Wiltshaw E, Fisher C, McKinna JA. Ifosfamide is an active drug for chemotherapy of metastatic cystosarcoma phyllodes. Cancer. 1992;69(9):2271-5.
66. Tan BY, Geza ACS, Apple SK, Badve S, Bleiweiss IJ, Brogi E, et al. Phyllodes tumours of the breast: a consensus review. Histopathology. 2016;68(1):5-21.

CHAPTER 15

Management of Thyroid Nodule

Roma Pradhan, Amit Agarwal

INTRODUCTION

Nodules of the thyroid are one of the most common problems encountered in endocrinology and endocrine surgery clinic world over. Thyroid nodules have been defined by the American Thyroid Association (ATA) as "discrete lesions within the thyroid gland, radiologically distinct from surrounding thyroid parenchyma." The concerns and clinical aspects which need to be addressed with it are thyroid cancer and thyroid dysfunction especially big goiters associated with hyperthyroidism. A thyroid nodule is of special concern in a child where the incidence of cancer is significantly high. In most patients arriving at a diagnosis in a solitary thyroid nodule poses no problems. The traditional evaluation included clinical examination, biochemical evaluation [thyroid stimulating hormone (TSH)/thyroxine (FT4)], imaging and fine needle aspiration cytology. The problem with traditional approach is that majority of these lesions may come out to be nondiagnostic or of indeterminate cytology leading to unnecessary surgeries as majority of them turn out to be benign. Hence, certain newer investigations have been added to the management of thyroid nodule.

The series of investigations now include:
- *Laboratory investigations:* TSH/FT4
  - Thyroid scan: Only *when TSH is low*
- *Imaging:* High resolution ultrasound with colour Doppler, strain/shear wave elastography, contrast enhanced computed tomography (CECT)
  - Thyroid Imaging, Reporting, and Data System (TIRADS)/Elastography
- *Cytology:* Fine needle aspiration cytology (FNAC)/Tru-Cut biopsy
  - Molecular testing.

HISTORY TAKING AND CLINICAL EXAMINATION

History and clinical examination still holds equal importance even after introduction of modern tools and tests. There are certain factors which raise suspicion of malignancy in history taking:
- Extremes of age (<20 or >70 years)
- Male gender (8% vs. female 4%)
- Size >4 cm

- Recent rapid growth (may suggest anaplastic carcinoma or lymphoma)
- Family history: Thyroid malignancy or genetic disorders such as syndrome of multiple endocrine neoplasia (MEN) type 2, familial polyposis coli and Cowden syndrome
- History of exposure to radiation, including RT to head and neck (e.g., previous treatment of Hodgkin's disease affecting neck).

Clinical features which point toward malignancy are following:
- Rapid growth
- Symptoms of invasion: Hoarseness
- Hard consistency
- Fixity **(Fig. 1)**
- Vocal cord paralysis
- Enlarged lymph nodes **(Fig. 2)**.

If all the features are present then there is 71% risk of malignancy.

Hormonal Evaluation

All the patients with thyroid nodule should undergo hormonal evaluation with minimum of serum TSH levels as most of these patients are euthyroid. T4 is usually ordered along with TSH if there is any suspicion of hyper- or -hypothyroidism on history or clinical examination.

IMAGING

Elastography and TIRADS

Traditionally, a thyroid disorder or thyroid nodule is evaluated with TSH, high frequency ultrasound and cytology which is then followed by surgery or conservative management. The problem with this approach is that we get

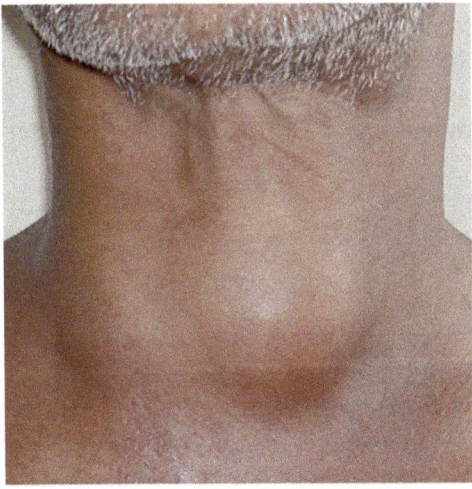

Fig. 1: Hard and fixed mass of thyroid (malignant).

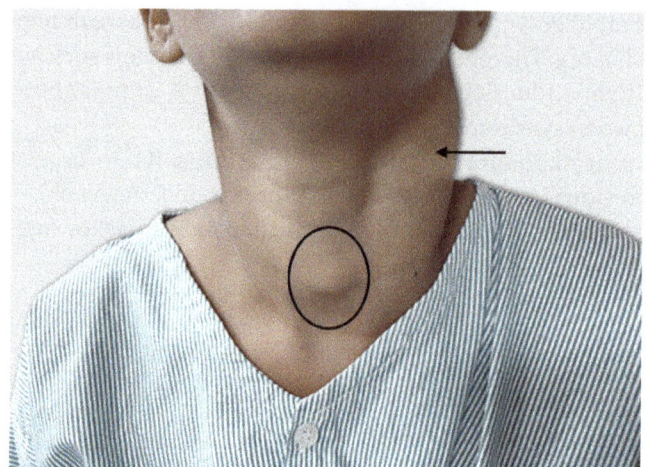

Fig. 2: Left solitary thyroid nodule with cervical lymphadenopathy (PTC).

indeterminate cytology in 10–15% of patients and nondiagnostic in 15%. In practice majority of these undergo surgery, but 80% turn out to be benign. Only 30% would harbor malignancy but due to risk/fear of malignancy, most patients with indeterminate nodules undergo surgery. Hence, thyroid ultrasound (TIRADS) and thyroid elastography can be used as a noninvasive investigation in such cases to decide for surgery.

Thyroid Imaging, Reporting, and Data System (TIRADS) classification was first introduced by Horvath et al.,[1] originating from the Breast Imaging Reporting and Data System.[2] TIRADS was based on 10 US patterns of thyroid nodules given by Horvath et al.[1] and they predicted the rate of malignancy according to the pattern. Due to its difficulty in use in clinical practice other TIRADS classification systems have been proposed.[3-6] No single ultrasound feature is adequately sensitive or specific to confirm or rule out malignancy. Multiple studies report ultrasound features in combination may better stratify malignancy risk. Pattern recognition may be more accurate for predicting a thyroid nodule is benign.

TIRADS assessment is based on five high-risk characteristics:
1. Hypoechoic
2. Irregular margins
3. Microcalcifications **(Fig. 3)**
4. Taller than wide
5. Predominantly solid.

The suspicious ultrasound features were classified and described in **Table 1**.

More recently, the usefulness of TIRADS score combined with the Bethesda System for Reporting Thyroid Cytopathology (BSRTC) for the stratification of malignancy risk of thyroid nodules in patients with indeterminate results on cytology has been addressed. The study by Maia et al.[8] demonstrated the high sensitivity and NPV of Bethesda III nodules with

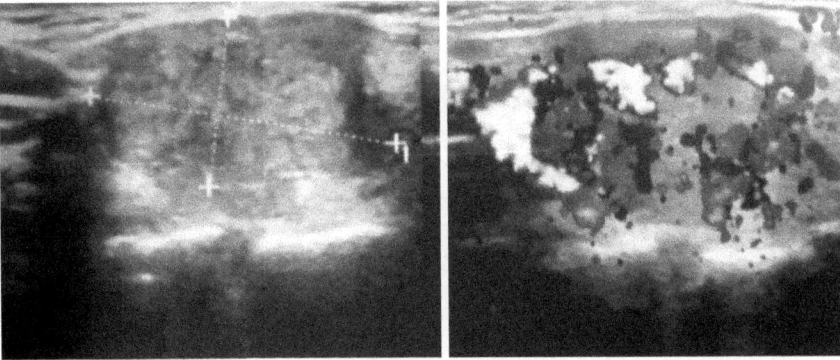

Fig. 3: USG showing solid nodule with microcalcifications with increased vascularity.

TABLE 1: TIRADS system of reporting thyroid nodules.

	No. of features	Risk of malignancy
TIRADS 3	No suspicious features	0%
TIRADS 4a	One suspicious feature	4%
TIRADS 4b	Two suspicious features	12.5%
TIRADS 4c	Three or four suspicious features	62.2%
TIRADS 5	Five suspicious features	100%[1,7]

a TIRADS score of 3/4A, which may suggest a conservative approach (follow-up and repeat US-FNAB) is appropriate. In contrast, TIRADS scores 4B and 5 in combination with Bethesda III, IV and V may suggest that proceeding directly to surgery is appropriate due to high rate of malignancy in such lesions.

Elastography

Clinical palpation is a practical diagnostic method for thyroid evaluation, and the presence of a hard thyroid nodule is usually associated with an increased risk of malignancy. As this method is subjective, a more objective newer technique known as elastography to evaluate the stiffness of the lesion was done. It is also known as "electronic palpation". Ultrasound elastography was first used in thyroid by Lyshchik et al. in 2005.[9]

There are two types of elastography:
1. *Strain elastography (SE)*: Strain elastography assesses tissue elasticity through tissue displacement induced by compression. Strain elastography can be with mechanic force (external or internal) or acoustic radiation force (ARF). Relative displacement (strain) is greater in soft compared to stiff tissues.
2. *Shear wave elastography (SWE)*: Focused acoustic impulses from the transducer induce laterally propagating shear waves, whose velocities are higher in stiffer tissues. Shear wave elastography assesses tissue elasticity by measuring the propagation speed of transverse shear waves.

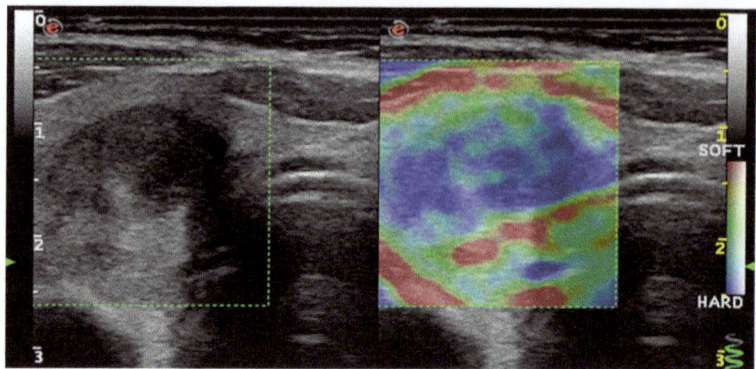

Fig. 4: Strain elastography: Harder tissue is represented by blue color while green represents softer tissue.

Assessment: Strain elastography is done by qualitative assessment using Rago 5 point score[10] or Asteria 4 point score.[11] Semiquantitative assessment can be done by measuring the parenchyma to nodule ratio or muscle to nodule ratio. Strain elastography can also be done using carotid artery as compression source. Pre- and postcompression signals are tracked and strain images are generated. The hardness is expressed as the thyroid stiffness index (TSI) or the elasticity contrast index (ECI).[12]

Strain elastography using ARF: Acoustic radiation force impulse (ARFI) imaging can image tissue deformation using focused ultrasound beams. Images are obtained before and after the application of force and displacement are measured. Strain changes are displayed as a gray-scale image. A bright shade indicates relatively soft-tissue, whereas a darker shade indicates relatively stiff tissue **(Fig. 4)**. Qualitative assessment is done by 6 point scale devised by Xu et al.[13]

Shear wave elastography: The acoustic pulses from the probe stimulate the target tissue, creating a shear wave (SW) traveling perpendicular to the conventional US waves. SWs are the transverse components of particle displacement that are rapidly attenuated by the tissue (1–10 m/sec). This transverse component is tracked and measured as a numerical value corresponding to the shear-wave speed (SWS). The elasticity index (EI) provides quantitative information about SWE (expressed in m/s) and the estimated tissue stiffness [expressed in kilopascals (kPa)].[14]

It relies on the degree of lesion stiffness. Malignant nodules have harder consistency or less elastic than benign ones due to the uncontrolled proliferation of cancer cells. The elasticity index (EI) provides quantitative information about SWE (expressed in m/s) and the estimated tissue stiffness [expressed in kilopascals (kPa)].[11] The modulus of elasticity, also known as Young's modulus (in kPa), is calculated based on the SWE. The Young's modulus increases as the tissue becomes harder.[15,16] In real clinical practice,

US elastography is usually performed as a supplement with conventional US and not as an independent test. This is supported by the results of Trimboli et al.,[17] who reported that the combination of these two modalities resulted in a sensitivity of 97% and negative predictive value (NPV) of 97%.

CECT

Whereas ultrasound is the imaging study of choice, CECT scan has more sensitivity for detecting central lymph node metastasis for all lesions. It is best used as an adjunct modality in imaging advanced thyroid pathology when there is aerodigestive tract invasion or where substernal, intrathoracic or retrotracheal extension of the gland is suspected.

CYTOLOGY

Fine needle aspiration cytology helps to distinguish between benign and malignant lesion and is the investigation of choice in thyroid nodules; however, in 15–20% of lesion it is unable to determine that. Although FNA and scanning are considered as important techniques for the diagnosis of thyroid nodules, there is still a large "gray zone" in these techniques. Therefore, USG-guided FNAC is advised in lesions which are nonpalpable, mostly cystic or posteriorly located. Traditionally, the cytology reporting was divided into four main categories: (1) nondiagnostic, (2) benign, (3) malignant and (4) indeterminate or suspicious of neoplasm. As more data was generated and with introduction of Bethesda reporting which was widely accepted among pathologist, the latest Bethesda system is followed which consists of six categories (*see* **Table 1**). A new pathological entity—noninvasive follicular thyroid neoplasm with papillary-like nuclear features (NIFTP) is the addition that has been considered in Bethesda reporting. The risk of malignancy in both these circumstances is mentioned in **Table 2**.

TABLE 2: The 2017 Bethesda System for Reporting Thyroid Cytopathology: Recommended Diagnostic Categories.[18]

	Diagnostic categories	Risk of malignancy NIFTP not considered malignancy	Risk of malignancy NIFTP considered as malignancy
BETHESDA I	Nondiagnostic or unsatisfactory	5–10	5–10
BETHESDA II	Benign	0–3	0–3
BETHESDA III	Atypia of undetermined significance or follicular lesion of undetermined significance	6–18	10–30
BETHESDA IV	Follicular neoplasm or suspicious for a follicular neoplasm	10–40	25–40
BETHESDA V	Suspicious of malignancy	45–60	50–75
BETHESDA VI	Malignant	94–96	97–99

Nondiagnostic Evaluation

For a thyroid cytology specimen to be satisfactory for evaluation (and benign), at least six groups of benign follicular cells are required, each group composed of at least 10 cells. The minimum requirement for group size allows one to determine (by the evenness of the nuclear spacing) whether it represents a fragment of a macrofollicle. The 2017 BSRTC[18] reinforces several exceptions to the numerical requirement of benign follicular cells. Any specimen that contains abundant colloid is adequate (and benign), even if six groups of follicular cells are not identified: a sparsely cellular specimen with abundant colloid is, by implication, a predominantly macrofollicular nodule and therefore almost certainly benign. Whenever a specific diagnosis can be rendered, and whenever there is any significant atypia, the specimen is, by definition is considered adequate for evaluation. For nondiagnostic lesions it is preferable to repeat ultrasound guided FNAC. Surgery is recommended in case of repeated nondiagnostic cytology.

AUS/FLUS: This category has two names—atypia of undetermined significance (AUS) and follicular lesion of undetermined significance (FLUS). These are synonyms and should not be used to denote two distinct interpretations. The rate of malignancy in these lesions is quite different when NIFTP is included or excluded from malignancy criteria (*see* **Table 1**). AUS/FLUS category is to be used as last resort by pathologist. According to original BETHESDA system an effort should be made to keep it to <7% of all thyroid FNA. The management for AUS/FLUS lesion now includes consideration of molecular testing for such lesions.

Follicular Neoplasm

This category again has two names: follicular neoplasm or suspicious for a follicular neoplasm. SFN is preferred by some pathologists because a major proportion of cases prove not to be neoplasms but rather hyperplastic proliferations of follicular cells. Similar to AUS/FLUS, if the ROM for FN/SFN is recalculated by removing NIFTPs from the tally of malignancies, the risk diminishes (*see* **Table 2**). Early data suggest that NIFTP constitutes a substantial proportion of the "malignancies" hidden in this category as well.[19,20] The recommended management of a patient with a diagnosis of FN/SFN is surgical excision of the lesion, most often a hemithyroidectomy or lobectomy, but molecular testing may be used to supplement risk assessment rather than proceeding directly to surgery.

Molecular Genetics

Molecular markers play a key role in taking decisions in thyroid surgeries. The efficiency and accuracy of diagnosis improves the surgery. So far the studies show a reduction in the hemithyroidectomies. There are broadly two types of molecular tests—rule-in and rule-out tests. Rule-out tests include the thyroid sequencing for common mutations such as BRAF, RET, etc., it could be 5-gene or 7-gene panel. Rule-in tests includes the gene expression classifier. There is some success with BRAFV 600E mutation in cytological specimens.[21] The GEC has been useful as a negative predictor of malignancy.[22] Galectin immunocytostaining in FNAC sample of thyroid is regularly used and help in discriminating benign from malignant thyroid lesions. Along with genetic markers, somatic mutation testing, mRNA gene expression platforms, protein immunocytochemistry and miRNA panels have improved the diagnostic accuracy of indeterminate thyroid nodules, and although no test is perfectly accurate.

Therefore, it is clinically important to have molecular markers that, in conjunction with FNA, can identify the subset of patients with subtypes and aggressive nature of tumor. Specific markers determine the type and aggressiveness of the cancer so that treatment will be targeted and efficient. The use of molecular markers for thyroid cancer diagnosis, prognosis, targeted therapy, and surveillance has been an exciting area of study and change; however, molecular testing needs significant amount of resources and in resource poor settings molecular testing must be used judiciously.

Isotope Scan

99mTc, ^{123}I, and ^{131}I are the isotopes commonly used for thyroid isotope scanning. Historically isotope scan was used in initial management of thyroid nodule to know if the nodule was cold as cold nodule may harbor malignancy. Now thyroid scan is indicated only if TSH is low and is especially useful in diagnosis of autonomously functioning thyroid nodule and its management **(Fig. 5)**.

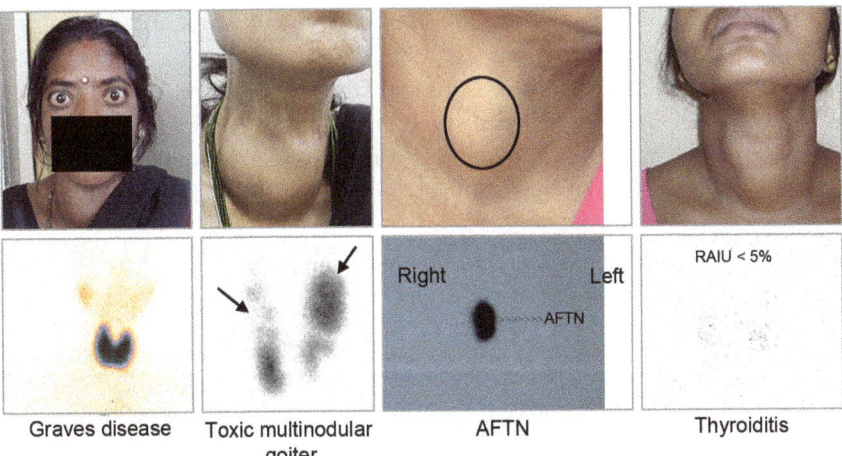

Fig. 5: Clinical and thyroid scan correlation of different etiologies of hyperthyroidism. (AFTN: autonomous functioning thyroid nodules).

SURGICAL MANAGEMENT OF THYROID NODULES

After proper assessment and diagnosis, several possibilities may arise, each requiring different management. Literature has many algorithms for management of thyroid nodules. The simplified algorithm for management of thyroid nodules is described in **Flowchart 1**.

Thyroid surgery in the 19th century carried a frightful mortality of 40% even in most skilled hands, mainly due to infection and hemorrhage. The French and German Academy of Medicine banned thyroid surgery. From that bloody and festering time, thyroid surgery is delivered to us, as we practice it, by seven successive surgeons[23] who brought down the mortality to less than 1%. Following refinements in surgery have now made modern thyroid surgery more precise, almost bloodless, with minimal complications in the hands of thyroid surgeons:

- Improved hemostasis by using energy devices
- Intraoperative detection of viable parathyroid glands
- Reduced incidence of severe hypocalcemia by early prediction of hypocalcemia
- Reducing incidence of recurrent laryngeal nerve (RLN) palsy by RLN neuromonitoring, and
- Improved cosmesis by endoscopic or robotic scar less thyroidectomy.

Improved Hemostasis

Thyroid surgery involves meticulous devascularization of the thyroid gland which has one of the richest blood supplies of all organs. Therefore, hemostasis is of paramount importance. One of the major concerns following thyroid surgery is the risk of life-threatening hematoma the incidence of which is 0.3–3%. Several randomized clinical studies have documented that the presence of a drain has no effect on the incidence of hematoma formation. Two of the most commonly used techniques for hemostasis are suture ligation and electrocoagulation. The disadvantage of these techniques is the prolonged operating time and possibility of stitch granuloma with the use of sutures. Evolutions in technology have allowed surgeons to achieve a better balance between hemostasis and tissue preservation. The advantages of the energy devices are:

- Minimal collateral damage for safe dissection near vital structure
- Less smoke formation
- No neuromuscular stimulation
- No electrical energy to or through the patient (ultrasonic)
- Cuts, coagulates, grasp, and dissects by same instrument, so no instrument exchanges
- Reliably seal and divide vessels up to 8 mm
- No possibility of suture granuloma formation.

Flowchart 1: Management of thyroid nodules.

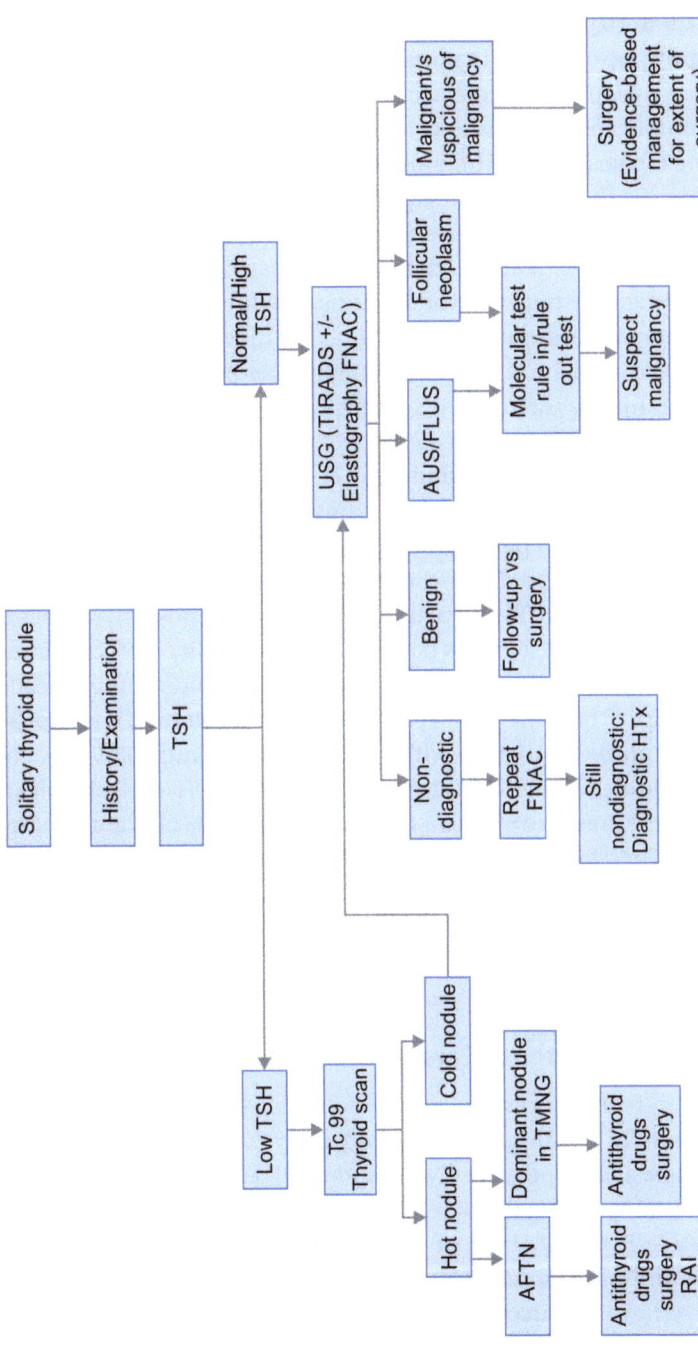

(AFTN: autonomous functioning thyroid nodules; AUS: atypia of undetermined significance; FNAC: fine needle aspiration cytology; FLUS: follicular lesion of undetermined significance; RAI: radioactive iodine; TMNG: toxic multinodular goiter; TSH: thyroid stimulating hormone; TIRADS: thyroid imaging, reporting, and data system; USG: ultrasonography)

Predictors of Hypocalcemia

The reported incidence of transient and permanent hypocalcemia ranging from 3 to 52% and 0.4 to 13%, respectively.[24,25] Various methods for diagnosing and managing postoperative hypocalcemia have been used. It is known that postoperative hypoparathyroidism leading to hypocalcemia is one of the most common complications after a total thyroidectomy. There are three methods of managing hypocalcemia. The most common approach used by surgeons is supplementing the calcium if the patient develops signs and symptoms of hypocalcemia by monitoring the serum calcium but thus increasing the days of hospitalization. This reactive method of managing hypocalcemia is still being used by many institutions worldwide because the nadir of hypocalcemia typically occurs within 48 hours after surgery. The routine use of postoperative oral calcium and/or vitamin D supplementation has been advocated by some surgeons to minimize the incidence of hypocalcemia and shorten hospital stays.

More recently, with the aim of finding an earlier predictor for hypocalcemia, the short half-life of the parathyroid hormone has led to increased interest in early postoperative intact parathyroid hormone (IPTH) as an early marker of hypocalcemia.[26] Various studies including a review[27] have evaluated the utility of postoperative intact PTH measurement to predict post-thyroidectomy hypocalcemia. Several researches have relied on the utility of PTH to foresee hypocalcemia after total thyroidectomy using hemithyroidectomy procedure as control group[28-30] but none could characterize an absolute PTH serum level or percentage hormone decline with 100% sensitivity and 100% specificity values. Some studies concluded that low perioperative PTH levels significantly correlate with the presence of postoperative hypocalcemia but cannot be used to predict it.[31] Therefore, iPTH done early in the postoperative period has the potential to allow early discharge from the hospital without the need of the patient undergoing serial calcium monitoring. Among the newer techniques, intraoperative parathyroid gland angiography during thyroidectomy can also be used to evaluate parathyroid gland perfusion and function.[32-34]

Intraoperative Detection of Parathyroid Gland

Parathyroid detection presents greatest difficulty in cases such as total thyroidectomy (TT), completion thyroidectomy (CT), central neck lymph node dissection, and reoperative thyroid surgery. The incidence of inadvertent parathyroidectomy during thyroidectomy ranges from 8 to 19%. For accurate intraoperative identification of the parathyroid glands, pathological examination and an intraoperative parathyroid hormone assay were reported to be effective; however, successful use depends on sufficient experience of the surgeon to locate the parathyroid glands precisely and quickly. There remains a clinical need for an intraoperative technique to detect the parathyroid gland instantly and with high accuracy.

There is, however, no objective intraoperative tool to determine if an ISPG (in-situ parathyroid glands) is well-perfused or not. Laser Doppler flowmetry was previously used for assessing parathyroid perfusion, but has not been widely practiced. Therefore, surgeons often have to rely on either visual inspection alone (i.e., by looking at the color changes in the ISPGs) or the "knife" test as ways of estimating parathyroid perfusion and viability. Indocyanine green (ICG) is an inert, water soluble, nonradioactive, and nontoxic contrast agent that has been approved by the US Food and Drug Administration since 1959. After intravenous injection, ICG is distributed throughout the intravascular space and rapidly bound to plasma proteins. When illuminated at 806 nm with a low-energy laser, these plasma-bound ICG molecules become fluorescent and this fluorescence is recorded by a charge-coupled device camera. Because the fluorescence intensity (FI) in a focused area is directly proportional to the perfusion in that area, the FI value of the ISPGs measured on the ICG fluorescence angiography (ICGA) may provide information regarding to the perfusion and the extent of viability of the ISPGs. This technology is actually not new and has been used in various clinical areas, including assessing perfusion of skin flaps, bowel anastomosis, and lower limbs. Although this technique has been used for assessing parathyroid remnant in subtotal parathyroidectomy, to our knowledge, its use in assessing parathyroid perfusion during thyroid operations has been is not commonly reported. It is hypothesized that the fluorescent intensity (FI) in the ISPGs may reflect not only the perfusion of the ISPGs, but also the residual parathyroid function and the subsequent risk of hypocalcemia. Given that parathyroid perfusion plays a vital role in normalizing early parathyroid function, perhaps patients with a greater FI value in their ISPGs (i.e., good parathyroid perfusion) have a lower chance of PH than those with a lower FI value.

Recurrent Laryngeal Nerve Monitoring

The relationship of RLN with voice has a fascinating story which dates back to sixth century BC written in Sushruta Samhita. Preservation of integrity of RLN seems to revolve around thyroid surgery. Injury to the RLN is the most feared injury in thyroid surgery. As external branch of superior laryngeal nerve supplies the cricothyroid muscle, the damage of the nerve has varied effect on voice and is less troublesome except in singers and teachers. Intraoperative neuromonitoring is considered a safe procedure to complement the traditional method of visualizing the nerve which is considered the gold standard. It can also be used to prognosticate the postoperative nerve function. Recurrent laryngeal nerve monitoring can be intermittent or continuous. Continuous neuromonitoring is the real time monitoring of RLN which warns the surgeon before actual injury takes place as happens when the thyroid is pulled stretching the nerve.

Robot Assisted Thyroidectomy

The traditional thyroidectomy technique produces a long scar on the neck that is difficult to conceal. Developments of "alternative" approaches were driven by patient-centered efforts to improve the cosmetic impact of thyroid surgery **(Fig. 6)**. Novel approaches developed along two divergent avenues of innovation: (1) minimally invasive anterior cervical approaches and (2) remote access approaches. Chest/breast approaches included: isolated anterior chest wall approach, bilateral transareolar approach and unilateral transareolar approach. However, despite the lack of cervical scars, they do involve incisions on the breast or anterior chest, subjected to hypertrophic scarring, and may be an unappealing alternative to some patients. Also, these approaches may also be limited by a narrow operative field and restriction of movement by the rigid endoscopic equipment. Then came the axillary approach. This approach is associated with improved cosmetic outcomes when compared to open surgery. However, it takes significantly longer to perform than a conventional open thyroidectomy. This approach is still subject to the constraints of CO_2 assisted dissection-relatively narrow corridors, the need for rigid specialized endoscopic equipment, and the risks of CO_2 related morbidity. Then came the hybrid approaches which included: axillobilateral breast approach (ABBA), bilateral axillobilateral breast approach (BABA). These were designed to capitalize on the cosmetic benefit of the axillary approaches while providing additional anterior chest working ports without producing a transverse parasternal scar. Then came the transoral approach for thyroidectomy, which was truly scarless. Application of robotic technology to thyroidectomy was a logical step to minimally invasive thyroidectomy. Potential advantages included: more precise dissection, improved visualization, surgeon controlled visualization and hand tremor filtering system. Different techniques are **(Fig. 7)**:

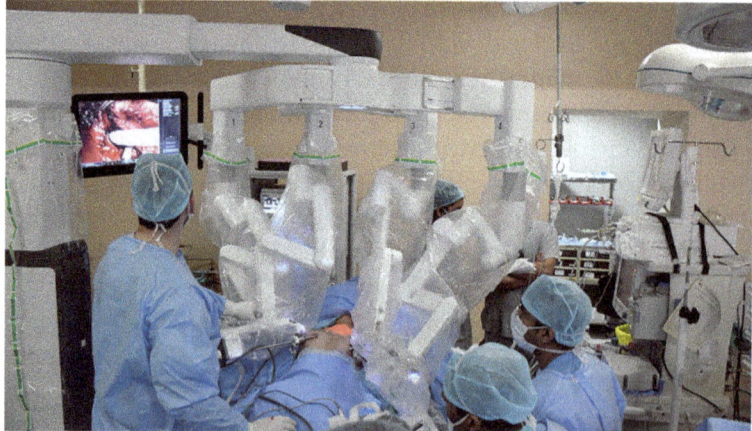

Fig. 6: Robot docked on patient.

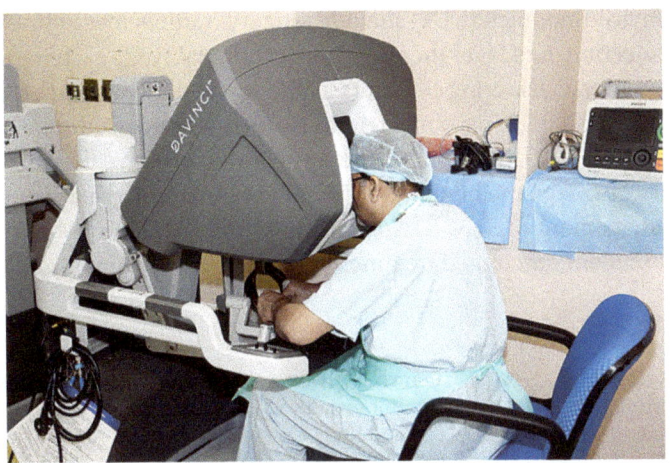

Fig. 7: Surgeon console in robotic surgery.

- Two-incision (axillary and anterior chest)
- Bilateral axillary
- Bilateral areolar
- Single incision
- Nonaxillary approach:
  - Robot face lift thyroidectomy (RFT)
  - Transoral.

An important consideration regarding robot assisted thyroidectomy (RAT) is that there is a considerable learning curve requiring at least 40 cases to master the technique. Comparing open and robotic thyroidectomy there is no difference in surgical outcome; however, there was longer operative time (232 vs. 109 min) in RAT.[35] Studies which objectively and subjectively analyzed found that there was no difference in complications.[36-39] In a systematic review and meta-analysis studies again seem to confirm that both endoscopic and RAT are procedures that can be performed safely with good outcomes in appropriately selected patients.[40]

CONCLUSION

Modern work-up of thyroid nodule now incorporates use of TIRADS and USG elastography along with molecular testing of thyroid aspirate. Various intraoperative adjuncts such as energy devices, use of Indocyanine green dye, using RLN/SLN neuromonitoring and IOPTH have made modern thyroid surgery almost bloodless and with minimal complications. Endoscopic and robotic approaches have made thyroid surgery cosmetically acceptable by either scarless surgery or by using remote incisions away from the neck. Also the treatment is now more personalized and tailored for individual patient. Sufficient data is now available to support the application of endoscopic and robotic surgery in a subset of thyroid patients. The modalities of treatment for solitary thyroid nodules (STN) include surgery, radioactive iodine therapy, ethanol injection, and laser therapy. The best modality for each patient must be decided after considering all factors including the patient's wishes, expertise and facilities available, cost considerations and the strategy must be guided by evidence. There is no role for blind therapy with suppressive dose of thyroxine as the risks outweigh the benefits. It should not be part of a treatment strategy in the management of STN. STN is an entity where majority of patients will have an excellent outcome if treatment is offered appropriately and wisely.

REFERENCES

1. Horvath E, Majlis S, Rossi R, Franco C, Niedmann JP, Castro A, et al. An ultrasonogram reporting system for thyroid nodules stratifying cancer risk for clinical management. J Clin Endocrinol Metab. 2009;94:1748-51.
2. Vanel D. The American College of Radiology (ACR) Breast Imaging and Reporting Data System (BI-RADS): a step towards a universal radiological language? Eur J Radiol. 2007;61:183.
3. Park JY, Lee HJ, Jang HW, Kim HK, Yi JH, Lee W, et al. A proposal for a thyroid imaging reporting and data system for ultrasound features of thyroid carcinoma. Thyroid. 2009;19:1257-64.
4. Kwak JY, Jung I, Baek JH, Baek SM, Choi N, Choi YJ, et al. Korean Society of Thyroid Radiology (KSThR); Korean Society of Radiology. Image reporting and characterization system for ultrasound features of thyroid nodules: multicentric Korean retrospective study. Korean J Radiol. 2013;14:110-7.
5. Russ G, Royer B, Bigorgne C, Rouxel A, Bienvenu-Perrard M, Leenhardt L. Prospective evaluation of thyroid imaging reporting and data system on 4550 nodules with and without elastography. Eur J Endocrinol. 2013;168:649-55.
6. Na DG, Baek JH, Sung JY, Kim JH, Kim JK, Choi YJ, et al. Thyroid Imaging Reporting and Data System Risk Stratification of Thyroid Nodules: Categorization Based on Solidity and Echogenicity. Thyroid. 2016;26(4):562-72.
7. Kwak JY, Han KH, Yoon JH, Moon HJ, Son EJ, Park SH, et al. Thyroid imaging reporting and data system for US features of nodules: a step in establishing better stratification of cancer risk. Radiology. 2011;260(3):892-9.
8. Maia FF, Matos PS, Pavin EJ, Zantut-Wittmann DE. Thyroid imaging reporting and data system score combined with Bethesda system for malignancy risk stratification in thyroid nodules with indeterminate results on cytology. Clin Endocrinol (Oxf). 2015;82(3):439-44.
9. Lyshchik A, Higashi T, Asato R, Tanaka S, Ito J, Mai JJ, et al. Thyroid gland tumor diagnosis at US elastography. Radiology. 2005;237:202-11.
10. Rago T, Santini F, Scutari M, Pinchera A, Vitti P. Elastography: new developments in ultrasound for predicting malignancy in thyroid nodules. J Clin Endocrinol Metab. 2007;92:2917-22.
11. Asteria C, Giovanardi A, Pizzocaro A, Cozzaglio L, Morabito A, Somalvico F, et al. US-elastography in the differential diagnosis of benign and malignant thyroid nodules. Thyroid. 2008;18:523-31.
12. Andrioli M, Persani L. Elastographic techniques of thyroid gland: current status. Endocrine. 2014;46:455-61.
13. Xu JM, Xu XH, Xu HX, Zhang YF, Zhang J, Guo LH, et al. Conventional US, US elasticity imaging, and acoustic radiation force impulse imaging for prediction of malignancy in thyroid nodules. Radiology. 2014;272:577-86.

14. Sebag F, Vaillant-Lombard J, Berbis J, Griset V, Henry JF, Petit P, et al. Shear wave elastography: a new ultrasound imaging mode for the differential diagnosis of benign and malignant thyroid nodules. J Clin Endocrinol Metab. 2010;95(12):5281-8.
15. Tanter M, Bercoff J, Athanasiou A, Deffieux T, Gennisson JL, Montaldo G, et al. Quantitative assessment of breast lesion viscoelasticity: initial clinical results using supersonic shear imaging. Ultrasound Med Biol. 2008;34(9):1373-86.
16. Bercoff J, Tanter M, Fink M. Supersonic shear imaging: a new technique for soft tissue elasticity mapping. IEEE Trans Ultrason Ferroelectr Freq Control. 2004;51(4): 396-409.
17. Trimboli P, Guglielmi R, Monti S, Misischi I, Graziano F, Nasrollah N, et al. Ultrasound sensitivity for thyroid malignancy is increased by real-time elastography: a prospective multicenter study. J Clin Endocrinol Metab. 2012;97:4524-30.
18. Cibas ES, Ali SZ. The 2017 Bethesda System for reporting thyroid cytopathology. Thyroid. 2017;27(11):1341-6.
19. Strickland KC, Howitt BE, Marqusee E, Alexander EK, Cibas ES, Krane JF, et al. The impact of non-invasive follicular variant of papillary thyroid carcinoma on rates of malignancy for fine-needle aspiration diagnostic categories. Thyroid. 2015;25:987-92.
20. Faquin WC, Wong LQ, Afrogheh AH, Ali SZ, Bishop JA, Bongiovanni M, et al. Impact of re-classifying non-invasive follicular variant of papillary thyroid carcinoma on the risk of malignancy in The Bethesda System for Reporting Thyroid Cytopathology. Cancer Cytopathol. 2016;124(3):181-7.
21. Jinih M, Foley N, Osho O, Houlihan L, Toor A, Khan JZ, et al. Redmond HP. BRAFV600E mutation as a predictor of thyroid malignancy in indeterminate nodules: a systematic review and meta-analysis. Eur J Surg Oncol. 2017;43(7):1219-27.
22. Ming Z, Oscar L. Molecular testing of thyroid nodules: a review of current available tests for fine-needle aspiration specimens. Arch Pathol Lab Med. 2016;12:1338-44.
23. Hannan SA. The magnificent seven: a history of modern thyroid surgery. Int J Surg. 2006;4(3):187-91.
24. Vescan A, Witterick I, Freeman J. Parathyroid hormone as a predictor of hypocalcemia after thyroidectomy. Laryngoscope. 2005;115(12):2105-8.
25. Pisaniello D, Parmeggiani D, Piatto A, Avenia N, d'Ajello M, Monacelli M, et al. Which therapy to prevent post-thyroidectomy hypocalcemia? G Chir. 2005;26(10):357-61.
26. Lombardi CP, Raffaelli M, Princi P, Santini S, Boscherini M, De Crea C, et al. Early prediction of post thyroidectomy hypocalcemia by one single iPTH measurement. Surgery. 2004;136 (6):1236-41.
27. Noordzij JP, Lee SL, Bernet VJ, Payne RJ, Cohen SM, McLeod IK, et al. Early prediction of hypocalcemia after thyroidectomy using parathyroid hormone: an analysis of pooled individual patient data from nine observational studies. J Am Coll Surg. 2007;205(6):748-54.
28. Alía P, Moreno P, Rigo R, Francos JM, Navarro MA. Postresection parathyroid hormone and parathyroid hormone decline accurately predict hypocalcemia after thyroidectomy. Am J Clin Pathol. 2007;127:592-7.
29. Di Fabio F, Casella C, Bugari G, Iacobello C, Salerni B. Identification of patients at low risk for thyroidectomy-related hypocalcemia by intraoperative quick PTH. World J Surg. 2006;30:1428-33.
30. Lo CY, Luk JM, Tam SC. Applicability of intraoperative parathyroid hormone assay during thyroidectomy. Ann Surg. 2002;236:564-9.
31. Ghaheri BA, Liebler SL, Andersen PE, Schuff KG, Samuels MH, Klein RF, et al. Perioperative parathyroid hormone levels in thyroid surgery. Laryngoscope. 2006;116:518-21.
32. Lang BH, Wong CK, Hung HT, Wong KP, Mak KL, Au KB. Indocyanine green fluorescence angiography for quantitative evaluation of in situ parathyroid gland perfusion and function after total thyroidectomy. Surgery. 2017;161(1):87-95.

33. Zaidi N, Bucak E, Yazici P, Soundararajan S, Okoh A, Yigitbas H, et al. The feasibility of indocyanine green fluorescence imaging for identifying and assessing the perfusion of parathyroid glands during total thyroidectomy. J Surg Oncol. 2016;113(7):775-8.
34. Vidal Fortuny J, Belfontali V, Sadowski SM, Karenovics W, Guigard S, Triponez F. Parathyroid gland angiography with indocyanine green fluorescence to predict parathyroid function after thyroid surgery. Br J Surg. 2016;N103(5):537-43.
35. Foley CS, Agcaoglu O, Siperstein AE, Berber E. Robotic transaxillary endocrine surgery: a comparison with conventional open technique. Surg Endosc. 2012;26(8):2259-66.
36. Lee J, Na KY, Kim RM, Oh Y, Lee JH, Lee J, et al. Postoperative functional voice changes after conventional open or robotic thyroidectomy: a prospective trial. Ann Surg Oncol. 2012;19:2963-70.
37. Lee J, Lee JH, Nah KY, Soh EY, Chung WY. Comparison of endoscopic and robotic thyroidectomy. Ann Surg Oncol. 2011;18(5):1439-46.
38. Yoo H, Chae BJ, Park HS, Kim KH, Kim SH, Song BJ, et al. Comparison of surgical outcomes between endoscopic and robotic thyroidectomy. J Surg Oncol. 2012;105(7):705-8.
39. Lee S, Ryu HR, Park JH, Kim KH, Kang SW, Jeong JJ, et al. Excellence in robotic thyroid surgery: a comparative study of robot-assisted versus conventional endoscopic thyroidectomy in papillary thyroid microcarcinoma patients. Ann Surg. 2011;253(6):1060-6.
40. Lang BH, Wong CK, Tsang JS, Wong KP. A systematic review and meta-analysis comparing outcomes between robotic-assisted thyroidectomy and non-robotic endoscopic thyroidectomy. J Surg Res. 2014;191(2):389-98.

CHAPTER 16

Surgical Practice in COVID Era

Sankha Shubhra Chakrabarti, RN Meena, SK Gupta

INTRODUCTION

Coronavirus disease-2019 (COVID-19) is a multisystem acute infectious disease caused by the severe acute respiratory syndrome coronavirus-2 (SARS-CoV-2), which originated in Wuhan, China in November-December 2019. It predominantly affects the respiratory, circulatory and coagulation systems of the body.[1] The virus has shown an exaggerated tendency to spread and despite an overall low mortality as compared to its predecessors—severe acute respiratory syndrome coronavirus (SARS-CoV) and Middle East respiratory syndrome coronavirus (MERS-CoV), SARS-CoV-2 has affected more than 90 million people worldwide as of January 11th, 2021. The World Health Organization (WHO) declared COVID-19 a pandemic on March 11th, 2020. Despite a mortality rate of around 3% or less worldwide, COVID-19 has accounted for in excess of 1.9 million deaths, mostly due to the large population affected.[2] Even in countries like India which have low mortality and a possible higher immunity to severe COVID-19, the absolute number of patients affected and dying have been significant.[1,2] Overall, COVID-19 has burdened the health system of the world and created unprecedented challenges to providing quality healthcare to both COVID and non-COVID patients. The major countries to have had maximum deaths per million population include Peru, Belgium, Spain, the United States and the United Kingdom, whereas the major countries with maximum cases per million population have been the United States, Belgium, Bahrain, Netherlands and Qatar. In absolute number of cases, the US (22.5 million), India (10.5 million), Brazil (8.1 million) and Russia (3.4 million) lead the field, whereas the US, Brazil, India, and Mexico have had the maximum gross number of deaths.[2] More significant has been the uncertainty about the ideal medical and socioeconomic response to the COVID-19 pandemic at country-level with administrators everywhere grappling with restrictive and mitigation strategies. Governments in major nations have adopted intensive testing of cases, isolation/quarantine, mask usage, social distancing, lockdown, and similar practices in an attempt to control the disease from spreading.

SARS-CoV-2 AND PATHOGENESIS OF COVID-19

Severe acute respiratory syndrome coronavirus-2 is the seventh coronavirus which infects humans. Among these, HCoV-229E and HCoV-NL63 are alpha coronaviruses whereas HCoV-OC43, HCoV-HKU1, SARS-CoV, MERS-CoV, and SARS-CoV-2 are beta coronaviruses. 229E, NL63, OC43, and HKU1 are endemic corona viruses which exist in the community, affect humans, and cause self-limited respiratory illnesses (common flu) in immunocompetent individuals. The three others, namely SARS-CoV, MERS-CoV, and SARS-CoV-2 are animal origin corona viruses which have evolved to be able to affect humans. These are known to cause severe disease.[3,4] SARS-CoV-2 is presumed to be of bat origin and has acquired mutations to enable it for human infection, while propagating through previous animal hosts. It shows 96% genomic similarity with RaTG13, found in the bat *Rhinolophus affinis*.[4] The pangolin coronavirus, Pangolin-CoV is 91% identical to SARS-CoV-2 and appears to be its second closest relative.[5] SARS-CoV-2, like other beta coronaviruses has a single strand positive sense RNA as its genomic material. There are two notable features of SARS-CoV-2. The first is the predilection of the receptor binding domain (RBD) of its spike (S) protein to bind to its predominant receptor angiotensin converting enzyme 2 (ACE2) on pulmonary epithelial and other human cells. This high affinity seems to be due to mutations in the RBD of SARS-CoV-2. The second novel feature is the presence of a polybasic furin cleavage site (RRAR) at the junction of the S1 and S2 subunits of its spike protein. This feature which is not found in other related beta coronaviruses, may have additional role in viral infectivity and host range.[4]

Severe acute respiratory syndrome coronavirus-2, being a virus, which predominantly affects the pulmonary and cardiac systems, is transmitted by the respiratory route. However, much controversy has emerged regarding whether it is solely transmitted through fomites or there is a significant component of airborne spread. Further, it is still unclear how long the virus can survive on different fomites and what is the potential for spread through packaged and open food items, and through alternative routes such as the eyes.[6,7] Major COVID-19 manifestations occur when the virus gains entry into its target cells in the lungs and heart and possibly other organs. ACE2 protein expressed on pulmonary epithelial cells and in other organs in humans such as the gastrointestinal tract, the pancreas, etc., is the primary receptor for SARS-CoV-2. Viral entry is initiated by the binding of the RBD of the viral S protein to ACE2. This is followed by cleavage and activation of the S protein by the transmembrane serine protease TMPRSS2 present on pulmonary epithelial cells. This activation enables the S2 subunit of the S protein to fuse with host (human pulmonary epithelial or other) cell, thus bringing about SARS-CoV-2 entry.[8,9] Although TMPRSS2 is the major activator of the viral S protein, some other host proteases may also play an accessory part. These include the extracellular trypsin, lysosomal cathepsins, and the predominantly intracellular furin.[10] Herein lies the importance of the unique polybasic furin cleavage site in the S protein of SARS-CoV-2, which may predispose it to cleavage and activation by host furin. The viral life cycle in the host cell is shown in **Figure 1**.

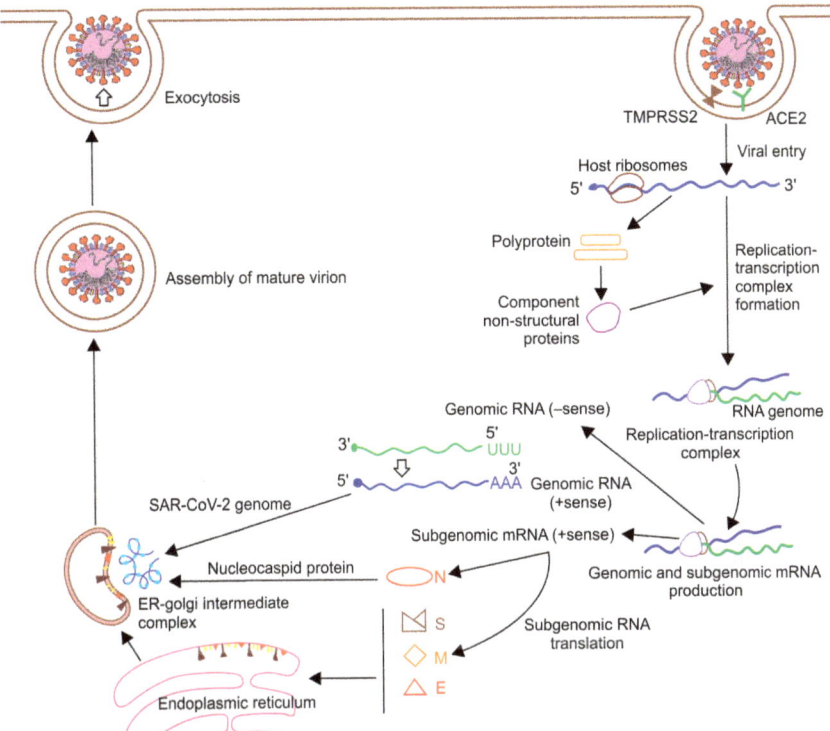

Fig. 1: Severe acute respiratory syndrome coronavirus-2 (SARS-CoV-2) life cycle. (Clockwise from top right) SARS-CoV-2 has Spike (S) protein on its surface which binds to ACE2 on human cells (mainly pulmonary epithelial cells) through the receptor binding domain of its S1 subunit. The S protein is then primed by TMPRSS2 present on the human cells following which the S2 subunit brings about viral fusion with host cell and viral entry. The viral genome which is a single strand RNA is then released into the host cell cytoplasm where, by making use of host cell machinery SARS-CoV-2 polyproteins pp1a and pp1ab are formed. These give rise to non-structural replication proteins of the virus and subsequently the replication-transcription complex is formed. The viral genomic RNA (+ sense) undergoes both replication through a – sense RNA intermediate and transcription to subgenomic RNAs which produce the four main structural proteins—nucleocapsid (N), membrane (M), envelope (E) and spike (S). The nucleocapsid protein directly moves to virion assembly along with the viral genomic RNA produced by replication. The other three structural proteins move through endoplasmic reticulum processing before proceeding to virion assembly. The assembled virions are released by exocytosis from the host cell.
Courtesy: Dr Bisweswar Ojha.

The chief pathological components of COVID-19 are acute respiratory distress syndrome (ARDS), disseminated intravascular coagulation (DIC) and myocardial injury leading to myocarditis and probable arrhythmias including sudden cardiac death.[9] An important entity that has been identified is intravascular coagulopathy limited to the lungs, referred to as diffuse pulmonary intravascular coagulopathy (DPIC).[11] The role of a cytokine storm in the adverse effects of severe COVID-19 has also been a matter of concern.

Cytokine storm which has been documented over the years in several acute infections refers to an upregulation of proinflammatory cytokines such as interleukin-6 (IL-6), IL-1β and tumor necrosis factor alpha (TNFα), and as a corollary several acute phase reactants. It occurs usually later in the disease course and proves to be detrimental to multiple systems.[12]

CLINICAL MANIFESTATIONS OF COVID-19

Similar to other common flus, COVID-19 also presents most commonly with fever, sore throat, and cough with or without expectoration.[13] Rhinorrhea and headache may also occur, and myalgia is often present, especially being complained of by patients in the author's clinical practice. Fatigue often continues in the post-acute illness phase and so does cough. This may, however, be true for most respiratory and other acute viral illnesses. Anosmia, ageusia and diarrhea are other major complaints in COVID-19 patients, reported from different settings worldwide but since large Indian observational studies are still lacking, how much these symptoms serve to have a discriminant value for diagnosis of COVID-19 is unclear.[13] Most viral diseases are multisystem in presentation, and hence the presence of symptoms outside the common ones does not rule out COVID-19. Especially, select groups such as the elderly may present as they do in other etiologies of sepsis, with fever being absent, and instead generalized weakness, delirium, and nonspecific features such as anorexia predominating. The presence of atypical symptoms and signs does not however call for unnecessary panic and should just guide physicians or surgeons toward having a broader diagnostic overview.

In around 10% patients, the disease progresses to severe form and mortality occurs in around 3% of symptomatic COVID-19 patients worldwide. The mortality rate calculation is not accurate in the middle of an epidemic and may need corrections in the future. The current Indian mortality ratio is around 1.44% only, which is much lower than most developed nations, and may be attributable to several biological and environmental factors.[1] Severe COVID-19 disease is characterized by diffuse viral pneumonia, ARDS, respiratory failure and thrombotic and bleeding manifestations due to DIC. Myocarditis resulting in shock and sudden cardiac deaths due to arrhythmias are also possible and a watch needs to be kept for these entities.[14,15] Several patients, especially in India have complained of sudden drops in arterial blood oxygen saturation levels. However, how much of these are true sudden falls, and how much can be attributed to panic, late consultation with doctors, improper use of pulse oximeters or downright faulty pulse oximeters, is unclear at present. Worsening has also been observed in patients who have recovered from the initial fever and respiratory illness. The role of immune phenomena, incomplete resolution, biphasic illness, or bacterial superinfection resulting in such complications needs to be elucidated in large scale studies. Other major severe forms of disease such as cerebral involvement, acute kidney injury, post-COVID autoimmune phenomenon such as Guillain-Barre syndrome, post-COVID pulmonary fibrosis, long COVID syndrome have also been reported but the presence of multiple confounding reports including autopsy studies makes it difficult to rely on these at present.[16-18] One complication noted in particular and reported from multiple countries is multisystem inflammatory syndrome (MIS) in the pediatric age group.[19] This is a syndrome akin to Kawasaki disease in children, but occurs following documented COVID-19 disease. The age group is also slightly higher (median age around 7 years) than that of Kawasaki disease (mostly below 5 years age). The syndrome is characterized by prominent gastrointestinal, cardiovascular, and dermatological involvement, an elevation in the levels of acute phase reactants and sometimes culminating in hyper-inflammatory shock.[19]

STRATIFICATION OF COVID-19 (INDIAN GUIDELINES) AND SETTINGS OF CARE

The Emergency Medical Relief (EMR) division of the Directorate General of Health Services of the Ministry of Health and Family Welfare (MoHFW) of the Government of India provides official guidelines for diagnosis and management of COVID-19 disease in India. These are simplified, periodically updated, and consider both western recommendations and indigenous data and country-specific characteristics of COVID-19 disease. These guidelines have been highly successful in managing the COVID-19 pandemic in India. The latest guidelines were provided in early July 2020. As per these guidelines, a person with laboratory confirmation of SARS-CoV-2 infection irrespective of signs and symptoms is considered to be a confirmed case of COVID-19. Patients more than 60 years of age and those with underlying noncommunicable chronic diseases are considered to be at high risk of severe COVID-19.

Patients are stratified into mild, moderate, and severe. Patients with signs and symptoms of uncomplicated upper respiratory tract infection without breathlessness or hypoxia are considered to have mild COVID-19. It is recommended that these patients should be managed at COVID Care Centers, First Referral Units (FRUs), Community Health Centers (CHC), sub-district, and district hospitals. Moderate COVID-19 cases are those with pneumonia but with no signs of more severe disease. For adults, the severity features which should be present include dyspnea and/or hypoxia, fever, cough, with an arterial blood oxygen saturation of less than 94% on room air or a respiratory rate ≥24 per minute. As per guidelines, these patients should be managed at dedicated COVID Health Centers (DCHCs) or district hospitals or medical college hospitals. Severe COVID-19 comprises three categories of patients, namely those with severe pneumonia, those with ARDS, and those with sepsis or septic shock. Patients with clinically diagnosed pneumonia with at least one of respiratory rate >30/min, severe respiratory distress and arterial blood oxygen saturation <90% on room air, are considered to have severe pneumonia whereas for ARDS and sepsis/septic shock, standard internationally accepted definitions are used. These patients need intensive care.[20]

MEDICAL MANAGEMENT OF COVID-19

The medical management of COVID-19 may be divided into prevention and prophylaxis, diagnosis, and treatment.

Prevention and Prophylaxis

The guidelines of the MoHFW emphasize strict adherence to infection prevention and control practices. These include use of triple layer surgical masks by suspect patients and healthcare practitioners, adequate hand hygiene and social distancing. Cleaning of potential contaminated surfaces should be frequent. Goggles and face shields should be used, and universal surgical and microbiological precautions should be adhered to by healthcare workers providing close contact care to COVID-19 suspects. Use of disposable or dedicated equipment has been proposed and adequate ventilation of rooms is a must. Healthcare workers have also been reminded frequently not to touch the eyes unnecessarily. N95 respirators (fit tested) should be used along with full personal protective equipment (PPE) while caring for laboratory confirmed COVID-19 patients, and also for suspect patients when performing aerosol generating procedures. Hydroxychloroquine and ivermectin have been recommended as prophylaxis against COVID-19 by some Indian organizations. The role of supplemental vitamins B complex, C and D has also been highlighted as immunity enhancers. Vaccines are also being launched after emergency use approval by many drug regulators worldwide. Since guidelines are ever changing, it is prudent to be aware of the latest official versions. Hence, exact regimens are not discussed here.[20]

Diagnosis

Reverse transcriptase polymerase chain reaction (RT-PCR) for SARS-CoV-2 is the gold standard diagnostic test recommended. PCR tests based on the cartridge based nucleic acid amplification test (CBNAAT) or TrueNat platforms may also be utilized for this purpose. Rapid antigen tests aid in screening but a patient with positivity in either of above tests is considered laboratory confirmed case of COVID-19. A patient with symptoms suggestive of COVID-19 but with a negative rapid antigen test should be subjected to RT-PCR based confirmation. Samples for these tests are collected by nasal and oropharyngeal swabs and transported in viral transport media (VTM). On demand testing of patients has now been approved by the government of India, and India is doing a commendable job of testing COVID-19 patients, being second only behind the United States in absolute number of tests performed. Additionally, COVID-19 patients undergo monitoring of fever and vital signs, testing of blood oxygen saturation using pulse oximeters, chest X-ray, routine blood investigations, as necessary. Arterial blood gas monitoring and advanced investigations such as high-resolution computed tomography (HRCT) of the chest may be performed on case by case basis. It is also advisable that patients with moderate to severe disease undergo electrocardiograms, complete blood counts, liver and renal function tests daily, and C-reactive protein, ferritin, and D-dimer levels every 48–72 hours.[21]

Treatment of COVID-19

Adequate rest, a healthy diet, and plenty of fluids are the cornerstone of the management of any acute viral illness, and COVID-19 is no exception to this. Early initiation of basic management results in less chances of complications. Mild cases should be administered symptomatic treatment in the form of antipyretics (paracetamol) and antitussives for cough. Multivitamins including B-complex and C may be prescribed. Hydroxychloroquine may be used in those with risk factors for severe disease after ensuring that there are no contraindications such as underlying cardiac disease, history of unexplained syncope or QT prolongation (>480 ms). Antibiotics are added if there is suspicion of secondary bacterial infection, and this remains a common practice in the Indian scenario.

Moderate and severe cases need escalation of oxygen therapy in steps and as per patient tolerance, in addition to the treatment rendered in mild cases. Broad spectrum antibiotics are often prescribed to these patients as many are managed in intensive care settings with predisposition to secondary infections. Oxygen is administered through face masks or nasal prongs; in case of non-improvement, face mask with reservoir bags, high flow nasal cannula (HFNC), noninvasive ventilation and finally invasive mechanical ventilation are resorted to. A blood oxygen saturation of 92–96% is targeted in patients, and up to 92% in those with chronic obstructive pulmonary disease (COPD). Awake proning should be practiced in those patients with an oxygen requirement of >4 liters/min who have a normal mental status, no hemodynamic instability, and an ability to change position with minimal assistance. Prone positioning is done only when close monitoring of patients is possible. Proning protocols involve 30–120 minutes each in prone position, left and right lateral decubitus, and upright sitting position. Low molecular weight heparin (LMWH) or unfractionated heparin are recommended in all patients with moderate to severe disease without any obvious contraindication to the same and if not at high bleeding risk. The dose of LMWH is 40 mg subcutaneous daily in moderate cases and twice daily in severe cases. Methylprednisolone 0.5–1 mg/kg or dexamethasone 0.1–0.2 mg/kg may be administered intravenously for 3 days with a decision of further continuation based on clinical response. Oral hydroxychloroquine 400 mg twice daily on 1st day followed by 200 mg twice daily for 4 days may be given in moderate cases. Fluid management, management of ARDS and septic shock, prevention of ICU related complications such as pressure sores, stress ulcers, ventilator associated pneumonia, deep venous thrombosis, and management of comorbidities should be as per existing internationally accepted protocols. Investigational agents which are being tried in moderate to severe cases but do not have definite proven value include remdesivir, tocilizumab, and convalescent plasma from patients who have recovered from COVID-19. Latest updates of MoHFW management protocols for COVID-19 should be referred to for dosing and other details of these therapies.[20]

Controversies in Medical Management of COVID-19

Information regarding COVID-19 is being continuously updated and management protocols are changing frequently in line with emerging evidence. The importance of home isolation has been realized with time in resource-constrained settings.[22] Steroids have undergone a paradigm shift in the management of severe COVID-19 after the success of the Recovery trial with dexamethasone.[23] Most proposed drugs such as hydroxychloroquine, remdesivir, favipiravir and tocilizumab have given confounding results in studies and meta-analyses but continue to be used in different setups based on diverse national guidelines and preferences of infectious disease experts. New information regarding the use of ACE inhibitors/angiotensin receptor blockers and benefits of vitamins C and D, ivermectin, zinc, host protease inhibitors such as bromhexine and ammonium chloride continue to emerge.[10,24-28] ICU management protocols, ventilator protocols, and personal safety protocols are also changing day by day. The role of asymptomatic carriers of the virus and the probability of air borne viral transmission are further areas of controversy.[29,30] With time, it has also become clear that mortality due to COVID-19 is indeed low in most developing countries such as in India.[31] It is much lower than that of other contemporary deadly viral diseases such as SARS, MERS, Ebola, Nipah, and even Japanese encephalitis and severe Dengue fever. However, there is a vulnerable subset of patients who easily develop complications and succumb to COVID-19. While initial focus was on elderly patients with comorbidities, in India, even young patients without comorbidities have been observed to die due to COVID-19. This raises the prospect of future research in immune factors and patient-specific factors which may result in aggravated COVID-19 and eventual fatality. Overall, one may say that the management of COVID-19 remains in flux till date. In such a situation, it would be prudent on part of doctors to not be overwhelmed by the media barrage of information and stick to relevant national and international guidelines, aided by clinical sense. It is expected that COVID-19 would stay for a long time and may become endemic gradually. Since we have to live with it, personal hygiene, safe and nutritious diet, and a healthy lifestyle would be the hallmarks of how we continue to deal with this disease.

COVID-19 AND THE SURGICAL PRACTICE

Surgical practice has undergone extensive changes during the COVID-19 crisis, mostly because of the close contact nature of surgical procedures putting surgeons at higher risk. In the past 3 months, almost 3 million surgeries have been cancelled worldwide. A Bayesian beta-regression model has projected that more than 70% surgeries were cancelled, of which more than 90% were for benign conditions. This is bound to have an impact on "life-saving surgeries" as almost 40% of cancer surgeries and 25% of cesarean sections may be postponed too.[32]

For safe global surgical treatment, the COVIDSurg Collaborative has described important points where practice should be updated during the COVID-19 pandemic.[33] These include:

- Prepare a surgical pandemic response plan to delay elective procedures, repurpose operating rooms (OR) as essential areas of treatment and create an organizational workflow.
- Developing a specific plan for emergency surgical services to be rendered.
- Education of workers on personal protective equipment (PPE) and COVID-19 management.
- Recognizing and controlling infections with COVID-19 thus reducing health care workers exposure.
- Developing a dedicated space for COVID-19 operations.[33]

Changes to Surgical Systems

Usage of Surgical Facilities

Hospitals are being reconfigured in expectation of surges in COVID-19 cases to provide more space for critically ill patients. Elective and other regular procedures are cancelled or deferred, allowing critical care units to be used as activity and recovery rooms.

Redeploying Staff

The need for qualified medical professionals to care for them has increased, given the large numbers of expected critically ill patients. The role of surgeons in this is valuable, as patients may perform line insertions and pronunciation while maintaining airway protection and infusion and line management. Critical care nursing may be provided by other healthcare professionals with OR expertise, such as nurses and allied healthcare staff.[34] **Figure 2** delineates the changing positions of qualified surgeons in the setting of the COVID-19 pandemic.

Strategies to use the surgical workforce efficiently are also important. One such technique to reduce the risk of contracting COVID-19 infection when overseeing patients' critical care includes reorganizing the surgical team into

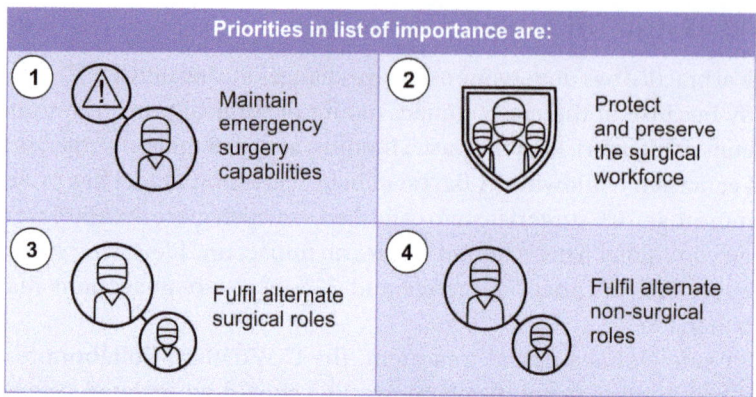

Fig. 2: The changing roles of surgeons in the coronavirus disease 2019 (COVID-19) pandemic.

two groups, one involved in hospitals and one operating remotely in isolation, with both groups rotating at 2-week intervals with each other. An alternative solution is to consolidate the surgical teams into two teams working long (e.g., 12 h) shifts for each day using each available OR in turn (rather than finishing the list of the entire day in a single OR). This gives maximum time for each OR to be deeply cleaned and minimizes the amount of workers who could be potentially exposed in a department.[35]

Prioritizing Patients

In order to prioritize the workload and provide the best possible care under the conditions, stratification of patients into groups is essential. For example, for cancer patients undergoing surgery, NHS England advises that patients should be graded according to clinical necessity into priorities 1–3.[36] It is important to further divide Priority 1 patients into 1a and 1b. 1a includes patients requiring an emergency operation to sustain life within 24 hours; 1b includes patients with acute conditions secondary to their underlying problem which if not operated urgently, may cause irreversible damage, i.e., within 72 hours (e.g., gastrointestinal obstructions, bleeding or compression of the spinal cord). In order to treat and avoid the progression of the disease to an inoperable stage, Priority 2 patients should be operated on within 4 weeks. Priority 3 patients are categorized as those whose operations without harmful effects can be delayed for 10–12 weeks.[36]

Outpatient Clinics and Telemedicine

Where appropriate, face-to-face outpatient appointments could need to be avoided during the COVID-19 pandemic to minimize infection risks. Where these are still relevant, the suggestion is to pursue a policy of "one patient, one place". However, with the exception of emergencies, telemedicine consultation by either telephone services or video conferencing services or applications should be the preferred form of consultation.

Procedural Considerations in Surgery in COVID Times

Five areas, including the use of PPE, minimizing preoperative risks, resolving particular operational risk concerns, mitigating postoperative risks, and keeping others secure, can be divided into considerations for optimum safety when working throughout COVID periods.

Use of Personal Protective Equipment

The US Centers for Disease Control and Prevention (CDC) and Public Health England (PHE) have advised the use of PPE for all procedures involving a patient with known or suspected COVID-19 infection.[37] A higher standard of safety, such as N95 respirators, is recommended for procedures involving aerosol generation (e.g., intubation and extubation) with strict focus on fit testing **(Fig. 3)**.[38] The basic method of discarding disposable PPE should be in line with local policy and strict hand hygiene should be followed.

Reducing Preoperative Risks

Significant concerns for surgical staff are the possibility of COVID-19 transmission by aerosolization and droplets. Bronchoscopy, endotracheal

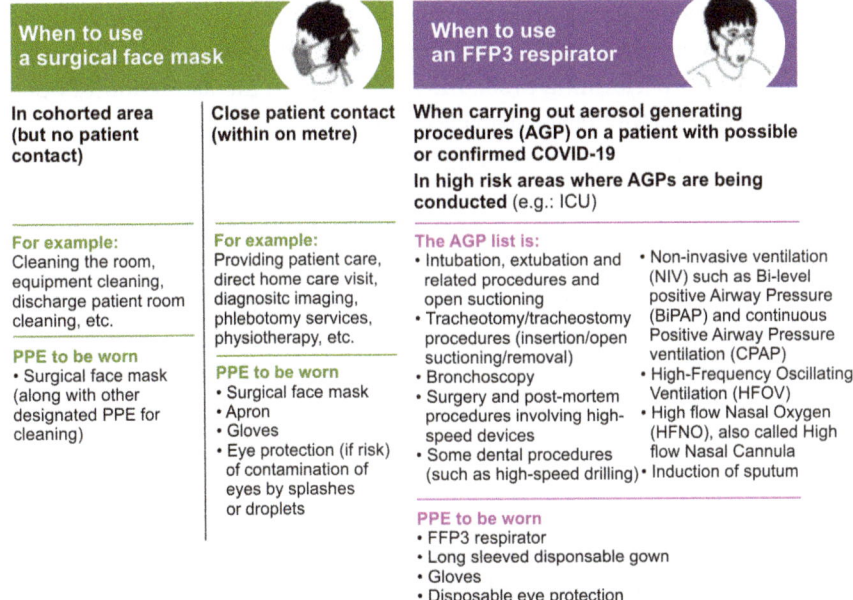

Fig. 3: Public Health England (PHE) guidance on appropriate use of personal protective equipment (PPE).

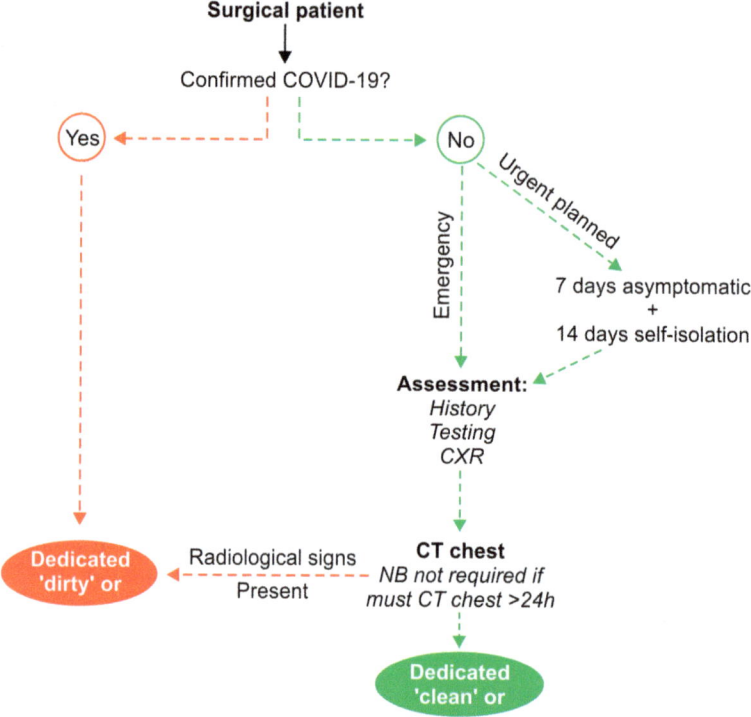

Fig. 4: Surgical preoperative pathway.

intubation, tracheostomy procedures, cardiopulmonary resuscitation, and diagnostic sputum induction are procedures which are believed to produce aerosols. When performing procedures that require the aspiration of body fluids, surgical personnel are at an elevated risk.[39]

The Royal Surgical Colleges of the United Kingdom recommends that all patients planned for priority procedure must have been asymptomatic for 7 days, self-isolated for 14 days, and then have a negative swab within 48 hours of scheduled admission **(Fig. 4)**.[40] COVID-19 using history, RT-PCR for SARS-CoV-2 conducted on swab samples and a chest X-ray should be examined for any patient presenting to the hospital and needing urgent or emergency surgery. In order to exclude COVID-19, any patient undergoing an emergency abdominal computed tomographic scan for acute pain should also undergo a HRCT chest at the same time (unless a prior scan was done in the past 24 hours).

In order to reduce the risk of transmission, the CDC recommends that during aerosol generation operations, non-essential surgeons and staff be excluded from the OR. For example non-essential staff should wait outside the OR while anesthesia induction and intubation are completed when dealing with a confirmed or suspected COVID-19 event. In addition, prior to entering the OR, even critical staff should be checked for temperature.[41]

Ergonomics is also important for the control of infections. Dexter et al. recommends double gloving during induction and putting alcohol or chlorhexidine hand rub on the IV pole to the left of the anesthetist and a wire basket lined with a zip closure plastic bag on the IV pole to the right as a designated dirty area to position infected instruments such as laryngoscopes, among other evidence-based perioperative recommendations. It is also advised to use an updated COVID-19 version of the WHO Safety Surgery Checklist. Cross-contamination can be avoided by designating dedicated PPE donning and doffing areas.

In order to avoid contaminating general equipment shops, another suggestion is to use pre-prepared bags of equipment. This might involve intubation sets (such as laryngoscopes and airway devices), intravenous access sets, monitoring sets for transportation (such as blood pressure and ECG equipment) and medication sets (such as muscle relaxants and sedatives) that are frequently used. To prevent frequent contamination, "high-touch" appliances such as displays, nursing stations and aesthetic workstations should be wrapped up.[42] In addition, to reduce risk, modifications can be made to the OR ventilation systems. The OR should be set to have a high frequency of air flow adjustments (about 25 per hour) during the activity of patients with COVID-19 to optimize viral load reduction. By incorporating low-velocity airflow directed toward exhaust outlets, contaminant diffusion is further reduced. In addition, as this acts as a filtration buffer, workers in neighboring areas will benefit from negative pressurization in ORs. An official CDC recommendation now is negative pressurization in ORs.

Tackling Specific Operative Risk Issues

During an operation on a COVID-19 patient, there are a range of steps that must be taken to protect critical operating team members. During these procedures, surgical practitioners should pay additional attention to any needle stick injuries or PPE injury. The lowest power setting should be used when using electrocautery, and a smoke evacuator should also be used to reduce exposure to surgical smoke and any possible aerosolized virus particles.[41]

For potentially infectious patients undergoing surgical procedures, the Public Health England has also proposed protocols.[43] This include the placing of a surgical mask on the patient during the transfer to and from the OR the anesthetization (and recovery) of the patient in the OR rather than the anesthetic space, the use of single-use instruments whenever practicable, the decontamination of surgical instruments by usual procedure, the reduction of personnel to a minimum and the placement of all operations on patients with COVID-19 verified or suspected at the end of the list.

Laparoscopy/Endoscopy

During laparoscopy, there is a potential possibility of SARS-CoV-2 transmission as it is an aerosol producing technique and as other viruses have also been found in surgical smoke.[44] In addition, it was proposed by Tao et al.[41] that laparoscopy should be avoided in patients with reduced lung volume due to artificial pneumoperitoneum, which may cause increased airway pressure, CO_2 retention, and decreased lung compliance. Zheng et al.[45] documented their experiences in China and Italy of minimally invasive surgery and suggested the use of minimally viable insufflation pressures and liberal intraperitoneal suction, as well as minimizing the use of the role of Trendelenburg. In addition, the Royal Surgical Colleges of Great Britain recommends that laparoscopy should only be conducted in select cases where the risk of viral transmission to surgical personnel may be clinically justified.[40] The Society of American Gastrointestinal and Endoscopic Surgeons advises that incisions should be made as minimal as possible to prevent leakage, that insufflation pressures should be held to a minimum, that smoke evacuation systems should be used, and that prior to extracting specimens, trocars or port closure, CO_2 insufflation should be switched off and vented via a philtre.[46-48]

Mitigating Postoperative Risks

As part of the modification of the normal patient flow, patients should be recovered in the OR, both to reduce the risk of spread and because of the repurposing of the regular surgical recovery area. A single dose of 5-HT3 antagonist (such as ondansetron) or metoclopramide should also be offered to patients to reduce postoperative nausea and vomiting that may result in further spread. It is important to mark surgical specimens as suspected COVID-19 and seal them in the OR. Furthermore all body fluids, disposable supplies, tubing, gowns and PPE should be double-bagged, identified with an OR sign with a confirmed/suspected COVID-19 patient and disposed of in compliance with local guidelines for infectious waste. Subsequently, according to local protocols, the OR must be disinfected, which can involve disinfection of high-touch surfaces such as the operating table and anesthetic system with at least 75% alcohol or chlorine disinfectant. In addition, with a neutral detergent accompanied by a chlorine-based solution with a minimum strength of no less than 1,000 ppm of chlorine, other surfaces in the OR should be thoroughly washed after each activity. This is particularly significant as the virus is known to live on surfaces for a long time without adequate decontamination.[49]

It is also important to reduce the number of staff involved in transporting confirmed or suspected COVID patients and to provide a dedicated route for the transfer of suspected COVID-19 patients. Then all transportation team members should wear different PPE to what was given during the operation, and a respirator should be given to the patient to wear according to local protocols. In the postoperative period, patients should be closely monitored because postoperative pulmonary complications are not unusual and late complications of COVID-19 should be treated as part of a differential diagnosis alongside aspiration pneumonia or pulmonary embolism.[50]

Keeping Others Safe

Many frontline employees share their places of residence with relatives or friends who live in the same apartment or flat. Therefore an understandable fear about passing on the infection occurs. Although hospitals and healthcare facilities may provide housing for staff living with vulnerable people (e.g., the elderly and the immunocompromised), this is not a viable choice for all. In addition, it is important to consider the total reduction in physical interaction with family and friends. If healthcare professionals are at all worried about potential SARS-CoV-2 infection, they should contact their occupational health service and begin monitoring their temperature and any other symptoms.

IMPACT OF COVID-19 ON SURGICAL EDUCATION, TRAINING, AND RESEARCH

It is expected that the pandemic would bring an unforeseen disruption to the provision of surgical education. Undoubtedly, with the suspension of regular training rotation, undergraduate medical education and training of surgical residents would suffer. Also several surgical educational conferences have been cancelled or postponed, reducing the amount of surgical trainee learning opportunities. Hospitals also enrolled surgical residents in nursing workshops for critical care, helping them to assist key allies. Before they begin new positions, ensuring safe practice, there has been a strong focus on deployed trainees having suitable induction and supervision. In order to compensate for the lack of experience, many national and international academic surgical organizations are coming up with modern and technology-aided learning programs.

Due to the COVID-19 pandemic, surgical testing, both laboratory and clinically focused, has been halted, with several academic surgeons being redeployed to the clinical environment to help treat COVID-19 patients.[39] Nevertheless, organizations such as the University of Birmingham and the Global Surgery Unit of the National Institute for Health Research (NIHR) are generating and making good use of international collaborative data in the real world in the process of developing new research areas, especially in the field of COVID-19.

Recovery of Surgical Services

A substantial backlog will eventually arise from the postponement of nonurgent surgical services. This has a huge effect, both on the surgical system's ability and at a personal level, causing patients to feel intense stress and anxiety. One study found that 30% of patients who had postponed operations during winter stresses complained of severe stress and anger, as well as considerable concern about their condition deteriorating.[51]

A plan for the resumption of normal services has been outlined by the Royal College of Ophthalmology. This consists of a provisional cycle of incremental resumption of activities while retaining surge capability over the next 12–18 months in the event of more COVID-19 peaks (Recovery phase 1: interim period) and a longer period (Recovery phase 2: the new normal). Additionally, nine main elements for the short-term recovery of surgical services have been developed by the Royal College of Surgeons (RCS) England.[52] These are:

- Main considerations before the resumption of elective services—decreasing numbers, adequate testing capability and PPE are identified
- Establishing unified leadership and regular contact mechanism with daily clinical feedback by a committed local recovery management team
- Evaluation of surgical workload and populations of patients—baseline demand assessment and patient prioritization
- Ensuring ample capacity and facilities for hospitals—temporary field hospitals and facilities for the private sector
- Staff capability enhancement—management of temporary redeployment
- Reconfiguring services: "Cold" free COVID-19 sites, patient testing protocols for COVID-19, triage protocols, virtual clinics and patient-initiated reviews
- Supporting the surgical workforce—sufficient PPE and testing, monitoring of burnout and well-being of the surgical workforce
- Communication with patients
- Training support: Development of trainees, cross-specialty learning from workers deployed.[52]

Surgical Specialty Guidelines

Oncological Surgery

In cancer patients it is routine that most complex elective surgical procedures receive ward-based care postoperatively. The NHS has identified cancer patients who are most at risk during the outbreak and who are likely to become seriously unwell if they were to contract the virus. These include patients on active chemotherapy or radiotherapy, immunotherapy or any antibody treatments, or immune system modulation therapy. Surgical teams are encouraged to offer telephone or video consultations when possible, cancel follow-ups which are deemed nonessential, limit the time patients spend on services, and follow a scheduled appointment time system.

Breast Cancer Surgery

Surgeons are encouraged to maximize breast conserving surgery when possible, as definitive mastectomy and/or reconstruction may be deferred if radiotherapy options are available. Surgeons should also consider alternative, nonsurgical therapy where possible.[53]

Colorectal Cancer Surgery

In locally advanced resectable colon cancer, surgeons are urged to consider neoadjuvant chemotherapy and revisit the idea of surgery in 2-3 months. Diverting stomas should be utilized or given preference to over anastomoses, to reduce the risk of postoperative complications such as anastomotic leaks.

General Surgery

An essential element of surgical service planning is the delivery of emergency general surgery. It is important to ensure that this continues as normal wherever possible for both patients infected with COVID-19 or not. Furong et al. have suggested that high ACE2 receptor expressions in the pancreas may be a cause of mild pancreatitis in patients infected with SARS-CoV-2 and advice clinicians to remain vigilant of this phenomenon. In cases of progression to necrotizing pancreatitis during the COVID-19 pandemic, percutaneous and interventional radiology (IR) drainage strategies should be favored.[54]

Trauma Surgery

Nonoperative management may be appropriate for certain hemodynamically stable trauma patients with solid organ injury. However, the surgeon needs to keep in mind coagulopathy including DIC that is seen often in COVID patients. In hemodynamically unstable trauma patients or those with ruptured abdominal aortic aneurysm, hollow viscus perforation, intestinal ischemia, and intestinal obstruction, an appropriate surgical approach should be wisely chosen.

Transplant Surgery

COVID-19 is having a significant impact on organ donation services worldwide. As the pandemic evolves, the transplant community faces various challenges, from allocation of resources and consenting patients, to optimizing immunosuppressive medication in patients with suspected COVID-19 infections.[55] Currently, there is a limited amount of data to draw firm conclusions on the effect of COVID-19 on organ transplantation.

Vascular Surgery

The Vascular Society of Great Britain and Ireland have issued guidance for clinicians on the impact of COVID-19 on vascular surgery services. Regarding outpatients, only urgent cases should be seen, and virtual clinics considered. Regarding surgical procedures, most arterial surgery is either classified as urgent or emergency and should therefore continue where possible. Elective procedures, venous surgery, and asymptomatic conditions requiring intervention should be deferred.[56]

CONCLUSION

The impact of COVID-19 on surgical practice and education has been profound. Elective surgeries have been cancelled or postponed widely. While this has enabled surgeons to take up a critical care role to manage the pandemic, their core areas of work have suffered. Conservative and radiologically guided minimally invasive procedures have started flourishing. Surgeons all over have however worked out of their skins to make unhindered emergency care a reality. With the possibility of SARS-CoV-2 becoming an endemic coronavirus, it is imperative for surgeons to function in close coordination with other medical and auxiliary staff to adequately address patient care during and after COVID-19.

REFERENCES

1. Chakrabarti SS, Kaur U, Banerjee A, Ganguly U, Banerjee T, Saha S, et al. COVID-19 in India: Are Biological and Environmental Factors Helping to Stem the Incidence and Severity? Aging Dis. 2020;11(3):480.
2. Worldometers. COVID-19 Coronavirus pandemic. Available from: https://www.worldometers.info/coronavirus/. [Last Accessed January, 2021].
3. Centers for Disease Control and Prevention. Human Coronavirus Types. Available from: https://www.cdc.gov/coronavirus/types.html. [Last Accessed January, 2020].
4. Andersen KG, Rambaut A, Lipkin WI, Holmes EC, Garry RF. The proximal origin of SARS-CoV-2. Nat Med. 2020;26(4):450-2.
5. Zhang T, Wu Q, Zhang Z. Probable Pangolin Origin of SARS-CoV-2 Associated with the COVID-19 Outbreak. Curr Biol. 2020;30(7):1346-1351.e2.
6. Patel KP, Vunnam SR, Patel PA, Krill KL, Korbitz PM, Gallagher JP, et al. Transmission of SARS-CoV-2: an update of current literature. Eur J Clin Microbiol Infect Dis. 2020;39(11):2005-11.
7. Olaimat AN, Shahbaz HM, Fatima N, Munir S, Holley RA. Food Safety During and after the Era of COVID-19 Pandemic. Front Microbiol. 2020:11.
8. Hoffmann M, Kleine-Weber H, Schroeder S, Krüger N, Herrler T, Erichsen S, et al. SARS-CoV-2 Cell Entry Depends on ACE2 and TMPRSS2 and is Blocked by a Clinically Proven Protease Inhibitor. Cell. 2020;181(2):271-280.e8.
9. Kaur U, Acharya K, Mondal R, Singh A, Saso L, Chakrabarti S, et al. Should ACE2 be given a chance in COVID-19 therapeutics: a semi-systematic review of strategies enhancing ACE2. Eur J Pharmacol. 2020;887:173545.
10. Kaur U, Chakrabarti SS, Ojha B, Pathak BK, Singh A, Saso L, et al. Targeting host cell proteases to prevent SARS-CoV-2 invasion. Curr Drug Targets. 2020;21.
11. McGonagle D, O'Donnell JS, Sharif K, Emery P, Bridgewood C. Immune mechanisms of pulmonary intravascular coagulopathy in COVID-19 pneumonia. Lancet Rheumatol. 2020;2(7):e437-45.
12. Clark IA, Alleva LM, Budd AC, Cowden WB. Understanding the role of inflammatory cytokines in malaria and related diseases. Travel Med Infect Dis. 2008;6(1-2):67-81.
13. Johnson KD, Harris C, Cain JK, Hummer C, Goyal H, Perisetti A. Pulmonary and Extra-Pulmonary Clinical Manifestations of COVID-19. Front Med. 2020:7.
14. World Health Organization. Clinical Management Novel Coronavirus. Available from: https://www.who.int/csr/disease/coronavirus_infections/ InterimGuidance_ ClinicalManagement_NovelCoronavirus_11Feb13u.pdf/. [Last Accessed January, 2020].

15. Shafi AMA, Shaikh SA, Shirke MM, Iddawela S, Harky A. Cardiac manifestations in COVID-19 patients—A systematic review. J Card Surg. 2020;35(8):1988-2008.
16. Cheng Y, Luo R, Wang K, Zhang M, Wang Z, Dong L, et al. Kidney disease is associated with in-hospital death of patients with COVID-19. Kidney Int. 2020;97(5):829-38.
17. Yuan W, Liu S, Lu L, Feng J, He X. Clinical interventions for severe and critical COVID-19: what are the options. Am J Transl Res. 2020;12(5):2110-7.
18. Ellul MA, Benjamin L, Singh B, Lant S, Michael BD, Easton A, et al. Neurological associations of COVID-19. Lancet Neurol. 2020;19(9):767-83.
19. Abrams JY, Godfred-Cato SE, Oster ME, Chow EJ, Koumans EH, Bryant B, et al. Multisystem Inflammatory Syndrome in Children Associated with Severe Acute Respiratory Syndrome Coronavirus 2: a systematic review. J Pediatr. 2020;226:45-54.e1.
20. Ministry of Health and Family Welfare Government of India. Updated Clinical Management Prootocol for COVID-19. Available from: https://www.mohfw.gov.in/pdf/UpdatedClinicalManagementProtocolforCOVID19dated03072020.pdf. [Last Accessed October, 2020].
21. Indian Council of Medical Research. Advisory on Strategy for COVID-19 Testing in India. Available from: https://www.icmr.gov.in/pdf/covid/strategy/Testing_Strategy_v6_04092020.pdf. [Last Accessed October, 2020].
22. Ministry of Health and Family Welfare Government of India. Revised guidelines for Home Isolation of very mild/pre-symptomatic/asymptomatic COVID-19 cases. Available from: https://www.mohfw.gov.in/pdf/RevisedHomeIsolationGuidelines.pdf?pfrom=home-coronavirus-drsadvice_live. [Last Accessed October, 2020].
23. The RECOVERY Collaborative Group. Dexamethasone in Hospitalized Patients with Covid-19 — Preliminary Report. N Engl J Med. 2020:2021436.
24. Kaur U, Chakrabarti SS, Patel TK. RAAS blockers and region-specific variations in COVID-19 outcomes: findings from a systematic review and meta-analysis. medRxiv. 2020:20191445.
25. Simonson W. Vitamin C and coronavirus. Geriatr Nurs (Minneap). 2020;41(3):331-2.
26. Bergman P. The link between vitamin D and COVID-19: distinguishing facts from fiction. J Intern Med. 2020:13158.
27. Kumar A, Kubota Y, Chernov M, Kasuya H. Potential role of zinc supplementation in prophylaxis and treatment of COVID-19. Med Hypotheses. 2020;144:109848.
28. Heidary F, Gharebaghi R. Ivermectin: a systematic review from antiviral effects to COVID-19 complementary regimen. J Antibiot (Tokyo). 2020;73(9):593-602.
29. Tan J, Liu S, Zhuang L, Chen L, Dong M, Zhang J, et al. Transmission and clinical characteristics of asymptomatic patients with SARS-CoV-2 infection. Future Virol. 2020;15(6):373-80.
30. Tang S, Mao Y, Jones RM, Tan Q, Ji JS, Li N, et al. Aerosol transmission of SARS-CoV-2? Evidence, prevention and control. Environ Int. 2020;144:106039.
31. Chakrabarti SS, Kaur U, Singh A, Chakrabarti S, Agrawal B, Mittal A, et al. Of Cross-Immunity, Herd Immunity and Country-Specific Plans: experiences from COVID-19 in India. Aging Dis. 2020;11(6):1339-44.
32. MedScape. Global COVID-19 Pandemic Could Lead to 28 Million Surgeries Canceled Worldwide. Available from: https://www.medscape.com/viewarticle/931548. [Last Accessed January, 2020].
33. Global guidance for surgical care during the COVID-19 pandemic. Br J Surg. 2020;107(9):1097-103.
34. NHS England. (2020). Clinical guide to adult critical care during the coronavirus pandemic: staffing framework. Available from: https://www.england.nhs.uk/coronavirus/wpcontent/uploads/sites/52/2020/03/C0087-specialty-guide-critical-care-standardoperating-procedure-and-coronavirus-v1-28-march.pdf. [Last Accessed January, 2020].

35. Dexter F, Parra MC, Brown JR, Loftus RW. Perioperative COVID-19 Defense: an Evidence-Based Approach for Optimization of Infection Control and Operating Room Management. Anesth Analg. 2020;131(1):37-42.
36. NHS England. Clinical guide for the management of noncoronavirus patients requiring acute treatment: Cancer. Available from: https://www.england.nhs.uk/coronavirus/wpcontent/uploads/sites/52/2020/03/specialty-guide-acute-treatment-cancer-23-march-2020.pdf. [Last Accessed January, 2020].
37. Centers for Disease Control and Prevention. Donning PPE. Available from: https://www.cdc.gov/vhf/ebola/hcp/ppe-training/n95respirator_gown/donning_01.html. [Last Accessed January, 2020].
38. Public Health England. When to use a surgical face mask or FFP3 respirator. Available from: https://www.gov.uk/government/publications/wuhan-novel-coronavirusinfection-prevention-and-control. [Last Accessed January, 2020].
39. American College of Surgeons. COVID-19: considerations for optimum surgeon protection before, during, and after operation. [online] Available from: https://www.facs.org/covid-19/clinical-guidance/surgeon-protection. [Last Accessed January, 2020].
40. Royal College of Surgeons of Edinburgh. Intercollegiate guidance for preoperative chest CT imaging for elective cancer surgery during the COVID-19 pandemic. Available from: https://www.rcsed.ac.uk/news-public-affairs/news/2020/april/intercollegiateguidance-for-pre-operative-chest-ct-imaging-for-elective-cancer-surgery-duringthe-covid-19-pandemic. [Last Accessed January, 2020].
41. Tao KX, Zhang BX, Zhang P, Zhu P, Wang GB, Chen XP, et al. Recommendations for general surgery clinical practice in 2019 coronavirus disease situation. Zhonghua Wai Ke Za Zhi. 2020;58(3):170-7.
42. Wong J, Goh QY, Tan Z, Lie SA, Tay YC, Ng SY, et al. Preparing for a COVID-19 pandemic: a review of operating room outbreak response measures in a large tertiary hospital in Singapore. Can J Anesth Can d'anesthésie. 2020;67(6):732-45.
43. Public Health England. Reducing the risk of transmission of COVID-19 in the hospital setting. Available from: https://www.gov.uk/government/publications/wuhan-novelcoronavirus-infection-prevention-and-control/reducing-the-risk-of-transmissionof-covid-19-in-the-hospital-setting. [Last Accessed January, 2020].
44. DesCôteaux JG, Picard P, Poulin ÉC, Baril M. Preliminary study of electrocautery smoke particles produced in vitro and during laparoscopic procedures. Surg Endosc. 1996;10(2):152-8.
45. Zheng MH, Boni L, Fingerhut A. Minimally Invasive Surgery and the Novel Coronavirus Outbreak: Lessons Learned in China and Italy. Ann Surg. 2020;272(1):e5-6.
46. Schultz L. Can Efficient Smoke Evacuation Limit Aerosolization of Bacteria? AORN J. 2015;102(1):7-14.
47. SAGES. Resources for Smoke and Gas Evacuation During Open, Laparoscopic, and endoscopic procedures. Available from: https://www.sages.org/resources-smoke-gas-evacuationduring-open-laparoscopic-endoscopic-procedures/. [Last Accessed January, 2020].
48. SAGES. SAGES and EAES recommendations regarding surgical response to COVID-19 crisis. Available from: https://www.sages.org/recommendations-surgical-response-covid-19/. [Last Accessed January, 2020].
49. van Doremalen N, Bushmaker T, Morris DH, Holbrook MG, Gamble A, Williamson BN, et al. Aerosol and Surface Stability of SARS-CoV-2 as Compared with SARS-CoV-1. N Engl J Med. 2020;382(16):1564-7.
50. Aminian A, Safari S, Razeghian-Jahromi A, Ghorbani M, Delaney CP. COVID-19 Outbreak and Surgical Practice. Ann Surg. 2020;272(1):e27-9.
51. Herrod PJJ, Adiamah A, Boyd-Carson H, Daliya P, El-Sharkawy AM, Sarmah PB, et al. Winter cancellations of elective surgical procedures in the UK: a questionnaire survey of patients on the economic and psychological impact. BMJ Open. 2019;9(9):e028753.

52. Royal College of Surgeons of England. Recovery of surgical services during and after COVID-19. Available from: https://www.rcseng.ac.uk/coronavirus/recovery-of-surgicalservices/. [Last Accessed January, 2020].
53. Zhao L, Zhang L, Liu JW, Yang ZF, Shen WZ, Li XR. The treatment proposal for the patients with breast diseases in the central epidemic area of 2019 coronavirus disease. Zhonghua Wai Ke Za Zhi. 2020;58(5):331-6.
54. Association of Coloproctology of Great Britain and Ireland. Urgent Intercollegiate General Surgery Guidance on COVID-19. Available from: https://www.acpgbi.org.uk/news/urgent-intercollegiate-general-surgery-guidance-on-covid-19. [Last Accessed January, 2020].
55. Moris D, Shaw BI, Dimitrokallis N, Barbas AS. Organ donation during the coronavirus pandemic: an evolving saga in uncharted waters. Transpl Int. 2020;33(7):826-7.
56. Vascular Society of Great Britain and Ireland. COVID-19 Virus and Vascular Surgery. Available from: https://www.vascularsociety.org.uk/professionals/news/113/covid19_virus_and_vascular_surgery. [Last Accessed January, 2020].

Index

Page numbers followed by *b* refer to box, *f* refer to figure, *fc* refer to flowchart, and *t* refer to table.

A

Abdominal sepsis 147, 149
  antimicrobial therapy for 149*t*
  guidelines for empirical antibiotics therapy in 148
  principles of management of 147
Abdominal surgery, antibiotics 137
Acardiac, cases of 40
Acinetobacter 142
Acland's test 222
Acral lentiginous melanoma 160*f*
Acute respiratory distress syndrome 275
Adenocarcinoma 77
Adsorbents 56
Ageusia 276
American College of Surgeons Oncology Group 174
American Joint Committee on Cancer 164, 166*t*, 232
American Medical System 64
American Society of Clinical Oncology 79
American Society of Gastrointestinal Endoscopy 123*t*
American Thyroid Association 256
Amitriptyline 56
Amniocentesis 39
Amniotic bands division 40
Amniotic cavity 45*f*
Amniotic fluid, complications of 46
Ampulla of Vater 118
Ampullary
  stenosis 119
  tumor 119
Amputated hand, replantation of 227*f*
Anal canal sensation 49
Anal manometry 55
Anal plug 57
Anal repair (post), result of 63*t*
Anal sphincter 66*f*
  anatomy of 49*f*
  artificial 64, 65*t*
  complex, anatomy of 48
  external 48
  internal 48

Anastomosis 220
  failure of 222
Angiogenesis inhibitors 73
Anidulafungin 149
Anomalous pancreatobiliary
  junction 120
  maljunction 119
Anorectal manometry 53
Anorectal surgery 50
Anosmia 276
Antibiotics
  broad spectrum 279
  de-escalation of 6
  resistance, emergence of 6
Anticoagulation agents 224
Antidiarrheals 56
Antimicrobial prophylaxis 140*t*
  duration of 139
  practice of 138
Antimicrobial therapy 148
  duration of 149
Antireflux mucosectomy 112
Antityrosine kinase 82
Antrum, posterior wall of 16*f*
Aortic stenosis 39
Apatinib 73
Appendicitis, acute 139, 143 145
  antibiotics for 143
  antimicrobial prophylaxis for 145*t*
Appetite, loss of 14
Areolar, bilateral 269
Artificial intelligence, advent of 113
Aspire Assist System 112
Atraumatic technique 222
Atropine 56
Autofluorescence imaging 92
Autoimmune phenomenon 277
Avibactam 148
Axillary
  adenopathy 233
  bilateral 269
Axillobilateral breast
  approach 268
  bilateral 268
Azoles 149

B

Bacterial infection
  diagnosis of 5
  differentiation of 5
Bacteroides 153
  fragilis 143, 152
  species accounts 148
Balanitis, chronic 194
Balloon dilatation 39
Barrett's esophagus 93
Basaloid carcinoma 199
Benign
  biliary stricture 119, 130
  follicular cells 262
  phyllodes tumor 246
Beta coronaviruses 274
Bethesda system 261*t*
Bethesda System for Reporting Thyroid Cytopathology 258
Bevacizumab 73, 80, 83, 86
Bile duct dilatation 124*f*
  causes of 129
Bile duct
  polyp 120
  radiological evaluation of 119
Bile salt binders 56
Biliary dilatation, causes of 120*t*, 125*f*
Biliary obstruction 129
Biliary procedures 141
  antibiotics for 139
Biliary strictures 128
Biliary system 118
Biliary tract
  cancer 86
  imaging, recent advances in 130
  procedures, antimicrobial prophylaxis for 142*t*
Biliary, type 120
Biofeedback training 56
Biomarkers 2
  associated with phyllodes 249
  newer 8
  role of 132, 210
Biopsy 164
  histopathologic examination 200
  Tru-Cut 256
  types of 165*t*
    excisional biopsy 165
    punch biopsy 165
    shave biopsy 165
  virtual 94

Bleomycin 210
Blood monocyte expression, circulating 10
Blumer's shelf 14
Body mass index 232
Bowel anastomosis 267
Bowel management 56
Bowel preparation 59
  mechanical 150
Bowel sphincter, artificial 64*f*, 65*t*
Bowen's disease 195
Brachytherapy 107
Breast approaches 268
Breast cancer, inflammatory 232, 235, 238
  clinical signs of 233*f*
  differential diagnosis 237
  genetics in 236
  imaging 233
  locoregional treatment for 238
  pathology 235
  prognosis 240
  significance in 237
  symptoms and signs 233
  treatment 237
Breast cancer, surgery 288
Breast cancer syndromes 236
Breast erythema 232
Breast lesion 234*f*
Breast reconstruction 226*f*
Breslow's thickness 172
Bursectomy, role of 20
Buschke-Löwenstein tumor 195

C

Cabozantinib 211
Calcific pancreatitis, chronic 119
Calcitonin gene-related peptide 1 4
Candida glabrata 149
Capecitabine 78
Carbapenems 147
Carboplatin 238
Carcinogenesis, role in 74*f*
Carcinoma in situ 194, 203
Carcinosarcomas 244
Caspofungin 149
Cediranib 73
Cefazoline 138, 145
Ceftazidime 148
Ceftolozane 148
Ceftriaxone 138

Celiac disease 93
Celiac plexus neurolysis 100
Cell death-ligand 1 77
Cell free DNA 8
Cell membrane 74*f*
Cell pathways 70
Cell proliferation, signaling pathways 74*f*
Cell-mediated 4
Centers for Disease Control and Prevention 137
Cervical lymphadenopathy 258*f*
Cetuximab 79-81, 86
Charged couple devices 92
Chemolabeled 71
Chemotherapy 69, 207
　for advanced disease 210
Chimeric monoclonal antibody 70
Cholangiocarcinoma 119, 120
　advanced 86
Cholangiography, intraoperative 125
Cholangiopancreatoscopy 131
Cholangioscopy 96
Cholecystitis 104
　acute 141, 143, 143*t*
　　antibiotics for 141
　mild acute 143
　severe 143
Choledochal cyst 119, 120, 127, 128*f*
Choledochoduodenostomy 101-103
Choledocholithiasis 122
　presence of 123*t*
　risk for 123
Chorion villus sampling 39
Chromoendoscopy, virtual 93
Cigarette smoking 193
Circumcision, role of 203
Cisplatin 210
Clindamycin 145
Clonorchis sinensis infection 119
Clostridium difficile infection 139
Clostridium species 141
Coagulase negative Staphylococci 137
Coagulation 223
Codeine 56
Coil and glue, combination of 106
Colonic mucus lining 151
Colonic transit time 49
Colorectal bowel malignancy 79
Colorectal cancer 79
　advanced 80*t*
　surgery 289

Colorectal, lateral spreading tumors 110
Colorectal surgery 150
　antibiotic prophylaxis for 151
　antibiotic therapy in 150
　emergency antibiotics for 152
　evolution of 150
Common bile duct 101, 103, 118, 120*f*, 124*f*
　dilatation 122, 126, 128, 130
Community Health Centers 277
Continuous sutures 221
Contrast-enhanced computed tomography 256
Contrast-enhanced endoscopic ultrasound 99
Convoluted neural network 113
Cordocentesis 39
Corpora cavernosa 206*f*
Corticotrophin 82
Coupling devices 228
COVID-19 273-289
　adverse effects of 275
　and surgical practice 281
　changes to surgical systems 281
　clinical manifestations of 276
　control of infections 285
　diagnosis 278
　endoscopy 285
　Indian guidelines 277
　infection 283
　laparoscopy 285
　medical management of 278, 280
　mitigating postoperative risks 286
　on surgical education, training, and research 287
　outpatient clinics and telemedicine 282
　pandemic 281, 282*f*
　prioritizing patients 282
　procedural considerations in surgery 283
　recovery of surgical services 287
　reducing preoperative risks 283
　risk of transmission 284
　surgical practice in 273
　surgical specialty guidelines 288
　suspects 278
　syndrome 277
　tackling specific operative risk issues 285
　treatment of 279

Cowden syndrome 257
C-reactive protein 3
Cutaneous melanoma, management of 176
Cystic adenomatoid malformation, congenital 44
Cytology 256, 261
Cytoreductive surgery 25
Cytotoxic chemotherapy 80, 177

D

Dacron-impregnated silastic sling 58
Damage-Associated Molecular Patterns 7
Deep inferior epigastric artery perforator flap 226f
Deep learning 113
Deep neural network 113
Defecography 54, 55
Dermal lymphatic
 emboli, presence of 232
 tumor emboli 236f
Dermal tumor emboli 233
Desmoplastic melanoma 161
Dexamethasone 279
Diaphragmatic hernia, congenital 34, 40, 43
Diarrhea-inducing foods 55
Diarrheal states 50
Diffuse pulmonary intravascular coagulopathy 275
Digital image analysis 132
Dilated bile duct, evaluation of 131
Diphenoxylate hydrochloride 56
Disseminated infection 3
Distal body 20
Distal fingertip replantations 225
Distal gastrectomy, open 26
Distal margin 24
Distal tumors 20
Distant metastases 198, 245
 assessment for 200
Diverticulitis 139
DNA proliferation, digital image analysis 132
DNA repair mechanisms 86
Docetaxel 210
Dopamine 82
Doppler flow patterns 222
Ductal system 101
Duodenal 25

Duodenal bypass 28
Duodenal mucosal resurfacing 113
Duodenal obstruction 102f

E

Echinocandins 149
Edema 232
EGFR (HER-1), targeting 73
Elasticity index 260
Elastography 259
Electromyography 54
Electronic chromoendoscopy techniques 92
Electronic cylindrical phased array 132
Embolectomy 223
Emergency medical relief 277
Endoanal ultrasonography 53f
Endocrine neoplasia, multiple 257
Endocytoscopy 94
Endoplasmic reticulum processing 275f
Endorectal ultrasonography 52
Endoscopic bariatric, advances in 112
Endoscopic equipment 268
Endoscopic findings, correlation of 93
Endoscopic full thickness resection 111
Endoscopic imaging, advances in 92
Endoscopic mucosal resection 16, 112
Endoscopic myotomy
 conventional 109
 per oral 107-109, 109f
 per rectal 108
Endoscopic resection 16
Endoscopic retrograde cholangiopancreatography 95, 103, 121
 advances in 95
 guided photodynamic therapy 96
 guided radiofrequency ablation 96
Endoscopic sleeve gastroplasty 113
Endoscopic submucosal dissection 16, 17, 110, 112
Endoscopic surgical approach to LND 209
Endoscopic tunneling, per oral 108
Endoscopic ultrasound 123
 choledochoduodenostomy 102f
 diagnostic, advances in 97
 elastography 98f
 elastography 98t
 guided 107f
 biliary drainage 100, 101

Endoscopic ultrasound-guided
  biliary drainage, techniques of 103*t*
  cancer therapy 106
  elastography 97
  gallbladder drainage 104
  gastrojejunostomy 105
  pancreatic duct drainage 104, 104*f*
  tissue acquisition, advances in 99
  vascular interventions 105
Endoscopic ultrasound,
    hepaticogastrostomy 101*f*
Endoscopy
  high-resolution, 93
  magnification 92
  recent advances in 92
  role of 92
  spectrum of "third-space" 107, 108*fc*
Endothelial proliferation 73
Enterobacter 142, 148
Enterobacteriaceae 148, 152
Enterococci 137, 140, 141
Enterococcus 143, 145
Enzyme-linked immunosorbent assay 9
Epidermal growth factor receptor 73, 74*f*, 236
Epidermis 159
Epithelial and stromal components 248
Epithelium, excision of 205
Equipment and accessories 108
Ergonomics 285
Erlotinib 81, 86
Erythrocyte sedimentation rate 3
Erythroplasia of queyrat 195
Escherichia coli 140
Esophageal cancer 76, 110
  management of 77
Esophageal malignancy 76
Esophagus, restoration of 108
European Association of Urology 199, 201
Everolimus 83
Ex utero intrapartum treatment 36, 39, 41, 41*t*, 42
Extended resections, role of 25
Extracellular domains 83
Extracellular-signal-regulated kinases 75
Extrahepatic bile duct 121*f*
Extrahepatic ducts 118

Extrahepatic portal vein obstruction 119
Eye strain 218

F

Fecal incontinence 50
  classification of 51
  common causes of 50
  diagnosis 51
  etiopathogenesis 48
  evaluation 51
  investigation 55
  management of 48
  surgical treatment for 59
  treatment 55
Fetal bleeding 43
Fetal, endoscopic surgery 39
Fetal, image-guided surgery 39, 39*t*
Fetal intervention
  indication of 44
  techniques of 38
Fetal skin biopsy 39
Fetal surgery 34
  applications of 43
  approach for 38*f*
  challenges in 43
  complication 43
  components of 34
  contraindications 38
  diagnosis 35
  history of 35*t*
  indications 38
  multidisciplinary approach in 37
  open 39, 41, 42*t*, 43
  potential of 43
  types of 39
Fetal therapy, evolution of 34
Fetoendoscopic surgery 40*t*
Fetoscopic endoluminal tracheal occlusion 40*f*
Fibroadenomas 247
Fine needle aspiration cytology 146, 172, 200, 261, 265
Flexible spectral imaging color enhancement 92
Fluorescein angiography 222
Fluorescence in situ hybridization 132
Fluorescent intensity 267
Fluorodeoxyglucose 16
FNB needles, different kinds of 99*f*
Follicular lesion of 265

Follicular neoplasm 262
Food and Drug Administration 77
Food intolerance, source of 55
Free latissimus dorsi muscle flap 227f
Free radial forearm flap 225f
Free survival
　progression 80, 82, 85
　recurrence 84, 85
Free-hand technique 106f
Functional utility 186
Fusobacterium 153

G

Gallbladder cancer 86, 119, 120
Gastrectomy
　proximal 19, 28
　subtotal 19
　total 19
Gastric cancer 13, 77, 110
　advanced 17
　clinical presentation 13
　complications of 27
　diagnosis and staging 14
　early 16
　endoscopic resection 17
　histological classification of 13
　management of 16, 27
　neoadjuvant chemotherapy 23
　perforation 28
　postgastrectomy care 28
　role of surgery 27
　surgery for 13, 20
　trastuzumab for 78
Gastric metaplasia 93
Gastric outlet obstruction 28
　causing 15f
Gastric per oral endoscopic myotomy 108
Gastric plication and suturing 112
Gastric variceal coiling 107f
Gastric varices 105
　endoscopic vision of 107f
Gastric wall thickening 15
Gastroenterology surgery, practice of 92
Gastroesophageal junction 14, 77
Gastroesophageal reflux disease 111
　advances in management of 111
Gastrointestinal
　bleed, advances in management of 111
　carcinoid tumors 82

　stromal tumor 83, 85t, 99
　surgery, practice of 92
Gastrojejunostomy 28
Gefitinib 81
Gene therapy 107
Genetic engineering 46
Genital warts 194
Genital warts, history of 194
Gentamicin 145
Giant condylomata acuminata 195
Glasgow Coma Scale 2
Glasgow revised seven point checklist 163
Glucose transporter-1 16
Gluteus maximus muscle 64
Glycosaminoglycans 7
Gracilaplasty therapy study group, dynamic 63
Gracilaplasty, dynamic 61, 63t
Gram-negative rods 137
Gram-positive bacteria 145
Granulocyte macrophage colony stimulating factor 175
Growth factor receptors 72
Growth factors, targeting 73

H

Haemobilia 120
Hand foot disease 82
Healing, mechanism of 219
Heat shock protein 7
Hedgehog pathway 86
Helicobacter pylori infection 93
Hemostasis 264
Heparin 224
Hepatic cyst 119
Hepaticogastrostomy 101, 103
Hepatitis B virus 72
Hepatitis C virus 81
Hepatobiliary ascariasis 119
Hepatocellular carcinoma 81, 106
　advanced 82t
　development of 72
Hepatocyte growth factor receptor 74f
HER-2, targeting 73
Heterogeneity of internal echo 131
Heterogeneous
　blue 98
　green 98
　red and green 98

Heterozygosity, loss of 236
High-mobility group B1 7
Hilar block vs distal obstruction 129
Hilar cholangiocarcinoma 120
Hirschsprung's disease 50, 109
Histamine 82
Hodgkin's disease 257
Homogeneous
 blue 98
 green 98
Hormonal evaluation 257
Hormone receptor 236
Hormone receptor expression 249
Host cell cytoplasm 275f
Human body's response 2
Human epidermal growth factor
 receptor 74f, 78
Human monoclonal antibody 70
Human papillomavirus infection 194
Humanized monoclonal antibody 70
Hydroxychloroquine 279
Hyperbaric oxygen therapy 224
Hyperthermic intraperitoneal
 chemotherapy 25
Hyperthermic isolated limb perfusion
 174, 175t
Hyperthyroidism, etiologies of 263f
Hypocalcemia
 nadir of 266
 predictors of 266
Hypothesis 151

I

Iatrogenic 59
Ifosfamide 210
Illness (acute), cause of 1
Immune checkpoint inhibitors 211
Immunotherapy 211
Immunotoxins 71
Incidental biliary dilatation, causes for
 118, 119b
Indocyanine green 267
Infected pancreatic necrosis, therapeutic
 antibiotics for 146
Infectious diarrhea 50
Infectious Diseases Society of America 6
Inflammation 3
 marker of 4
Inflammatory bowel disease 50
Inflammatory cytokines 237
Inflammatory process 9

Inguinal lymph node 199
 dissection 208
Inguinal metastases 198
Inguinal nodes 204t
 clinical staging 199
Injectable biomaterials 58
Injury, accidental 50
Intensive care units 182
Interleukin-27 8, 9
Interleukin-6 3
International Consensus Definitions for
 Sepsis and Septic Shock 147
International Fetal Medicine and
 Surgery Society 34
International Union for Cancer Control
 232
Intestinal ischemia 152
 occlusive type of 152
Intracellular domains 73
Intraductal cholangioscopy 131
Intraductal echogenic focus 125f
Intraductal papillary mucinous tumor
 120
Intraductal stones 97f
Intragastric balloons 112
Intrahepatic biliary dilatation 128f
Intralesional therapies 175
Intrauterine procedures 38
Invasive penile carcinoma 194
Ipilimumab 211
Irish node 14
Isolated bile duct 118
Isolated limb infusion 175
Isotope scan 263

J

Jaundice, symptoms of
Jejunal loops, dilated 106f
Juxtamembrane domain 83
Juxtapapillary diverticulum 119

K

Kinase domains 83
Kinases 72
Klebsiella 148
 pneumoniae 152
 species 140-142
Korean Laparoscopic Study Group 26
Krukenberg tumor 14

L

Laparoscopic
  appendectomy 144
  cholecystectomy 139, 140t
  surgery 26
Laryngeal nerve
  monitoring 267
  recurrent, incidence of 264
Laser-assisted anastomosis 228
Laser coagulation of vessels 40
Laser Doppler flowmetry 267
Laser endomicroscopy, confocal 92, 94, 132
  in evaluation of dilated bile duct 132
Laser endomicroscopy, needle-based confocal 100
Lauren classification, features of 14t
Lentigo maligna melanoma 160f
Lethal malignancy 212
Levatorplasty, anterior 62f
  repair with 60
Lichen sclerosus 195f
Li-Fraumeni syndrome 244
Lobectomy 42
Local tumor staging 1
Locoregional radiation therapy 239
Low-molecular-weight heparin 224, 279
Lumen-apposing metal stents 100
Lung malformation 42
  congenital 36
Lymph nodal dissection, extent of 21
Lymph node
  disease 168
  dissection 21f, 168, 200
  enlarged 257
  management of 172
  metastasis, left axillary 170f
Lymphatic metastasis 166, 167
Lymphatic surgery 225
Lymphedema, management of 228
Lymphoma 120
Lymphovascular invasion, presence of 205

M

Macroscopic disease 173
Magnetic anal sphincter 65
Magnetic resonance cholangiopancreatography 121, 124f, 128f
Magnetic resonance imaging 37, 52
  advantages of 37
  risks of 37
Malignancy 86
Malignant lymphoma 119
Malignant melanoma 159
  surgical management 169
  surveillance after treatment 178
Malignant phyllodes 249
Mammograms, bilateral 234f
Matrix metalloproteins 75
Mean arterial pressure 2
Medigus ultrasonic surgical endostapler 112
Mega rectum 50
Megaloblastic anemia 28
Melanoma 159
  ABCDE of 162f
  advanced 176
  amelanotic 161
  clinical diagnosis 161
  clinical progression of 159
  difficult 163
  excision specimen of 171f
  in children 163
  locoregional therapies in 174
  management of 176fc, 169
  pigment synthesizing (animal-type) 161
  prognostic factors and staging 164
  progression of 159f
  subtypes of 160
    acral lentiginous melanoma 161
    lentigo maligna melanoma 161
    nodular melanoma 160
  superficial spreading 160
  thickness 173
  tumor-node-metastasis staging of 166t
  various thicknesses of 172t
Meningomyelocele 42
  surgery for 46f
Metabolic therapies, advances in 112
Metal stents 28
Metastases 120
Metastatic penile cancer (T4, N2-3, M1) 209
Metastatic phyllodes 251
Methotrexate 210
Methylcellulose 55
Methylprednisolone 279

Metronidazole 145, 148
Microcalcification 258, 259f
  extensive 233
Microlithiasis 119
Microsatellite instability 77
Microsurgery 220, 223
  contraindication of 223
  failure of 223
  field of 228
  limitation for 225
  masters of 218
  refinement of 217
Microvascular
  clamps 219f
  procedure 222
  surgery 217, 223
    applications of 225
Minimally invasive fetal endo-surgery 40
Minimally invasive surgery 26
Minimally symptomatic biliary dilatation 129
Minimum inhibitory concentration 138
Ministry of Health and Family Welfare 277
Mirizzi's syndrome 120
Mitochondrial DNA 7
Mitogen activated protein kinase 73, 74f
Mitotic stromal, activity 247, 250
Mixed carcinoma 199
Mohs micrographic surgery 205
Molecular
  genetics 262
  signatures 81
  targets in cell pathway 74f
  tests, types of 263
  therapy 69
    development of 86
Momab 70
Monoclonal antibodies 70, 71, 71f
  mouse 70
  production of 71f
Mucinous cystic neoplasm 119
Mucosa 226f
Mucosal incision 108
Multidrug resistance, development of 6
Multikinase inhibitors 83
Multisystem inflammatory syndrome 277
Multivisceral resections 25
Murine Int-1 gene 248

Muscle plasty, dynamic 63
Muscle transfer procedures 58
Myeloid cells-1 8, 10
Myotomy 108, 109f

N

N95 respirators 283
Narrow-band imaging 92, 93
Nasojejunal tube 28
National Cancer Registry Programme 13
National Comprehensive Cancer Network 23, 199, 201, 251
  guidelines 173t
National Healthcare Safety Network 144
National Institute for Health Research 287
National Institute of Care and Excellence 138
Neural network, artificial 113
Neuroendocrine cells 82
Neuroendocrine tumor 119
Neurogenic integrity 49
Neurological conditions 50
Neurotensin 82
Neutralizing antibodies 73
Nipple retraction 245
Nitric oxide synthase 74f
Nivolumab 211
Nodular melanoma 160f, 164, 171f
Nonpalpable ILNs, surgical treatment of 207
Nucleocapsid protein 275f
Nutritional
  rehabilitation 28
  supplements 28

O

Obstetric trauma 50, 59
Obstetrical injury 50
Obstruction, level of 129
Obstructive pulmonary disease, chronic 279
Olaparib 86
Omentectomy, total 20
  for early tumors 20
Opium
  derivatives 56
  tincture of 56
Optical biopsy 93, 94
  concept of 92

Optical coherence tomography 94
Oral malignancy reconstruction 225f
Orbera Intragastric Balloon System 112
Oslen's theory 170
Ovarian masses 14
Overall survival 85

P

p53, expression of 249
p53 germline mutation 244
Paclitaxel 210
Paget's disease of penis 195
Palliative hemostatic radiotherapy 27
Palpable ILNs, surgical treatment of 208
Pancreas 104
 head of 15f
Pancreatic cancer 84, 102f, 119, 120
 familial 86
 prognosis of 84
Pancreatic cyst 119
Pancreatic infiltration 25
Pancreatic necrosis 146
Pancreatic pseudocyst 120
Pancreatic rendezvous 104
Pancreaticobiliary malignancy 119
Pancreaticoduodenectomy 24, 25
Pancreatitis
 acute 120, 144, 145
  pathogenesis of infection in 145
 chronic 119, 120
 recurrent 128f
Pancreatoscopy 96
Panitumumab 79, 80, 81, 86
Papilla, accessibility of 101
Papillary carcinoma 199
Papillary stenosis 119, 120
Papillary surface 131
Parasites 120
Parathyroid detection 266
Parathyroid gland 266
 in situ 267
 intraoperative detection of 266
Parathyroid hormone 266
Parathyroidectomy, subtotal 267
Parenchymal edema 233
Parenchymal thickening 235f
Partial penectomy 206f
Peau d'orange 232, 233
Pelvic floor denervation 50
Pelvic INS, surgical treatment of 209
Pelvic lymph nodes 197, 198

Penile cancer 192, 195f-197f, 207, 212, 213t
 diagnosis of 198, 201t
 epidemiology 192
 etiopathology of 193
 higher risk of 194
 histological, subtypes of 199t
 in situ, surgical treatment of 203
 majority of 198
 management of 192
 palliation in advanced 212
 risk factors 193
 spread of 197
 staging in 201t
Penile intraepithelial neoplasia 195
Penile stump 206
Penile trauma, chronic 194
Penis 194
Penoscrotal junction 206, 206f
Peptide receptor nucleotide therapy 83
Percutaneous transhepatic
 cholangiography 121
 drainage 100, 103
Periampullary cancer 120
Periampullary diverticulum 120, 126
Perianal
 sensation 52
 examination 51
Peritoneal carcinomatosis 25
Peritonitis
 primary 149
 secondary 149
 tertiary 149
Personal protective equipment 283f
Pertuzumab 238
Phimosis 193
Phosphoinositide 3-kinase 74f
Phospholipase C 74f
Photodynamic therapy 96
Phyllodes 249
 biology of 248
 borderline 250
 molecular classification of 249
 tumor 250
  borderline 247
  breast of 244
  chemotherapy 251
  clinical presentation 245
  diagnosis 245
  epidemiology 244
  grading of 246

histological grading of 247t
histopathology 246
hormone therapy 251
malignant 248
mammography 246
management 249
MRI of breast 246
radiology 246
radiotherapy 251
recurrence of 244, 245f
Plasma-bound ICG molecules 267
Plasma cell neoplasm 119
Platelet derived growth factor receptor 74f
Plate-reinforced suture 112
Pleural shunts 39
Polyadenosine diphosphate 86
Polydioxanone 59
Polyposis coli, familial 257
Polytetrafluoroethylene 112
Portal biliopathy 119
Portal vein 106
Positron emission test 235
Positron emission tomography 170f, 200
Postanal repair 61
Premalignant lesions 194
Premature rupture of membrane 41
Prenatal surgery 34, 38
Presepsin 8
Procalcitonin 4, 5
  guidance study 6
  in postoperative period 7
  in renal failure 8
  levels 8
    interpretation of 5t
  utility of 5
Prognostication 8
Programmed cell-death ligand-1 10
Proinflammatory cytokines, upregulation of 276
Prophylactic antibiotic
  general principles 137
  role of 145
Prophylactic measure 26
Proteins
  kinase B 73, 74f
  main structural 275f
Proteus 148
Proteus mirabilis 152
Proton-pump inhibitor 27, 112
Pseudoepitheliomatous 195
Pseudointima 219

Pseudomembranous colitis 139
Pseudomonas 142
Psoralen plus ultraviolet therapy 161
Psychological motivation 49
Psyllium products 55
Public Health England, guidance 283f
Puborectalis muscle 48, 49
  testing 52
Pudendal nerve terminal motor latency 54
Pulmonary airway malformation, congenital 44
Pulmonary epithelial cells 274, 275f
Pulmonary fibrosis 277
Pylorus 20

Q

Qualitative assessment 98
Quinolones 147

R

Radial and linear scanning 132
Radial sector scan system, mechanical 132
Radiation 207
  therapy 176, 177, 239
Radiation Therapy Oncology Group 84
Radical gastrectomy, principles of 18
Radioactive iodine 265
Radiofrequency ablation 39f, 71, 96
Radiolabeled 71
Radiotherapy 69
  for advanced penile cancer 211
Ramucirumab 73
Rapamycin, mechanistic target of 74f
Rapidly accelerated fibrosarcoma 73, 74f
Rat sarcoma 74f
  signals of 73
Reactive-oxygen species 96
Rectal
  examination 14
  prolapse 50
  sensory testing 54
Regional lymph node 179
  surgical management of 207
Rendezvous 101, 103
Reservoir bags, high flow nasal cannula 279
Respiratory illnesses 274
Respiratory infections, antibiotic therapy in 7

Reverse transcriptase polymerase chain reaction 278
Rhinolophus affinis 274
Ribose polymerase inhibitor 86
Rituximab 70
RNA-binding proteins 84
RNA, single strand 275*f*
Robot-assisted thyroidectomy 268, 269
Robot face lift thyroidectomy 269
Robotic-assisted endoscopes 113
Robotic gastrectomy 27
Robotic surgery, surgeon console in 269*f*
Roux-en-Y reconstruction 19
Royal Surgical Colleges 284

S

Sacral nerve stimulation system 57, 58*f*
Sacrococcygeal teratoma 39, 39*f*, 42
Saga of development
  advancing frontiers 217
  giant leap in surgery 217
  microsurgery everywhere 218
  preparation 217
  small stitch on tissue 217
Sarcomatoid carcinoma 199
SARS-CoV-2
  infection 277
  life cycle 275*f*
  polyproteins 275*f*
Scanning electron microscopes 103
Sclerosing cholangitis, primary 119
SECCA procedure 65
Sentinel lymph node 177
  biopsy 169, 173*t*
Sentinel node biopsy, dynamic 201, 207
  technique of 207
Sepsis 3
  biomarkers of 1
  diagnosis of 5
Sequential organ failure, assessment score 2*t*, 147
Serotonin 82
Serum lactate dehydrogenase 167, 169
Severe acute respiratory syndrome coronavirus-2 273, 274
Shear-wave 260
  elastography 259, 260
  speed 260
Short gut syndrome 50
Sister Mary Joseph node 14

Skeletal muscle flaps 58
Skin flaps 267
Skin grafting 227*f*
Small bowel adenocarcinoma 81
Small bowel malignancy 79
Small intestinal malignancy 81
Small molecule inhibitors 72
Somatic mutations of KRAS 86
Sorafenib 73, 83
Sorafenib Hepatocellular Carcinoma Assessment Randomized Protocol trial 82
Sphincter, normal and damaged 49*f*
Sphincter of Oddi 118
  dysfunction 127, 129
  resulting in dilatation 122
Sphincter repair 58, 59
  direct, result of 60*t*
Sphincteroplasty 58
  overlapping 60, 60*t*, 62*f*
Spina bifida 45
Spindle cell metaplastic carcinomas 244
Spitzoid melanoma 161
Splenectomy 23
Squamous cell carcinoma 76, 192, 198, 199
  pathogenesis of 194
Staphylococcus aureus 137
Staphylococcus spp. 143
Steatohepatitis, nonalcoholic 81
Steatorrhea 28
Stent placement, antegrade 103
Stone 120, 125*f*
Stool consistency 49
Strain elastography 259, 260*f*
Streptococcal species 137
Streptococci 143
Stromal atypia 247
Stromal cellularity 246, 247
Stromal overgrowth 247
Subepithelial connective tissue 205
Submucosal
  bleb, formation of 108
  endoscopy 107
  injection 109*f*
  tunneling 109
    and myotomy 109
    endoscopic resection 108
Subungual melanomas 164
Succinate dehydrogenase mutations 83
Sunitinib 73, 83

Supermicrosurgery 228
Surgical antimicrobial prophylaxis 137
Surgical margins, adequacy of 23
Surgical metastasectomy 176
Surgical Patient Safety System 184
Surgical preoperative pathway 284f
Surgical safety checklist 182, 185f
   communication 185
   compliance of 188
   contents of 183
   disadvantages of 188
   history of 183
   implementation 188
   need for 182
   teamwork enhancement 186
   validity of 189
Surgical site infection 137
Surviving Sepsis Campaign 6
   guidelines 148
Sutures, number of 220
Systemic inflammatory response syndrome 1, 1b

T

T2-T4 disease, surgical treatment of 206
Talimogene laherparepvec 175
Targeted agents 76, 177, 211
   challenges 76
   classes of 70
   hepatocyte growth factor 75
   in gastrointestinal malignancy 69
   matrix metalloproteins 75
   PI3K-Akt-mTOR pathway 75
   targeting gene fusion 75
Taxane 238
Tazobactam 148
Therapeutic endoscopic ultrasound, advances in 100
Thiersch procedure 58
Thyroid cytopathology 261t
Thyroid imaging, reporting, and data system 256, 258
Thyroid malignant, mass of 257f
Thyroid nodule 259t
   autonomous functioning 263f, 265
   clinical examination 256
   imaging 257
   management of 256, 265fc
   surgical management of 264
Thyroid ST 265
Thyroid stimulating hormone 256

Thyroidectomy technique produces 268
TIRADS
   assessment 258
   system 259t
Tissue injury 3
Tissue sampling techniques, advances in 132
TNM staging system 202
Tobacco
   chewing 193
   consumption 193
Toxic multinodular goiter 265
Trachea, balloon occlusion of 40
Tracheal stenosis 42f
Transabdominal ultrasonography 119
Transanal ultrasound 55
Transarterial chemoembolization 82
Transient, incidence of 266
Transluminal drainage 104
Transoral incisionless fundoplication 112
Transplant surgery 289
Trastuzumab 70, 238
Trauma surgery 289
Tricyclic antidepressant 56
Tropomyosin receptor kinase 75
Tumor
   bleeding 27
   invades corpus cavernosum 202
   necrosis factor alpha 4, 276
   node metastasis 202
   of papilla of vater 119
   proximal margin for 23
   superficial 159
   surgery by site of 19
Twins
   acardiac 40
   anomalous 39
   cord cauterization in 39
Twin-to-twin transfusion syndrome 40
Tyrosine kinase inhibitors 81
Tyrosine kinase pathway, targeting 84

U

Ugly duckling sign 163
Ultrasound
   advances, utility of 36
   development in 36
   limitation of 37
Umbilical nodule 14

Urethral
 dissection 206f
 flap glanuloplasty 206f
 stump 206f
 valves, posterior 44
Urinary bladder 45f
Urinary tract obstructions, lower 44
Urological malignancies 198

V

Vaccines 72
Vaginal delivery 50
Vaginal introitus 61
Vascular endothelial growth factor
 receptor 17, 73
Vascular surgery 289
Vasculoendothelial growth factor
 receptor 74f
Vasopressin 9
Vasospasm 222
Vater's papilla 129
Venous thromboembolism 224
Ventral phalloplasty 206
Ventral urethral spatulation 206f
Verrucous carcinoma 199
Vesicoamniotic shunt 45f
Vessel repair, triangulation technique
 of 221f
Vessels, milking of 222
Video capsule endoscopy 95, 95f
Vinci Xi Surgical System 27
Viral entry 274, 275f
Viral genome 275f
Viral genomic RNA 275f
 produced 275f

Viral infections, differentiation of 5
Viral transport media 278
Virchow node 14
Visual examination 162
Vitamin D supplementation 266
Vocal cord paralysis 257

W

Warm breast 232
Warty-basaloid carcinoma 199
Warty carcinoma 199
Weight loss 82
White blood cell 3
Wieberdink toxicity grading system 174t
Wnt gene 248
World Health Organization 70, 138, 244
 melanoma program trial 171
 surgical safety checklist 184f
World Society for Emergency Surgery
 146
Wound infection, higher risk of 137

X

Ximab 70

Y

Young's modulus 260
Yttrium-aluminum garnet 203
Yttrium-90 labeled 83

Z

Zenker's diverticulum 109, 110f
Zumab 70

EU GSPR Authorised Reprsentative
Logos Europe, 9 rue Nicolas Poussin
1700, La Rochelle, France
Phone: +33 (0) 6 67 93 73 78
E-mail: contact@logoseurope.eu

www.ingramcontent.com/pod-product-compliance
Ingram Content Group UK Ltd.
Pitfield, Milton Keynes, MK11 3LW, UK
UKHW051846210426
5322IPUK00019B/279